Management of Neck Pain Disorders: a Research-Informed Approach

Management of Neck Pain Disorders: a Research-Informed Approach

GWENDOLEN JULL, PhD, MPhty, GradDipManipTher, DipPhty, FACP

Emeritus Professor, Physiotherapy, School of Health and Rehabilitation Sciences, The University of Queensland, Australia

DEBORAH FALLA, PhD, BPhty

Professor; Chair in Rehabilitation Science and Physiotherapy, School of Sport, Exercise and Rehabilitation Sciences, The University of Birmingham, UK

JULIA TRELEAVEN, PhD, BPhty

Senior Research Officer in Physiotherapy, School of Health and Rehabilitation Sciences, The University of Queensland, Australia

SHAUN O'LEARY, PhD, MPhty, BPhty, FACP

Senior Research Fellow in Physiotherapy, School of Health and Rehabilitation Sciences, The University of Queensland, Australia

FOREWORD BY
JEREMY S LEWIS, PHD, FCSP

Consultant Physiotherapist, MSK Sonographer, Independent Prescriber, Professor of Musculoskeletal Research, Department of Allied Health Professions and Midwifery, School of Health and Social Work, University of Hertfordshire, UK

ELSEVIER   Edinburgh   London   New York   Oxford   Philadelphia   St Louis   Sydney   2019

ELSEVIER

First edition 2019

ISBN: 978-0-7020-7477-6

Notices

Practitioners and researchers must always rely on their own experience and knowledge in evaluating and using any information, methods, compounds or experiments described herein. Because of rapid advances in the medical sciences, in particular, independent verification of diagnoses and drug dosages should be made. To the fullest extent of the law, no responsibility is assumed by Elsevier, authors, editors or contributors for any injury and/or damage to persons or property as a matter of products liability, negligence or otherwise, or from any use or operation of any methods, products, instructions or ideas contained in the material herein.

Content Strategist: Poppy Garraway
Content Development Specialist: Helen Leng
Project Manager: Anne Collett
Design: Bridget Hoette
Illustration Manager: Karen Giacomucci
Illustrator: Robert Britton
Marketing Manager: Emily Wall

 your source for books, journals and multimedia in the health sciences

www.elsevierhealth.com

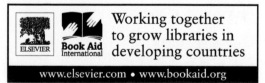

Working together to grow libraries in developing countries

www.elsevier.com • www.bookaid.org

The publisher's policy is to use **paper manufactured from sustainable forests**

Printed in Great Britain

Last digit is the print number: 9 8 7 6 5 4

CONTENTS

FOREWORD

■ ■

I t remains an on-going challenge to keep up to date with advances in science and changes in clinical practice to provide the best care for people experiencing neck pain disorders. The amount of new knowledge available is bewildering not only for patients, but also for clinicians. This is due to the rate at which new ideas, philosophies and research are published and disseminated across a vast range of communication systems, traditional and new. Gwen Jull, Deborah Falla, Julia Treleaven and Shaun O'Leary have, in a unique and uncompromised manner, brought together, between the covers of this wonderful text book, the knowledge and understanding any clinician from any discipline, and from any level of experience and knowledge, would require to confidently guide and support the management of a person experiencing neck pain. The breadth and depth of information contained within these pages is unparalleled, and this text would make an invaluable resource to any personal or public library.

The Global Burden of Disease Study has ranked neck pain, along with low-back pain, as the main health conditions associated with the longest number of years lived with disability (1). For some, musculoskeletal pain is associated with a reduction in the subjective quality of life that is comparable to complicated diabetes mellitus, chronic liver disease requiring transplantation, and those diagnosed with terminal cancer (2). Knowledge of this should encourage and inspire all clinicians entrusted with the unassailable privilege of caring for a member of their society to learn more, know more and do better. Through its 19 chapters, presented in 4 sections, *Management of Neck Pain Disorders* supports clinicians to realise these important goals taking them through a truly biopsychosocial journey of discovery that synthesises the research evidence and clinical knowledge that has taken many, many decades to acquire.

Section 2 of *Management of Neck Pain Disorders* covers the Clinical Sciences and the text synthesises modern pain science in the context of pain experienced in the region of the neck and explores in-depth the psychosocial factors that may influence the perception of pain. Uncertainties surrounding the relationship between cervical posture and symptoms are explored. The anatomy and biomechanics of the region, as well as adjacent regions, are expertly presented, as are injuries and pathology of the neural tissues and their impact locally and more distally. Currently, there is no better synthesis of the research evidence available for clinicians with detailed information exploring changes in motor output, muscular co-ordination and activity, temporal characteristics of neck muscle activity, and pathological changes within muscle tissue and disturbances in sensorimotor control, for those that experience neck pain.

Section 3 skilfully guides the clinician through every stage of the clinical-assessment process, from interview though the physical examination, and comprehensively supports the clinician's ability to clinically reason and conduct a state-of-the-art examination. Pertinent issues such as the patient–clinician relationship, language, outcome measures, psychosocial factors, lifestyle factors and sleep, and red-flag recognition are presented. The physical examination includes provocative movement testing, comprehensive movement assessment procedures, neurological and vascular testing methods, all-inclusive muscle testing in multiple positions, ligament tests, balance, and a battery of methods of assessing a wide range of sensorimotor disturbances including oculomotor assessment. The importance of differential diagnosis is emphasised throughout the text and includes sections on headache, and the differential diagnosis of dizziness, including minor brain injury, benign paroxysmal positional vertigo, peripheral vestibular lesions, tinnitus and visual disturbances, and much, much more.

Section 4 provides the reader with the most comprehensive system of care imaginable, and is uncompromising in its patient-centred approach to management. It includes sections on communication, education, and work and life-style advice. Guidance on selection of interventions, together with comprehensive exercise strategies, including sensorimotor exercise and virtual-reality exercises, balanced and wide-ranging manual-therapy procedures, the management of nerve tissue, home-based rehabilitation, and a detailed section on self-management, will prove invaluable for all clinicians caring for people with neck pain disorders. The penultimate chapter presents the reader with a series of five comprehensive case studies aiming to support clinical reasoning and clinical decision-making strategies. The final chapter discusses the role of prevention in neck pain disorders.

For *Management of Neck Pain Disorders* to achieve its intended purpose, as an essential clinical resource, it should not remain in the unspoiled condition in which it was delivered. In order for this text to support clinical practice and to provide the best possible care to the most important person in healthcare, the patient, the pages in this textbook should quickly become well thumbed, reflected upon, annotated with reference tabs, discussed with colleagues, and its information compared to new and emerging research. Providing care for people with musculoskeletal conditions, including neck pain disorders, is not only a privilege but also comes with a responsibility. It demands that you conduct your practice with understanding, empathy and knowledge, translated from the best possible resources. *Management of Neck Pain Disorders* will assist you in achieving these goals, and should quickly become the go-to resource for every clinician, newly qualified or experienced. Currently, there is no better resource for the management of neck pain disorders and all will find value within its pages.

JEREMY LEWIS
2018

REFERENCES

1. Global Burden Disease 2015 Disease and Injury Incidence and Prevalence Collaborators. Global, regional, and national incidence, prevalence, and years lived with disability for 310 diseases and injuries, 1990-2015: a systematic analysis for the Global Burden of Disease Study 2015. Lancet 2016;388:1545–602.
2. Taylor W. Musculoskeletal pain in the adult New Zealand population: prevalence and impact. N Z Med J 2015;118:U1629.

PREFACE

It is certainly not enjoyable to have neck pain. It is a common and recurrent disorder characterized by episodes over many years, if not a lifetime. For some persons, it is of nuisance value but for many others it affects their work and leisure activities and for a few, especially in association with trauma from a motor vehicle crash, its onset may substantively change their quality of life and work well into the future. Our clinical and research interests over the past 15 to 20 years have been in neck pain where we have worked in a "laboratory to bedside" framework to better understand the pathophysiology of neck pain disorders, the person with neck pain and the interrelationships of these features in the context of the biopsychosocial model. The overarching aim of our work has been to improve the outcomes for people with neck pain disorders by utilising and developing best practice, research informed assessment and management strategies. The aim of this text is to inform clinicians and assist them to provide optimal management for their patients presenting with neck pain disorder.

We previously presented our work in the text, *Whiplash, Headache and Neck Pain*, published by Elsevier in 2008. This current book is, in part, a second edition reflecting the advances in research and clinical practices in the last 10 years, but it has been completely rewritten. Its new title reflects a new structure and emphasis, and it presents a more comprehensive coverage of the features we contend need to be considered in the assessment and management of patients with neck pain disorders. We discuss some contemporary issues in patient presentation, assessment and management across a range of cervical disorders and hope to stimulate clinicians' and researchers' thinking about current and future practices in both research and patient management.

In particular, we stress the importance of regarding each patient as an individual with each person's management guided by a clinically reasoned and comprehensive patient-centred assessment. We stress the importance of regarding neck pain as a recurrent disorder for many, if not most, individuals. Patient management should not focus only on relieving the presenting episode of pain (although this an important aspect): rather, management must also be concerned with rehabilitation of movement, neuromuscular and sensorimotor function. The aim of management should be to try to prevent or lessen the frequency of recurrent episodes and, as with degenerative joint disease in other regions of the body, try to slow disease progression. It is critical to provide the patient with the knowledge, understanding and tools to empower them to self-manage their necks. This might sound an idealistic approach and certainly more expensive than administration of a generic programme of exercise or advice. However, thinking about the cost of one episode of care is narrow thinking because the costs are not in a single episode. The real costs and burden of neck pain are in its recurrent nature with the costs of repeated occasions of care, reduced work productivity, reduced quality of life and the cost of harms (e.g., the significant harms of prolonged use of nonsteroidal antiinflammatory drugs). Prevention at primary, secondary and tertiary levels must be the focus of research and practice into the future.

Research is a collaborative venture. In writing this text, we acknowledge the assistance we have received from our numerous multidisciplinary research and clinical collaborators, who are too many to name, as well as the work and stimulation provided by our many doctoral students and postdoctoral fellows. These collaborations have not only ensured quality and productive work, but have cemented friendships all over the world. We also wish to thank Susan Davies and Dominic Truong who modelled for the photographs in the text and Helen Leng and Poppy Garraway of Elsevier for their support in bringing the text to publication.

GJ, DF, JT, SO'L

Section 1 INTRODUCTION

This chapter introduces the topic of neck pain disorders and, as background to the text, presents some of the contemporary issues that are impacting on decisions for assessment and management of persons with neck pain disorders. From the outset, clinicians are challenged to change their thinking from a focus on relieving a presenting episode of neck pain, to a focus on the real challenge in management which is lessening or preventing the potential years of recurrent episodes of neck pain.

1 NECK PAIN DISORDERS

Neck pain is common. In the main it is not a catastrophic condition, but it can have a significant impact on a person's work, recreation and quality of life. Neck pain spares no age group, gender or culture.[1] Following a first episode of neck pain, there is a high chance of repeated episodes, which may extend over a lifetime.[2] Recovery from an acute episode is frequently incomplete.[3] Neck pain is a condition characterized by recurrence, or in some cases, persistent pain. Recent findings of the Global Burden of Disease Study indicated that neck pain along with low-back pain, ranked as number one of 310 chronic medical conditions in terms of years lived with a disability. Neck pain is a problem worldwide, it ranked as number one in the majority of the 195 countries surveyed.[1] The burden of neck pain for the individual manifests not only in the symptoms and physical complaints, but in its impact on their work and social participation and the related financial, family and emotional consequences.[4]

Neck pain disorders are heterogeneous in presentation.[5] Symptom intensities range from "nuisance value" to disabling pain, as evident in some cases of whiplash-associated disorder and cervical radiculopathy. In tandem, the impact on function is variable, ranging from a negligible impact, to a particular activity or action being difficult, to activity restriction to such an extent that it limits a person's participation in activities of daily living and work. Not all people with neck pain seek treatment and many self-manage either relying on time, over-the-counter medication or self-management strategies commonly gleaned from the internet. When treatment is sought from a health practitioner, conservative management is the first line of management. Recurrence is common whether the neck disorder begins as a minor or significant pain.[6] Clinicians and researchers across public health, medical and rehabilitation fields must assume the responsibility to further develop and deploy effective preventative and management strategies to assist and empower people to reduce the incidence, recurrence and consequent burden of neck pain globally.

BASIC TENETS OF NECK PAIN

Neck pain is a symptom of various origins. Musculoskeletal causes are by far the most common, but neck pain can also be a symptom of non-musculoskeletal sources such as infection, neoplasm, vascular disorders (carotid or vertebral arterial dissection), metabolic bone disease, inflammatory, neurological and visceral diseases, causes for which a clinician must always remain vigilant. From a musculoskeletal perspective, all structures of the cervical spine are innervated so all may be a source of peripheral nociception contributing to a primary neck pain disorder. Pain from a cervical musculoskeletal disorder is typically felt in the posterior neck. Depending on the segmental source and structure, it may spread to the head, shoulder, upper thoracic region or down the arm.[7] Although cervical musculoskeletal dysfunction usually underlies neck pain, there are other presentations. Neck pain and dysfunction may be secondary or comorbid features of pain syndromes in the craniomandibular complex, the shoulder or upper limb. Alternately, the neck itself may be a site of referred pain, rather than a pain source, as encountered in disorders such as migraine,[8] cardiac disease[9] or cervical arterial dissections.[10] Such presentations emphasize the necessity for a skilled physical examination. Clinicians need to be able to identify the presence or absence of a cervical musculoskeletal source to neck pain and, when present, if it is a primary cause, a secondary cause or comorbid problem.

Neck pain of musculoskeletal origin initially arises from a nociceptive source such as a local injury or mechanical stress or strain, from inflammation, or from injury or irritation of nerve structures, i.e., a neuropathic pain. Very simply, signals from the periphery travel to the central nervous system and are processed and modulated in various regions of the spinal cord and brain. There is much contemporary interest in sensitization and neuroplasticity at all levels of the nervous system and their possible role in persistent pain.[11] It is well recognized that pain is not merely a sensory event but a multidimensional experience with emotional reactions or psychological moderators, which all input into the plastic nervous system. Likewise, there can be social drivers and moderators in work and lifestyle that can impact on the pain experience and the neck pain disorder. The necessity for a skilled and comprehensive clinical examination is again evident to ensure a broad consideration of the patient and their neck pain disorder to inform a best practice management program.

Pain is an important consideration and patients usually seek pain relief as a primary goal of treatment. As important as pain relief may be, it is but one consideration. Pain and injury to any region of the musculoskeletal system have profound effects on the neuromuscular system. The cervical region is no exception where changes in both muscle behaviour and structure have been clearly demonstrated.[12] There is no evidence that neuromuscular function will always automatically return to normal when an episode of neck pain resolves. Indeed, there is evidence to the contrary.[13–16] The burden of neck pain to many individuals is in its recurrent or persistent nature, with numerous years lived with pain and disability. Recurrent neck pain impacts on physical health related quality of life.[17] Although pain relief is an important outcome, best practice management must also focus on decreasing the recurrence rate. Rehabilitation to restore neuro-

muscular function is a logical component of the management program.

Pain is not the only symptom of neck disorders. Other symptoms may include feelings of light headedness and unsteadiness, visual disturbances and cognitive difficulties such as problems concentrating.[18] The cervical spine is an important proprioceptive sensory organ. Together with input from the vestibular and ocular systems and somatosensory input from the rest of body, proprioceptive input from the neck muscles plays an important role in the control of posture, locomotion and oculomotor control. When cervical afferentation is disturbed, the mismatch in information processed in the central nervous system from all component systems is reasoned to underlie symptoms. Together with symptoms, deficits in cervical joint position and movement sense, balance, eye movement control and eye-head, trunk-head coordination are variously present. Symptoms of light headedness and unsteadiness, visual disturbances and cognitive difficulties can be functionally debilitating. Management must also focus on addressing these symptoms and sensorimotor deficits when present. There are many treatments that may help symptoms, but again, decreasing symptoms does not automatically mean the somatosensory impairment has resolved.[19] Best practice management should include specific rehabilitation of the impairments if sights are on decreasing recurrence rates as well as alleviating symptoms.

The biopsychosocial model

Neck pain disorders are multidimensional. Some 30 years ago, Waddell[20] adapted Engel's[21] biopsychosocial model for the field of psychiatry to apply it to low-back pain. Consideration of biological features in the traditional medical approach could not alone explain the disability associated with low-back pain and it was not logical to separate the person from their condition. Subsequently, the biopsychosocial model was adopted for neck pain and other musculoskeletal disorders. The biopsychosocial model, as its names implies, encourages simultaneous consideration of all potential biological, psychological and social determinants of a patient's neck pain presentation. The model accords with other frameworks such as the International Classification of Functioning, Disability and Health (ICF). It promotes consideration and assessment not only of multiple domains, but also of the potential moderating and mediating characteristics of features within and between the different domains. The model has limitations. It does not indicate which features should be evaluated in any domain and consequently cannot inform or guide selection of interventions. It is not an interventional model.[22]

The biopsychosocial model is often depicted as three symmetrical circles suggesting "equal" contributions of biological, psychological and social domains to every person's neck pain disorder. This is an inaccurate picture. The contribution of each domain varies between patients (Fig. 1.1). Even within a patient, the contribution of each domain is likely to change throughout the course of their disorder. The model provides a philosophy underpinning a comprehensive consideration of a patient's neck pain disorder in assessment and management. Lack of appreciation of the variable contribution of each domain in the individual patient, and relative importance of each domain at initial and subsequent time points will negate or compromise patient-centred

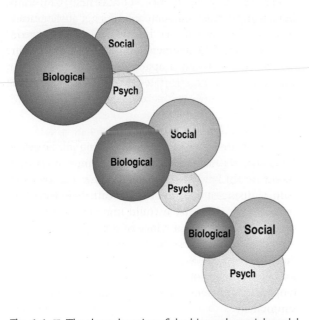

Fig. 1.1 ■ The three domains of the biopsychosocial model are fluid and will vary in their contribution between different patients and in different stages of a patient's neck pain disorder. Three examples of relative contributions of domains are presented in order of their probable frequency based on contemporary evidence.

management. It leads to the erroneous belief of a "one size fits all" treatment.

CONTEMPORARY ISSUES

No approach whether medical, physiotherapeutic, chiropractic, psychological, educational or any alternate or complementary therapy has as yet met the idealist challenge of successful primary and secondary prevention of neck pain. Controversies continue around the management of neck pain disorders. Although conservative physical therapies are not proving the answer for all with a neck pain disorder, there are positives. The majority of individual patients gain some if not considerable relief from physical therapies. The challenges are in selecting appropriate interventions and identifying likely responders and non-responders so that inappropriate treatment is not delivered. Although not a pure science, progress is being made to meet these challenges. This text will overview and explore neck pain disorders from the basic and applied clinical sciences in a biopsychosocial context. It will overview our and others research, which is increasing the understanding of neck pain disorders and which is informing patient assessment, management and prognosis. A research informed, comprehensive management and rehabilitation approach will be presented, which will emphasize the indications for and application of individualized multimodal management and, as relevant, multidisciplinary management. However, in the first instance, some of the issues and debates in the field of neck pain disorders will be presented to stimulate thought as the reader progresses through the text.

Classification of neck pain

Classification is a popular topic in physiotherapy research and clinical practice. It is well recognized that neck pain disorders as with most musculoskeletal disorders, have great variety in their presentations. Classification aims to group similar individuals. Its main purposes are to define diseases, to help direct management or to allocate resources to provide care. There are many criteria on which neck pain has been and may be defined. It would be ideal to have one classification system that could define neck pain disorders and direct appropriate management. Towards such an ideal, it is relevant to briefly overview some of the current criteria on which neck pain disorders are defined and explore whether or not they should be retained or discarded in a classification system.

Defining the neck pain disorder by mechanism of onset

Historically, neck pain disorders have been grouped or classified into one of three major domains: mechanical (or idiopathic or non-specific) neck pain; traumatic onset neck pain (e.g., whiplash associated disorders, sporting injuries, falls, blunt trauma to the head or neck); and degenerative (spondylosis) disorders, which can range from minor disc narrowing to acquired stenosis (lateral canal stenosis—cervical radiculopathy; central canal stenosis—cervical myelopathy). Two domains relate to mechanism of onset and the third to pathoanatomy, (which is discussed in the next section). Traumatic onset neck pain is self-explanatory. Mechanical neck pain is a descriptor term, predominantly of exclusion, for pain not arising from an incident of trauma, an inflammatory disease process or any other identifiable intrinsic or extrinsic pathology. The catchment for the term *mechanical neck pain* is large and variously includes pain induced by an unaccustomed movement or activity, postural strain or accumulated adverse strains from repetitive, static or high-load activity.

It would be easy to dismiss this onset-based classification as too unrefined, but there are differences between the groupings. In the first instance, the sites and nature of pathology could be expected to differ. Trauma from a motor vehicle crash or blunt trauma can result in lesions of several cervical structures of a greater variety and to a greater range with attendant bleeding and inflammation than may occur with accumulated postural or activity strain.[23] There are many similarities in the presentation of insidious onset mechanical neck pain and traumatic onset neck pain from the musculoskeletal impairment perspective. Yet there are differences. Taking comparative population averages, patients with whiplash-associated disorders, on average, present with higher pain and disability than patients with mechanical neck pain.[24] Furthermore, cohorts of patients with whiplash-associated disorders are more likely to exhibit central nervous system sensitization,[25] have greater physical impairments,[26,27] exhibit distinctive changes in cervical muscle morphology[28–30] and have

impaired somatosensory function of greater magnitude than insidious onset neck pain.[31] Emotional responses are also often more pronounced in whiplash-associated disorders. As will be illustrated in this text, such differences have implication for designs and components of patient-centred, management programmes. Hence this first basic classification, mechanism of onset, contributes to patient characterisation and makes a contribution to patient assessment and management planning. It should not be discarded.

Defining the neck pain disorder by pathoanatomy

The terms *mechanical* or *non-specific neck pain* and *whiplash-associated disorders* have been adopted in place of nominating a particular lesion, pathoanatomy or pathological process in the cervical musculoskeletal system. Even today, imaging methods such as standard x-rays or magnetic resonance imaging (MRI) are often not sensitive enough to identify relevant lesions.[32,33] Often there is little relationship between x-ray findings and pain.[34] This insensitivity has led to advice against routine imaging of the cervical spine as a first assessment in neck pain presentations. Guidelines (Canadian Cervical Spine Rule; National Emergency X-Radiography Utilization Study [NEXUS] Low-Risk Criteria) have been developed to designate specific indications for imaging especially in the case of traumatic onset neck pain to avoid unnecessary x-rays.[35] The absence of a lesion on x-ray does not necessarily mean there is no lesion. It could mean that the imaging method or the time it was used, was unable to detect a relevant lesion.[23,32] Care is needed when conveying information to patients regarding radiological findings. Although patients should be reassured that a lack of radiological findings does not question or discredit their report of symptoms, at the other extreme, patients should also be reassured that the presence of marked radiological findings does not necessitate marked levels of pain and disability. Poor communication of radiological findings can compromise patient clinician relationships. Explanation and qualification of x-ray findings should always be provided.

Recent decades have seen a move away from attempting to define a precise lesion, reflecting the challenges of identifying the lesion and differentiating it from age changes.[34] Furthermore, x-ray findings provide limited direction in management of the majority of persons with neck pain disorders. The previous emphasis on "biology" was a main driver for the adoption of the biopsychosocial model. Knowing that a patient has C2–3 osteoarthritis on x-ray, does not inform on pain mechanisms, reactions in the neuromuscular or somatosensory systems or emotional responses to the disorder which could direct treatment. Yet should attempts to make a pathoanatomic diagnosis be abandoned entirely? Surgeons operate on pathoanatomy, so for them a pathoanatomic diagnosis cannot be abandoned. Likewise, it might be premature to discard changes seen on x-rays as not relevant. Recent MRI research in low-back pain suggests that the presence of three or more changes in lumbar structures (as opposed to a single sign), is associated with a higher risk of future recurrence of low-back pain.[36,37] These findings encourage continued consideration of pathoanatomy. A similar line of research is warranted for cervical disorders because neck pain too is a recurrent disorder. Having a way to identify, quantitatively, those at high risk of recurrence would be a major advance in management planning. It would be unwise to dismiss identifying pathoanatomy in future research and practice, thus it cannot be discarded.

Identifying or nominating the precise lesion in a cervical structure may be difficult, but a symptomatic cervical segment can be identified with considerable accuracy in a clinical examination of patients with neck pain. Manual examination is not without its controversies, but there is now a considerable body of evidence indicating that manual examination is an accurate clinical method to locate a symptomatic cervical segment.[38–42] This should not be surprising because even at a very basic level, palpating for tender areas is a fundamental medical examination technique and is a minimum expectation of patients. Identifying the symptomatic cervical segment(s) is important to define the disorder and cannot be discarded.

Defining the neck pain disorder by time

It is common to define pain on the basis of time into acute, subacute and chronic. The criteria for chronic pain in these terms is pain which persists past the normal time of tissue healing which is customarily, greater than 12 weeks. This definition based on tissue healing is well recognized as flawed.[43] Healing may occur well within or well outside this timeframe or it may never occur (e.g., as in osteoarthritis, or spinal stenosis). Neck pain

is recognized as an episodic disorder with pain free periods of months or even years between episodes— periods where tissues had apparently healed. Is recurrent neck pain over years the same as chronic neck pain? Using time alone to classify chronic pain tends to portray a "sameness" across all pain states lasting greater than 12 weeks, which is far from reality.

What is chronic pain? Chronic pain may involve, in any combination, physical disorders both peripheral and central, biochemical disturbances in various body systems, local disease processes, psychological responses or unhelpful personal beliefs. The International Association for the Study of Pain[43] discourages the use of the term *chronic pain syndrome* because it usually implies persisting pain, which is driven by behavioural changes induced by psychological and social problems. They contend that the term helps clinicians evade the requirement for all patients to have accurate physical and psychological diagnoses, and that the term is often used disparagingly. Until there is better taxonomy for chronic pain, it behoves researchers and clinicians alike to clearly define the physical and psychological characteristics of the chronic pain presentation of the patient or patient group under discussion to facilitate accurate communication and importantly, management prescription. Time-based classification certainly contributes to defining the disorder. It should not be discarded, but its substantial limitations must be appreciated.

Defining the neck pain disorder by mechanisms

A diagnostic label is limited in the extent to which it can help direct management. The mechanisms underpinning symptoms and other functional limitations on the other hand, can direct management.

There is great interest in the mechanisms underlying various clinical pain presentations, the plasticity of the nervous system and how it can be modulated by both endogenous and external features. Knowledge is growing and constantly developing. Treatments can be guided by several features, such as whether pain is nociceptive, inflammatory or neuropathic in origin, if local or widespread mechanical or thermal hyperalgesia are present suggesting peripheral or central nervous system sensitization and by the extent to which emotional or psychological features might be moderating symptoms. Several studies have shown that patients cluster into groups on the basis of outcomes of quantitative sensory testing, which might indicate different pain mechanisms.[5,44,45] Understanding pain mechanisms can guide assessment protocols and treatments towards all levels of the nervous system.

Knowledge of the neurophysiological mechanisms underpinning symptoms of cervical dizziness such as light-headedness and visual disturbances is growing rapidly as is knowledge of the manifestations of impaired proprioception (position, movement and force sense), balance and eye, head and trunk coordination.[46,47] Understanding mechanisms of cervical somatosensory dysfunction helps define the condition and can guide assessment and management approaches.

Functional impairments such as poor control of posture, poor patterns and control of movements and inabilities to perform or sustain performance of an activity reflect deficits in the neuromuscular system. There is now a wealth of knowledge about the changes in the neuromuscular system with neck pain and injury in the acute, recurrent and persistent pain states. Understanding these changes defines the condition in neuromuscular terms and guides assessment and management approaches.

Defining the condition in terms of mechanisms clearly and precisely directs patient assessment and management planning and cannot be discarded.

Defining the neck pain disorder by predictors

Knowledge is increasing about predictors of neck pain as well as predictors of recovery and future neck pain in the general, occupationally induced neck pain and whiplash populations.[48–53] More studies are needed to explore predictors of neck pain of occupational, sporting, traumatic and insidious origins, so that certainty for a feature can be established by a critical number of studies.[52] Likewise, more studies need to consider all domains within the biopsychosocial context simultaneously, rather than focus on one domain. This provides a clearer picture of the relative predictive roles of features within and across all domains.

Knowledge of predictors for the development of, or recovery from neck pain informs our understanding of a patient's neck pain disorder. How useful it is to use predictors to direct management is yet to be explored in any detail.[54] Many predictors of persisting or recurrent episodes of neck pain cannot be modified, for example, age, gender or previous episodes of neck pain. However other features are possibly modifiable, for instance social features at work such as job control or physical features such as reduced neck muscle endurance.[50,51,53] Initial high-pain intensity and disability are strong risk factors for persistent pain following a whiplash injury.[52] Knowing this fact is important. Nevertheless, not all patients with initial high-pain intensity have a poor prognosis. For some, their condition resolves in a straight forward way. Likewise at this time, no treatment approach (physical, medical or psychological) has been successful in reducing the risk of transition to persistent pain for this small but difficult group of patients. At this point, there is little evidence or research to inform whether targeting risk factors for persistent neck pain improves outcomes. Yet risk factors help define neck pain and should not be discarded at this time.

Defining the neck pain disorder by clinical prediction rules

There has been interest over the past decade in developing clinical prediction rules (CPRs) to identify the characteristics of patients who may respond to a certain treatment technique or approach. CPRs have been developed to indicate the use of cervical or cervicothoracic manipulation for neck pain and for shoulder pain, for the use of cervical traction as well as the use of neurodynamic techniques in the management of arm pain and carpal tunnel syndrome.[55–59] However, most CPRs to direct treatment have remained in the first stage of development. CPRs that have been tested in validation studies to date have failed to gain support.[60–62] The use and indeed the future of CPRs to direct a particular treatment regime is uncertain. At this time their clinical use is not supported.[63]

Defining the neck pain disorder by subgrouping

The heterogeneity in presentation of neck pain disorders is recognized. There is widespread acknowledgement that a one size fits all treatment approach is ineffective. Subgrouping is a means to address the issue by grouping patients with similar clinical characteristics with the aim to better tailor treatments. Subgrouping has been explored for neck pain, but to a far lesser extent than for low-back pain. There are perhaps only two specific subgrouping systems for neck pain at this time. One is based on the overall goal of treatment.[64] Patients are allocated to one of five groups depending on whether the treatment intent is to increase mobility, to centralize pain, to condition the patient and increase exercise tolerance, to assist pain control or to reduce headache. There has been some preliminary research supporting the potential benefit of this classification system[65,66] but more research is required to determine whether this subgrouping method clearly improves treatment outcomes overall. A similar classification system has been incorporated in the Clinical Practice Guidelines for neck pain presented by the Orthopaedic Division of the American Physical Therapy Association.[67,68] The groups here are: neck pain with mobility deficits; neck pain with headaches; neck pain with movement coordination impairments; neck pain with radiating pain. The other system, Mechanical Diagnosis and Therapy, which was originally devised for the low back, has been applied to the neck.[69,70] Depending on the response to repeated movement, patients can be classified into four basic syndromes: posture, dysfunction, reducible derangement, irreducible derangement or "other" category. At the current time, this subgrouping has not proved to have resulted in any superior treatment effects.[71] Although subgrouping may have promise, it is considered that research and achievements in this field (whether neck or low-back pain) are far from optimal. Evidence does not as yet support their widespread adoption in clinical practice.[72]

This brief overview illustrates the breadth of factors that need to come under consideration to define or classify neck pain to direct management. Few can be dismissed. At this current time, and especially in research and clinical trials, the most common grouping is by mechanism of onset, that is, insidious onset (mechanical neck pain), traumatic onset (e.g., whiplash) and degenerative onset (including radiculopathies), reflecting some recognisable differences in these disorders within and between biopsychosocial domains. Perhaps this is the best starting point in developing a hierarchical classification algorithm to guide management. Nevertheless, the algorithm should incorporate all defining features of neck pain disorders, including stepped rankings of their importance, influence and dominance, and the potential interdependence or independence of the various features. In other words, it should reflect the high-level clinical reasoning processes that will define the patient's particular neck pain disorder and direct appropriate management.

Management of neck pain disorders

A considerable portion of the text will be devoted to describing conservative management options for patients with neck pain disorders. Many issues will be discussed in relation to best practice in the model of evidence-based practice. In this first instance, three issues are highlighted to stimulate thought before they receive fuller attention in the text.

Effectiveness and ineffectiveness; responders and non-responders

Recent updates of systematic reviews by the Bone and Joint Decade Task Force on interventions for neck pain and whiplash-associated disorders found evidence of benefit for manual/manipulative therapy, exercise, multimodal management, with some evidence of cost-effectiveness of conservative management.[73–76] Evidence points to the use of education as an adjunct but not a sole therapy.[77] There was neither evidence for or against the use of psychological interventions for neck pain disorders.[78] This evidence for conservative physical therapies is encouraging, but effect sizes are often at best moderate if not small.[79,80]

Small effect sizes have been associated with the heterogencity of mechanical neck pain, which is often not considered in participant selection in randomized controlled trials (RCTs). This challenge has fuelled the move to have better classification or subgrouping of neck pain disorders. A part of the complex process of optimizing classification to guide management is to recognize the characteristics of patients who are likely and who are not likely to respond to conventional physical therapies or conventional physical therapies alone. Understanding the characteristics of patients who do not respond is equally important as identifying responders. These patients need to be identified as early as possible so that alternate management strategies can be explored both in research and clinical practice in a multiprofessional manner.

Single or multimodal interventions

Often single treatment modalities are tested in RCTs and evaluated in systematic reviews. There is scientific merit in trying to discover the effects of a particular intervention. However, it is an unrealistic expectation that one modality/intervention will be a "cure all" for all abnormal, impaired or maladaptive features within and between each domain of the biopsychosocial model. There are criticism of practitioners of any discipline who focus predominantly on biological domains, resulting in many "hands on, hands off" debates.[81,82] Even within a biological focus, it is a flawed expectation that relieving pain will resolve automatically, any motor or proprioceptive impairment.[13–16] Equally, it is quite illogical to expect that interventions focussing on behavioural or central nervous system processes alone will automatically "fix" all abnormal, impaired or maladaptive features within each biopsychosocial domain. Outcome measures must be chosen to represent each impaired feature within each domain, so that clear knowledge is built about the effects of an intervention on each and every impairment. Such knowledge will further inform multimodal management approaches. This is the challenge in both clinical and research environments.

Neck pain—an episodic or a recurrent disorder

Neck pain is a recurrent disorder, the episode of pain returns again and again over the following months or years.[2,3] Neck pain (along with low-back pain) results in more years lived with a disability than any other chronic condition.[1] A review of RCTs of acute neck pain quickly reveals that pain is the primary outcome. The aim is to relieve that single episode of neck pain. There is no apparent interest in whether or not the neck pain recurs. Cost effectiveness is almost a mandatory feature of current RCTs. There seems to be a trend, not only to judge cost effectiveness, but to find the cheapest intervention. Yet it can be argued that the cost of neck pain is not in a single episode. Rather the financial, social and personal burdens are in repeated episodes of pain, repeated episodes of care, lost work productivity and costs of harm (e.g., side effects of nonsteroidal antiinflammatory drugs).

Relief of pain is an important clinical outcome and certainly patient centred. Yet this focus on pain seems to have dulled or eliminated a focus on rehabilitation to reduce recurrences. A major divide has developed between rehabilitation of a neck pain disorder and rehabilitation of an extremity disorder. A rehabilitation program for a knee or ankle disorder is usually inclusive of a comprehensive exercise program to train neuromuscular, proprioceptive and functional deficits to a normal functional level. Patients with neck pain are given exercises and numerous RCTs have tested exercise regimes for neck pain disorders. Yet the primary outcome is their effect on pain. Attention is usually not given to the neuromuscular impairment for which the exercise program was prescribed and whether or not that neuromuscular impairment was trained successfully. If a primary aim is to decrease the burden of neck pain, there needs to be a focus not only on pain relief but on the return of physical function towards decreasing recurrence rate. Restoration of normal neuromuscular function and proprioception, especially in the early stages of the disorder should contribute to this aim. Indeed, primary, secondary and tertiary preventative rehabilitation programs deserve equal attention to pain relief.

CONCLUSION

The statistic that neck pain along with low-back pain is the world's leading cause of years lived with a disability sends a major challenge to clinicians and researchers alike. Research has progressed knowledge at a remarkable pace particularly over the last 2 decades and this research is informing assessment and management. This text will synthesize knowledge relevant to the clinical sciences underpinning neck pain disorders and present a comprehensive approach to patient assessment and management, as well as commentary on key issues for defining neck pain disorders and primary, secondary and tertiary prevention. The approach is informed by our and others research and clinical expertise and patient experiences. Clinical relevance and application are key themes.

REFERENCES

1. Global Burden Disease 2015 Disease and Injury Incidence and Prevalence Collaborators. Global, regional, and national incidence, prevalence, and years lived with disability for 310 diseases and injuries, 1990-2015: a systematic analysis for the Global Burden of Disease Study 2015. Lancet 2016;388:1545–602.
2. Haldeman S, Carroll L, Cassidy JD. Findings from the Bone and Joint Decade 2000 to 2010 Task Force on neck pain and its associated disorders. J Occup Environ Med 2010;52:424–7.
3. Hush J, Lin C, Michaleff Z, et al. Prognosis of acute idiopathic neck pain is poor: a systematic review and meta-analysis. Arch Phys Med Rehabil 2011;92:824–9.
4. van Randeraad-van der Zee CH, Beurskens A, Swinkels R, et al. The burden of neck pain: its meaning for persons with neck pain and healthcare providers, explored by concept mapping. Qual Life Res 2016;25:1219–25.

5. Walton D, Kwok T, Mehta S, et al. Cluster analysis of an international pressure pain threshold database identifies 4 meaningful subgroups of adults with mechanical neck pain. Clin J Pain 2017;33:422–8.

6. Lee H, Nicholson L, Adams R. Neck muscle endurance, self-report, and range of motion data from subjects with treated and untreated neck pain. J Manipulative Physiol Ther 2005;28:25–32.

7. Cooper G, Bailey B, Bogduk N. Cervical zygapophysial joint pain maps. Pain Med 2007;8:344–53.

8. Kaniecki R. Migraine and tension-type headache: an assessment of challenges in diagnosis. Neurology 2002;58:S15–20.

9. Foreman R, Garrett K, Blair R. Mechanisms of cardiac pain. Compr Physiol 2015;5:929–60.

10. Thomas L. Cervical arterial dissection: an overview and implications for manipulative therapy practice. Man Ther 2016;21:2–9.

11. Siddall P. Neuroplasticity and pain: what does it all mean? Med J Aust 2013;198:177–8.

12. Falla D, Hodges P. Individualized exercise interventions for spinal pain. Exerc Sport Sci Rev 2017;45:105–15.

13. Jull G, Trott P, Potter H, et al. A randomized controlled trial of exercise and manipulative therapy for cervicogenic headache. Spine 2002;27:1835–43.

14. Lee H, Nicholson LL, Adams RD. Cervical range of motion associations with subclinical neck pain. Spine 2004;29:33–40.

15. Sterling M, Jull G, Vicenzino B, et al. Development of motor system dysfunction following whiplash injury. Pain 2003;103:65–73.

16. Uhlig Y, Weber BR, Grob D, et al. Fiber composition and fiber transformations in neck muscles of patients with dysfunction of the cervical spine. J Orthop Res 1995;13:240–9.

17. Nolet P, Côté P, Kristman V, et al. Is neck pain associated with worse health-related quality of life 6 months later? A population-based cohort study. Spine J 2015;15:675–84.

18. Treleaven J, Takasaki H. Characteristics of visual disturbances reported by subjects with neck pain. Man Ther 2014;19:203–7.

19. Reid S, Callister R, Snodgrass S, et al. Manual therapy for cervicogenic dizziness: long-term outcomes of a randomised trial. Man Ther 2015;20:148–56.

20. Waddell G. 1987 Volvo award in clinical sciences. A new clinical model for the treatment of low-back pain. Spine 1987;12:632–44.

21. Engel G. The need for a new medical model: a challenge for biomedicine. Science 1977;196:129–36.

22. Ghaemi S. The rise and fall of the biopsychosocial model. Br J Psychiatry 2009;195:3–4.

23. Taylor J. The Cervical Spine. An atlas of normal anatomy and the morbid anatomy of ageing and injuries. Australia: Elsevier; 2017.

24. Anstey R, Kongsted A, Kamper S, et al. Are people with whiplash-associated neck pain different from people with nonspecific neck pain? J Orthop Sports Phys Ther 2016;46:894–901.

25. Scott D, Sterling M, Jull G. A psychophysical investigation of pain processing mechanisms in chronic neck pain. Clin J Pain 2005;21:175–81.

26. Ris I, Juul-Kristensen B, Boyle E, et al. Chronic neck pain patients with traumatic or non-traumatic onset: differences in characteristics. A cross-sectional study. Scand J Pain 2017;14:1–8.

27. Stenneberg M, Rood M, de Bie R, et al. To what degree does active cervical range of motion differ between patients with neck pain, patients with whiplash, and those without neck pain? A systematic review and meta-analysis. Arch Phys Med Rehabil 2017;98:1407–34.

28. Elliott J, Jull G, Noteboom J, et al. Fatty infiltration in the cervical extensor muscles in persistent whiplash associated disorders (WAD): an MRI analysis. Spine 2006;31:E847–55.

29. Elliott J, Pedler A, Jull G, et al. Differential changes in muscle composition exist in traumatic and nontraumatic neck pain. Spine 2014;39:39–47.

30. Elliott J, Pedler A, Kenardy J, et al. The temporal development of fatty infiltrates in the neck muscles following whiplash injury: an association with pain and posttraumatic stress. PLoS ONE 2011;6:e21194.

31. Treleaven J, Clamaron-Cheers C, Jull G. Does the region of pain influence the presence of sensorimotor disturbances in neck pain disorders? Man Ther 2011;16:636–40.

32. Jonsson H, Bring G, Rauschning W, et al. Hidden cervical spine injuries in traffic accident victims with skull fractures. J Spinal Disord 1991;4:251–63.

33. Knackstedt H, Kråkenes J, Bansevicius D, et al. Magnetic resonance imaging of craniovertebral structures: clinical significance in cervicogenic headaches. J Headache Pain 2012;13:39–44.

34. Hogg-Johnson S, van der Velde G, Carroll LJ, et al. The burden and determinants of neck pain in the general population - Results of the Bone and Joint Decade 2000-2010 Task Force on Neck Pain and its Associated Disorders. Spine 2008;33:S39–51.

35. Stiell I, Clement C, McKnight D, et al. The Canadian C-Spine Rule versus the NEXUS low-risk criteria in patients with trauma. N Engl J Med 2003;349:2510–18.

36. Hancock M, Kjaer P, Kent P, et al. Is the number of different MRI findings more strongly associated with low back pain than single MRI findings? Spine 2017;42:1283–8.

37. Hancock M, Maher C, Petocz P, et al. Risk factors for a recurrence of low back pain. Spine J 2015;15:2360–8.

38. Hall T, Briffa K, Hopper D, et al. Reliability of manual examination and frequency of symptomatic cervical motion segment dysfunction in cervicogenic headache. Man Ther 2010;15:542–6.

39. Howard P, Behrns W, Martino M, et al. Manual examination in the diagnosis of cervicogenic headache: a systematic literature review. J Man Manip Ther 2015;23:210–18.

40. Jull G, Bogduk N, Marsland A. The accuracy of manual diagnosis for cervical zygapophysial joint pain syndromes. Med J Aust 1988;148:233–6.

41. Schneider G, Jull G, Thomas K, et al. Derivation of a clinical decision guide in the diagnosis of cervical facet joint pain. Arch Phys Med Rehabil 2014;95:1695–701.

42. Zito G, Jull G, Story I. Clinical tests of musculoskeletal dysfunction in the diagnosis of cervicogenic headache. Man Ther 2006;11:118–29.

43. Taxonomy Working Group. Classification of Chronic Pain, Second Edition (Revised). International Association for the Study of Pain (IASP) 2012; http://www.iasp-pain.org/PublicationsNews/Content.aspx?ItemNumber=1673.

44. Maier C, Baron R, Tolle TR, et al. Quantitative sensory testing in the German Research Network on Neuropathic Pain (DFNS): somatosensory abnormalities in 1236 patients with different neuropathic pain syndromes. Pain 2010;150:439–50.

45. Pedler A, Sterling M. Patients with chronic whiplash can be subgrouped on the basis of symptoms of sensory hypersensitivity and posttraumatic stress. Pain 2013;154:1640–8.

46. Clark N, Röijezon U, Treleaven J. Proprioception in musculoskeletal rehabilitation. Part 2: clinical assessment and intervention. Man Ther 2015;20:378–87.

47. Röijezon U, Clark N, Treleaven J. Proprioception in musculoskeletal rehabilitation. Part 1: basic science and principles of assessment and clinical interventions. Man Ther 2015;20:368–77.

48. Carroll L, Hogg-Johnson S, van der Velde G, et al. Course and prognostic factors for neck pain in the general population. Results of the Bone and Joint Decade 2000-2010 Task Force on Neck Pain and Its Associated Disorders. Spine 2008;33:S75–82.

49. Christensen J, Knardahl S. Work and neck pain: a prospective study of psychological, social, and mechanical risk factors. Pain 2010;151:162–73.

50. Christensen J, Knardahl S. Time-course of occupational psychological and social factors as predictors of new-onset and persistent neck pain: a three-wave prospective study over 4 years. Pain 2014;155:1262–71.

51. Shahidi B, Curran-Everett D, Maluf K. Psychosocial, physical, and neurophysiological risk factors for chronic neck pain: a prospective inception cohort study. J Pain 2015;16:1288–99.

52. Walton D, Macdermid J, Giorgianni A, et al. Risk factors for persistent problems following acute whiplash injury: update of a systematic review and meta-analysis. J Orthop Sports Phys Ther 2013;43:31–43.

53. Walton D, Carroll L, Kasch H, et al. An overview of systematic reviews on prognostic factors in neck pain: results from the International Collaboration on Neck Pain (ICON) Project. Open Orthop J 2013;7(Suppl. 4:M9):494–505.

54. Sterling M. Does knowledge of predictors of recovery and nonrecovery assist outcomes after whiplash injury? Spine 2011;36: S257–62.

55. Mintken P, Cleland J, Carpenter K, et al. Some factors predict successful short-term outcomes in individuals with shoulder pain receiving cervicothoracic manipulation: a single-arm trial. Phys Ther 2010;90:26–42.

56. Nee R, Vicenzino B, Jull GA, et al. Baseline characteristics of patients with nerve-related neck and arm pain predict the likely response to neural tissue management. J Orthop Sports Phys Ther 2013;43:379–91.

57. Puentedura E, Cleland J, Landers M, et al. Development of a clinical prediction rule to identify patients with neck pain likely to benefit from thrust joint manipulation to the cervical spine. J Orthop Sports Phys Ther 2012;42:577–92.

58. Raney N, Petersen E, Smith T, et al. Development of a clinical prediction rule to identify patients with neck pain likely to benefit from cervical traction and exercise. Eur Spine J 2009;18:382–9.

59. Tseng Y-L, Wang W, Chen W-Y, et al. Predictors for the immediate responders to cervical manipulation in patients with neck pain. Man Ther 2006;11:306–15.

60. Cleland J, Mintken P, Carpenter K, et al. Examination of a clinical prediction rule to identify patients with neck pain likely to benefit from thoracic spine thrust manipulation and a general cervical range of motion exercise: multi-center randomized clinical trial. Phys Ther 2010;90:1239–50.

61. Fernández-de-Las-Peñas C, Cleland J, Salom-Moreno J, et al. Prediction of outcome in women with carpal tunnel syndrome who receive manual physical therapy interventions: a validation study. J Orthop Sports Phys Ther 2016;46:443–51.

62. Mintken P, McDevitt A, Michener L, et al. Examination of the validity of a clinical prediction rule to identify patients with shoulder pain likely to benefit from cervicothoracic manipulation. J Orthop Sports Phys Ther 2017;47:133–49.

63. Kelly J, Ritchie C, Sterling M. Clinical prediction rules for prognosis and treatment prescription in neck pain: a systematic review. Musculoskelet Sci Pract 2017;27:155–64.

64. Childs J, Fritz J, Piva S, et al. Proposal of a classification system for patients with neck pain. J Orthop Sports Phys Ther 2004;34:686–96.

65. Fritz J, Brennan G. Preliminary examination of a proposed treatment-based classification system for patients receiving physical therapy interventions for neck pain. Phys Ther 2007;87: 513–24.

66. Fritz J, Thackeray A, Brennan G, et al. Exercise only, exercise with mechanical traction, or exercise with over-door traction for patients with cervical radiculopathy, with or without consideration of status on a previously described subgrouping rule: a randomized clinical trial. J Orthop Sports Phys Ther 2014;44: 45–57.

67. Blanpied P, Gross A, Elliott J, et al. Neck pain: revision 2017. J Orthop Sports Phys Ther 2017;47:A1–83.

68. Childs J, Cleland J, Elliott J, et al. Neck pain: clinical practice guidelines linked to the International Classification of Functioning, Disability, and Health from the Orthopedic Section of the American Physical Therapy Association. J Orthop Sports Phys Ther 2008;38:A1–34.

69. Clare H, Adams R, Maher C. Reliability of McKenzie classification of patients with cervical or lumbar pain. J Manipulative Physiol Ther 2005;28:122–7.

70. Hefford C. McKenzie classification of mechanical spinal pain: profile of syndromes and directions of preference. Man Ther 2008;13:75–81.

71. Takasaki H, May S. Mechanical diagnosis and therapy has similar effects on pain and disability as 'wait and see' and other approaches in people with neck pain: a systematic review. J Physiother 2014;60:78–84.

72. Saragiotto B, Maher C, Hancock M, et al. Subgrouping patients with nonspecific low back pain: hope or hype? J Orthop Sports Phys Ther 2017;47:44–8.

73. Southerst D, Nordin M, Côté P, et al. Is exercise effective for the management of neck pain and associated disorders or whiplash-associated disorders? A systematic review by the Ontario Protocol for Traffic Injury Management (OPTIMa) Collaboration. Spine J 2016;16:1503–23.

74. Sutton D, Côté P, Wong J, et al. Is multimodal care effective for the management of patients with whiplash-associated disorders

or neck pain and associated disorders? A systematic review by the Ontario Protocol for Traffic Injury Management (OPTIMa) Collaboration. Spine J 2016;16:1541–5165.

75. van der Velde G, Yu H, Paulden M, et al. Which interventions are cost-effective for the management of whiplash-associated and neck pain-associated disorders? A systematic review of the health economic literature by the Ontario Protocol for Traffic Injury Management (OPTIMa) Collaboration. Spine J 2016;16: 1582–97.

76. Wong J, Shearer H, Mior S, et al. Are manual therapies, passive physical modalities, or acupuncture effective for the management of patients with whiplash-associated disorders or neck pain and associated disorders? An update of the Bone and Joint Decade Task Force on Neck Pain and Its Associated Disorders by the OPTIMa collaboration. Spine J 2016;16:1598–630.

77. Yu H, Côté P, Southerst D, et al. Does structured patient education improve the recovery and clinical outcomes of patients with neck pain? A systematic review from the Ontario Protocol for Traffic Injury Management (OPTIMa) collaboration. Spine J 2016;16: 1524–40.

78. Shearer H, Carroll L, Wong J, et al. Are psychological interventions effective for the management of neck pain and whiplash-associated disorders? A systematic review by the Ontario Protocol for Traffic Injury Management (OPTIMa) collaboration. Spine J 2016;16: 1566–81.

79. Gross A, Langevin P, Burnie S, et al. Manipulation and mobilisation for neck pain contrasted against an inactive control or another active treatment. Cochrane Databae Syst Rev 2015;(9): doi:10.1002/14651858.CD004249.pub4.

80. Gross A, Paquin J, Dupont G, et al. Exercises for mechanical neck disorders: a Cochrane review update. Man Ther 2016;24:25–45.

81. Jull G, Moore A. Hands on, hands off? The swings in musculo-skeletal physiotherapy practice. Man Ther 2012;17:199–200.

82. Roth R, Geisser M, Williams D. Interventional pain medicine: retreat from the biopsychosocial model of pain. Transl Behav Med 2012;2:106–16.

Section 2

CLINICAL SCIENCES

The chapters in this section present key clinical sciences in biopsychosocial domains that underpin musculoskeletal practice to manage patients with neck pain disorders. The neurosciences and clinical sciences that underlie symptoms commonly reported by patients with neck pain disorders are discussed, as is the pathophysiology of the sensory, articular, nervous, neuromuscular and sensorimotor systems. The basic and clinical sciences provide the foundation for clinical practice. They provide the basis on which clinicians can undertake informed clinical reasoning in the clinical assessment, diagnosis and management of patients who will present with the infinite variety of neck pain disorders.

2 NOCICEPTION AND PAIN PERCEPTION

INTRODUCTION

Pain, as currently defined by the International Association for the Study of Pain (IASP), is "an unpleasant sensory and emotional experience associated with actual or potential tissue damage, or described [by the patient] in terms of such damage".[1] This definition carries within it several important points for the clinician. Firstly, pain is not always associated with tissue injury or damage. As such, it should be realized that pain is distinct from nociception; a physiological term, defined as "the neural process of encoding noxious stimuli".[2] Nociception is commonly associated with pain, yet it is neither necessary nor sufficient for the perception of pain. The second important point to be gained from the definition is that pain is not a sensation that simply reflects the state of peripheral tissues. Pain is, by definition, a multidimensional sensory and emotional experience; its unpleasant nature always bringing with it negative affect, notably distress.[3,4] This multidimensionality is also the route through which psychological factors, stress and immune responses may modulate and intensify a painful experience.

There are additional definitions that categorize pain by location (space), and some that do so by chronology (time). Cervical spinal pain is defined by the IASP as "arising from anywhere within the region bounded superiorly by the superior nuchal line, inferiorly by an imaginary transverse line through the tip of the first thoracic spinous process, and laterally by sagittal planes tangential to the lateral borders of the neck".[1] Cervical spinal pain can be further categorized into upper versus lower cervical pain by subdividing the region caudocephalically into two equal halves.[1] In addition, pain perceived between the superior nuchal line and an imaginary transverse line through the spinous process of the second cervical vertebra is defined as suboccipital pain.[1]

Chronic pain is considered that which "persists beyond normal tissue healing time";[1] 3 to 6 months is generally accepted as the period within which "normal tissue healing" should have occurred and has therefore been used to define chronic pain,[5] accepting its limitations. Pain has an adaptive (useful), protective role in that it can alert an organism to threatening circumstances, which could lead to real bodily harm if ignored. However, when pain persists beyond such threatening circumstances for some people it may no longer be adaptive or protective, instead becoming a source of poor quality of life, low mood, reduced function and even shortened life.[6,7]

This chapter will briefly review the different mechanisms that can lead to a perception of pain:[8,9] nociceptive, neuropathic, inflammatory and central hypersensitivity. These distinct pain mechanisms are clinically important for neck pain because they have implications for management.

THE NOCICEPTIVE PATHWAY: FROM NOXIOUS STIMULI TO PAIN PERCEPTION

The nociceptive pathway consists of four main processes: transduction, encoding, conduction and transmission.[10] Transduction is the process where a damaging or potentially damaging noxious stimulus (mechanical, thermal, chemical or electrical) is converted into electrical signals within specialized receptors of nerve endings that are embedded in the stimulated tissues. Encoding is the process of signal formation that contains information relevant to the nature and intensity of the stimulus. Consequences of encoding may be autonomic (e.g., elevated blood pressure) or behavioural (motor withdrawal reflex), however pain perception is not necessarily implied.[1] Transmission is the process whereby this encoded information is passed on from one nociceptive neuron to another, via synapses, toward higher brain centres. Perception is the conscious experience that follows the decoding of nociceptive information by higher brain centres.[10] At every stage along this nociceptive pathway, it is possible to interrupt, reduce or amplify the passage of encoded information; this is known as modulation, and is exploited by many therapeutic interventions.[10]

The high-threshold sensory neurons that respond to noxious stimuli are called nociceptors. They encode and transmit sensory information from the periphery to the central nervous system (CNS). Nociceptors include small-diameter, slow conducting, predominantly unmyelinated neurons known as *C fibres* and thinly myelinated neurons known as *Aδ fibres*.[10,11] They terminate as free, unencapsulated peripheral nerve endings in most tissues of the body including skin, muscles, joints and viscera and respond to various different stimuli. When stimulated, C fibres act almost like a gland, releasing a range of proinflammatory substances, such as prostaglandins, cytokines, bradykinin, from their peripheral terminals into the surrounding tissues.[10] These substances directly stimulate nearby nociceptors, proliferating the effect.[12] Simultaneously, nociceptor thresholds of activation reduce, in a process known as *peripheral sensitization*, so that less stimulation is needed to further activate the nociceptor receptors.[13]

The synaptic transmission of encoded signals is complex. The primary neurotransmitter of nociceptors appears to be glutamate, but multiple other chemicals are also released.[14] Nociceptors terminate in the dorsal horn of the spinal cord, predominantly within spinal lamina I and outer lamina II.[10,14] They pass their encoded signal on to relay nociceptive neurons, and local interneurons that are important for signal modulation.[14] This contrasts to low-threshold Aβ fibres, which transmit innocuous touch signals and synapse onto neurons primarily in lamina III.[15] A loss of this separation is intrinsic to the phenomenon of allodynia, in which pain is evoked as a result of innocuous stimuli such as light touch.[16]

The encoded signal can be modified within the dorsal horn. Local inhibitory and excitatory interneurons, in addition to descending pathways, can modulate the transmission of nociceptive signals.[14] These might, for example, facilitate the prioritization of pain perception over other competing demands, or block such perception if chances of survival are increased by doing so.[14] Second order neurons then transmit nociceptive signals through ascending pathways in the spinal cord, to higher centres in the brain.[10,13] The spinothalamic tract (also known as *anterolateral system*) transmits nociceptive signals to nuclei within the thalamus where third order neurones then ascend to terminate in the primary somatosensory cortex as well as other regions such as the cingulate cortex.[10] This pathway is particularly relevant for the localization of painful stimuli.[10,13] In contrast, the spinoreticular pathway is involved in the emotional aspects of pain.[10,13] Here fibres reach the brainstem reticular formation, before projecting to the thalamus and hypothalamus with further projections then to the cortex. The spinomesencephalic tract terminates primarily in the superior colliculus and the periaqueductal grey and is likely to be involved in multisensory integration and in behavioural reactions and orientating to painful stimuli.[13]

There are a number of brain regions activated during the experience of acute pain. They are collectively referred to as the *pain matrix*, which includes the primary and secondary somatosensory cortex, insular cortex, anterior cingulate cortex, prefrontal cortex and the thalamus.[10,13] This distributed cerebral activation likely reflects the multifaceted nature of pain involving discriminative, affective, autonomic and motor components.[13] The perception of pain is then subjective and can be modified or affected by numerous influences including distraction/attention and beliefs/attitudes.[10,17]

The brain is able to modulate nociceptive processing via descending pathways and descending inhibitory connections project back to the spinal cord to decrease the activity of nociceptive neurons thereby providing pain relief.[18] The descending pain control system includes the dorsolateral prefrontal cortex, periaqueductal grey, locus coeruleus of the pons and the nucleus raphe magnus of the medulla oblongata. Studies have revealed a correlation between the amount of pain relief reported and the extent of both activation and functional connectivity between these regions.[18–20] Descending pain inhibition is largely facilitated through endogenous opioids;[20,21] however, other neurotransmitters such as cannabinoids and dopamine can contribute.[12,18,19,22,23]

NOCICEPTIVE PAIN

Damage or threatened damage to non-neural tissue, which results in activation of nociceptors can lead to nociceptive pain.[1] Many structures within the cervical region are innervated by nociceptors and can therefore provide nociceptive input, including muscles, zygapophysial joint capsules, intervertebral discs and ligaments.[24] All too often a "pathoanatomic" lesion cannot be demonstrated with imaging for people with neck pain,[25] and it is often not possible to make a definitive pathoanatomic diagnosis, but that does not negate the existence of a physical cause. Several cadaveric studies have demonstrated the presence of subtle pathoanatomic

lesions in cervical structures, which have so far evaded detection by current imaging techniques.[26,27] In the case of motor vehicle accidents and whiplash trauma, there may be subtle lesions in the intervertebral discs and the zygapophysial joints,[25,28] with biomechanical studies confirming that even minor loads can lead to lesions of the latter.[29,30]

Zygapophysial joint capsules contain low-threshold mechanoreceptors, mechanically sensitive nociceptors and silent nociceptors[31,32] confirming them as a potential source of ongoing nociceptive pain. Various studies have described the area of experienced pain following noxious stimulation of individual cervical structures[33–35] (Fig. 2.1). Notably, the distribution of pain may become even larger when already symptomatic structures (e.g., zygapophysial joints) are stimulated.[33]

Controlled diagnostic blocks of the medial branches of cervical posterior primary rami can be used to determine the prevalence of cervical zygapophysial joint pain in a given population.[36] Typically, a positive test is awarded when at least one-half of the pain is reduced soon after the medial branch block. In one study,[33] of 194 patients with chronic neck pain lasting more than

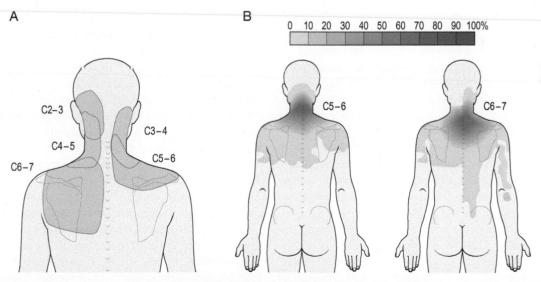

Fig. 2.1 ■ (A) The patterns of referred pain reported in healthy volunteers following stimulation of cervical zygapophysial joints by distending the joint capsule with injections of contrast medium. (From Dwyer A, Aprill C, Bogduk N. Cervical zygapophysial joint pain patterns I: a study in normal volunteers. Spine 1990;15:453–457.) (B) Representative examples of pain referral maps generated for the C5-6 and C6-7 disc levels from patients undergoing cervical discography. (From Slipman CW, Plastaras C, Patel R, et al. Provocative cervical discography symptom mapping. Spine J 2005;5:381–388.)

6 months (with a total of 347 diagnostic blocks performed), 134 patients (69%) presented with at least one symptomatic level. A recent review determined that the prevalence of zygapophysial joint pain varies from 36% to 67% with C5/C6 the most common joint affected.[37] In those involved in high-speed motor vehicle accidents, the prevalence may be as high as 74%.[38]

Recent studies have also demonstrated that radiofrequency denervation, a technique that reduces peripheral nociception from a zygapophysial joint by removing the sensory innervation of the joint, leads to enhanced neck range of motion, decreased psychological distress and reduced signs of central hyperexcitability in people with whiplash-associated disorders,[39,40] thus supporting the opinion that the zygapophysial joint is a continuing source of neck pain for many with chronic neck pain.

NEUROPATHIC PAIN

The IASP defines neuropathic pain as "pain caused by a lesion or disease of the somatosensory nervous system".[1] Neuropathic pain can be further divided into central or peripheral components. Central neuropathic pain is that "caused by a lesion or disease of the central somatosensory nervous system" whereas peripheral neuropathic pain is "caused by a lesion or disease of the peripheral somatosensory nervous system".[1] Nerve compression, nerve trauma, infection and diabetes are all examples of conditions that may lead to neuropathic pain, typically described by patients as burning, shooting and/or pricking and prickling in nature.[41,42] Neuropathic pain is attributed to an imbalance of activity in pathways resulting from actual loss or a disturbance to the physiological inputs caused by lesions in neurons.[41] More specifically, disparities between excitatory and inhibitory signalling, changes in ion channels and modification to the modulation of nociception are mechanisms associated with neuropathic pain.[41]

Neuropathic pain may be associated with dysesthesia (defined as unpleasant abnormal sensations), allodynia (which is the sensation of pain to non-noxious stimulation such as light touch) and hyperalgesia (which is an increased response to a normal noxious stimulus).[42,43] Cold hyperalgesia in particular is a common feature of neuropathic pain attributed to peripheral nerve injury.[44,45] Aberrant temporal summation of pain and

pain continuing after stimulation has ceased are other regular features observed in people with neuropathic pain.[42]

A neuropathic pain mechanism is commonly implied in cervical radiculopathy, although it is likely that these patients present with a combination of both nociceptive and neuropathic pain; that is, a mixed pain syndrome.[46,47] Signs of neuropathic pain may be present in some people following a whiplash trauma suggesting that there may be nerve injury as part of their presentation. For instance, cold hyperalgesia has been observed in people with moderate to severe pain following a whiplash injury and its presence is associated with poor recovery.[48] Moreover, loss of sensitivity or increased detection thresholds (hypoesthesia) to vibration, electrical and thermal stimuli have been observed in people following whiplash trauma[49] as they are in patients with cervical radiculopathy.[47,50,51] In addition, studies have confirmed neural tissue mechanosensitivity in patients with whiplash-associated disorders (WAD)[52,53] which could be an indication that nerve injury is a contributor to persistent symptoms seen in this condition. These findings are supported by cadaveric investigations which have revealed nerve damage (e.g., nerve roots and dorsal root ganglia) following motor vehicle accidents.[27]

Certain self-reported questionnaires can be used to help identify neuropathic pain. One such questionnaire, the Self-Administered Leeds Assessment of Neuropathic Symptoms and Signs (S-LANSS),[54] was completed by people with acute pain following a whiplash injury; around 20% were identified as having a likely neuropathic component.[55] The painDETECT questionnaire[56] can also be used to facilitate the identification of neuropathic pain, with convergent validity demonstrated with similar neuropathic pain screening tools[56] and to pain severity.[57] Although this questionnaire has been commonly applied to identify a neuropathic pain component in people with low-back and leg pain,[58,59] it has been less frequently applied in neck pain populations. One study showed that 30% of participants with cervical radiculopathy demonstrated the likely presence of neuropathic pain as identified by the painDETECT questionnaire, whereas neuropathic pain components were not identified in the enrolled participants with non-specific neck-arm pain.[47] The participants with cervical radiculopathy also displayed significant side-to-side differences in mechanical and vibration detection in their maximal pain area, the symptomatic side being less sensitive to the stimuli than the control side, consistent with observations in patients with peripheral nerve injury.[47] Approximately 50% of the participants also presented with cold hyperalgesia, another common feature following peripheral nerve injury.

INFLAMMATORY PAIN

Inflammatory pain is facilitated by an abundance of substances released following tissue damage in addition to the surge of inflammatory processes which follows. Inflammation following tissue injury results from plasma extravasation and infiltration of immune cells into the injured region including macrophages and neutrophils.[60] These immune cells, in addition to resident cells, release numerous inflammatory mediators including prosta-glandins, bradykinin, nerve growth factors, proinflam-matory cytokines, interleukin-1β and proinflammatory chemokines.[60,61] Some of these inflammatory mediators will directly activate and sensitize nociceptors, which changes their response characteristics[14] and may acti-vate "sleeping" or "silent" nociceptors, which do not usually respond to noxious stimulation but can be woken as a result of chemical mediators related with tissue damage.[14,62,63] Inflammation-induced nociceptor hyperactivity can also facilitate the release of neurotrans-mitters (e.g., glutamate) and neuromodulators (e.g., substance P) leading to hyperactivity of postsynaptic nociceptive neurons which contributes to the process of central sensitization.[64,65] Some proinflammatory cytokines, including tumour necrosis factor alpha (TNF-α) and interleukin-1β, have been implicated in the development of chronic pathological pain and both proinflammatory cytokines and chemokines can modulate the activity of both peripheral and central neurons.[61]

C-reactive protein (CRP) is an acute-phase reactant released by hepatocytes and the production of CRP may be regulated by proinflammatory cytokines including TNF-α and interleukin-1β.[66] Levels of CRP are typi-cally elevated following traumatic injury, infection and autoimmune disease, but have also been observed to increase in some conditions including acute sciatica[67] and whiplash.[68,69] CRP typically peaks within 48 hours of injury but usually falls rapidly, whereas persist-ing elevated levels of CRP is indicative of ongoing inflammation.[70,71]

There has been little investigation of inflammatory biomarkers in people with neck pain and this will likely become an area of future research. One study by Kivioja et al.[69] showed the presence of an immune response within 3 days of a whiplash trauma as evidenced by elevated TNF-α and interleukin-10-secreting blood mononuclear cells however, this had resolved by 14 days. This finding suggests an initial but resolving inflammatory response following whiplash injury. In another study, elevated CRP levels were identified in people when measured 2 to 3 weeks after a whiplash trauma[68] suggestive of ongoing inflammation of injured tissues. Interestingly, when tested 3 months after the injury, CRP levels had returned to normal in those who considered themselves recovered or only with mild disability whereas CRP remained elevated in those continuing to experience moderate to severe pain and disability likely because of unresolved tissue lesions.[68]

PERIPHERAL AND CENTRAL SENSITIZATION

Sensitization is defined as "increased responsiveness of nociceptive neurons to their normal input, and/or recruitment of a response to normally subthreshold inputs";[1] a process that can include a drop in thresh-old and an increase in suprathreshold response. It is important for the clinician to note that sensitization processes are physiological and adaptive, selected via evolutionary processes to confer protection to the organism. However, like many protective adaptations, sometimes the apparatus and processes underlying the mechanism can malfunction leading to problems; specifically, disproportional pain for somatosensory sensitivity.

Sensitization can occur after tissue injury or nerve damage and generally results in a heightened perception of pain for a given stimulus. When the painful stimulus is noxious, a heightened response is known as *hyper-algesia*; when the painful stimulus is innocuous, the phenomenon is *allodynia*. Spontaneous discharges and spatial expansion of the receptive field size also typically result.[1] Moreover, these consequences can outlast the stimulus considerably, almost like a "pain memory"; a process known as long-term potentiation.[10,13] As a result, spontaneous continuous pain, spontaneous intermittent pain and abnormally evoked pain (e.g., by light touch or movement) may occur.[72]

Sensitization may develop both through central and peripheral mechanisms. Peripheral sensitization is attributed to sensitization of the peripheral primary sensory neurons located within the dorsal root ganglia and trigeminal ganglia and can be caused by a number of mechanisms including inflammatory mediators (e.g., prostaglandins) and the release of substances from damaged cells.[42] In contrast, central sensitization comprises increased excitability of central nociceptive neurons in the cortex, brain stem, trigeminal nucleus and spinal cord.[65] A number of mechanisms have been implicated in long-term central sensitization, including cortical reorganization and maladaptive neuroplasticity, alterations in neurochemistry, loss of inhibitory neurons, alerted glial activity, dysfunction of endogenous pain control mechanisms, alterations in grey-matter volume and altered structural integrity and connectivity of white matter.[16,65,73]

One of the first studies to demonstrate central sensitization and widespread hypersensitivity in people with chronic WAD was performed by Koelbaek-Johansen et al.[74] In this study, hypertonic saline was injected into the tibialis anterior muscle of healthy controls and people with chronic WAD, and the participants were asked to draw their perceived pain on a body chart. Larger areas of referred pain were identified for the patient group with both distal and proximal referred pain areas.[74] Since then, a number of studies have applied quantitative sensory testing (QST) to evaluate both peripheral and central sensitization in people with neck pain disorders. QST involves the assessment of responses to controlled and quantifiable physical stimuli, typically either pressure or temperature. The pain threshold is commonly measured and is defined as the minimum amount of stimulation required to evoke pain. For instance, in the case of the pressure pain threshold, increasing amounts of pressure is applied at a standardized rate over a point (e.g., over a muscle belly) using an algometer and the patient is instructed to push a button as soon as the sensation changes from one of pressure to one of pain. Less commonly assessed is the pain tolerance, which measures the maximum stimulation a person is willing to bear. Temporal summation and conditioned pain modulation are also established ways of quantifying sensitivity, measuring excitability of afferent nociceptive

pathways and evoked descending pain inhibition, respectively.[75,76]

Mechanical hyperalgesia locally over the neck region is often detected in people with neck pain regardless of the aetiology of their pain.[77–81] However, mechanical hyperalgesia at remote sites (indicative of central sensitization) has been observed in people with WAD, especially those with greater pain severity,[77–79,82] or in some cases, people with non-traumatic neck pain of greater severity.[83] Thus this feature of widespread sensitivity to mechanical stimuli is not usually present in people with milder symptoms or those with neck pain of insidious onset.[77,78] Sensitivity to both heat and cold stimuli has also been seen in people with moderate to severe pain following a whiplash trauma and this has been found both at local and remote sites[48,51,78,84] with cold hyperalgesia having moderate evidence as a prognostic indicator of poor recovery following a whiplash injury.[48,85] Similar sensory disturbances have been shown in people with chronic cervical radiculopathy presenting with higher pain and disability levels.[47,51] However, sensitivity to thermal stimuli was not demonstrated in people with neck pain of non-traumatic origin[47,78] (Fig. 2.2). The nociceptive withdrawal reflex has been used to study the excitability of spinal cord neurons with evidence that people with chronic WAD have significantly lower thresholds compared with asymptomatic people, indicative of spinal cord hyperexcitability.[82,86] Recent systematic reviews have confirmed the presence of sensitization as a common feature in WAD[87] whereas it is not a characteristic feature of chronic idiopathic and non-traumatic neck pain.[88]

Studies have also examined hypoesthesia by evaluating detection thresholds for non-painful stimuli and, consistent with thermal pain threshold testing, sensory hypoesthesia was detected in people with chronic WAD[49,77] whereas it was not a feature of chronic idiopathic neck pain.[77] The widespread and generalized nature of hypoesthesia seen in people with WAD is again suggestive of central sensitization.

THE INFLUENCE OF PSYCHOLOGICAL FACTORS

The pain literature over the last two decades, particularly relating to low-back pain, has been dominated by the

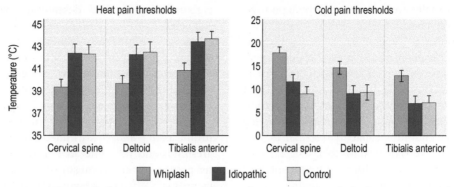

Fig. 2.2 ■ Temperature pain thresholds measured over the cervical spine, deltoid and tibialis anterior muscle in people with chronic whiplash associated disorders, chronic idiopathic neck pain and healthy controls. Note the significant change in temperature pain thresholds for the whiplash group only. (From Scott D, Jull G, Sterling M. Widespread sensory hypersensitivity is a feature of chronic whiplash-associated disorder but not chronic idiopathic neck pain. Clin J Pain 2005;21:175–181.)

influence of psychological factors. The development of "yellow flags" for psychological risk factors initially focused around chronicity and disability related to low-back pain. However, it has gradually become apparent that the same risk factors act across a wide variety of musculoskeletal pain conditions, including neck pain. In addition, event-related distress can be a consequence following a whiplash injury.[89,90]

Psychological factors, such as anxiety and distress create very real, measurable activity in the CNS. It is within this CNS activity that signals from the peripheral nervous system converge and interact to produce the effects we see in patients. Indeed, psychological factors (e.g., depression) that are known to increase the longevity of pain conditions increase activity of similar brain regions known to be involved in the processing of pain signals.[91,92]

Acute stressors activate the adrenomedullary hormonal system (AHS), hypothalamic-pituitary-adrenocortical (HPA) axis and sympathetic nervous system (SNS), which can induce transient stress-induced analgesia as part of the flight-or-fight response.[93] These processes also help to remember the stressful event in a process referred to as *memory consolidation*.[94] It is thought that an exaggerated stress response may actually lead to over consolidation of memories contributing to the development of posttraumatic stress disorder.[95]

There is accumulating evidence suggesting that the stress response may become maladaptive and

can contribute to ongoing pain and progression to chronicity.[96,97] Moreover, activation of the stress systems can contribute to hyperalgesia and allodynia after stressful events[98] and in neck pain, in the case of a motor vehicle accident.[48,99] Posttraumatic stress disorder has been detected in some people within just weeks of a whiplash injury which can persist and contribute to greater perceived pain and disability and poor recovery.[85,90] In this case, the initial and ongoing stress response becomes maladaptive and can facilitate the transition to chronicity.

Some evidence suggests that cortisol secretion may become dysfunctional in people with chronic pain, and reduced cortisol levels have been observed in chronic WAD[100] as well as other chronic pain conditions such as low-back pain and fibromyalgia.[101–104] Studies have also demonstrated altered activations of the HPA axis in response to experimentally induced pain.[97,105]

There may be a genetic predisposition to stress-induced pain; genetic variations with the capacity to influence responses of the stress system could explain the vulnerability of some people developing ongoing pain following a stressful/traumatic event such as a whiplash injury.[98,106] The catechol *O-methyltransferase* (*COMT*) gene is one such example. The *COMT* gene provides commands for producing the enzyme called COMT which degrades catecholamines, including epinephrine, norepinephrine and dopamine.[107] Studies have shown that variants of the *COMT* gene are linked to greater sensitivity to experimentally induced pain[108,109] and chronic pain.[108,110] A recent study evaluated the association between neck pain intensity and the COMT genotype immediately following a motor vehicle accident.[107] Interestingly, those with a COMT pain vulnerable genotype had more severe neck pain, headache and dizziness. Moreover, they estimated that a longer time would be needed for both their physical and emotional recovery. Thus genetic variations affecting the stress response have the capacity to influence both symptoms and psychological status following a motor vehicle accident.[107] No doubt future studies will shed more light on these influences.

Psychosocial influences on pain perception

When a person experiences acute pain, it is highly likely that they will have some degree of psychological distress. Chronic pain, by its very nature, can be associated with ongoing psychological distress but also with other features including negative beliefs, fear and depression. Psychological factors can have a powerful influence on pain perception and can play a key role in the transition from acute to chronic pain for some people. The social and environmental context, cultural background, socioeconomic status, attitudes, expectations and beliefs can also have a powerful influence on pain perception and can amplify peripheral sensations. As an example, when a patient receives a negative diagnosis and/or prognosis, it can amplify their pain.[111] Imaging studies have confirmed that a negative expectation increases the activity of the prefrontal cortex, anterior cingulate cortex and insula areas associated with pain processing and emotional regulation.[112,113] As a neck-specific example, poor expectations for recovery following a whiplash injury is associated with poor recovery even when accounting for potential cofounders such as initial pain and health status.[114–116] Other work has shown that a negative treatment experience can impede subsequent unrelated treatment effects.[117]

Anxiety and fear can also accentuate pain.[118] People presenting with pain-related anxiety and fear report greater attention to pain sensations and predict that they will experience a greater amount of pain during a physical assessment.[119] Fear can contribute to behavioural avoidance, inactivity, disability, and an increased focus on pain avoidance as described by the fear avoidance model.[120] Another relevant feature for some patients is pain catastrophizing, which is an exaggerated focus

on the pain experience in addition to negatively evaluating the ability to deal with pain.[17] Pain catastrophizing has been identified as a prognostic factor for poor outcome following a whiplash injury[121,122] and people who catastrophize present with greater disability, higher pain medication use and higher rates of health care usage.[17]

Depression has been consistently associated with chronic pain[92] and is associated with decreased pain thresholds and pain tolerance levels, reduced activity and passive coping strategies (e.g., withdrawing from activities).[114,123,124] The use of passive versus active coping strategies (e.g., exercising) is associated with poor recovery following a whiplash injury especially in those also presenting with depressed mood.[123] Depression may also be associated with larger pain areas. For instance, in a study that examined factors associated with larger pain extent in people with chronic WAD, we found that when accounting for age, sex, education, insurance status, financial status and neck pain intensity, pain extent remained associated with depression and self-efficacy.[125] That is, people with depressed mood presented with more widespread pain. Interestingly, this was not the case in a cohort with cervical radiculopathy.[126]

Lower socioeconomic status is associated with greater symptom severity[127] and in both whiplash-induced neck pain as well as cervical radiculopathy, lower socioeconomic status is associated with larger pain extent.[125,126] Social factors including poor social support, low job control, low skill discretion and job dissatisfaction are all identified risk factors for higher levels of neck pain.[128,129] Moreover, the interactions between job demands, decision authority and supervisor support are linked to higher perceived pain and disability in office workers.[130] As an example, if an employer remains in regular communication with employees off work with back pain, then the employees take less time off work and are more positive about recovering.[131] Likely, this would hold true also for neck pain. Support from family and friends is also highly relevant. For instance, measures of sensitivity as well as pain intensity scores are lower when taken in the presence of the family and friends versus when the patient is alone.[132] Thus both psychological and social factors can influence pain perception and can modify both the severity and distribution of pain and can modify patient behaviour. These factors can be relevant for the transition to chronicity and maintenance of a chronic pain disorder.

CONCLUSION

The experience of pain is not a direct representation of the state of peripheral tissues, but rather is shaped by the context in which it is experienced. People with neck pain will present with different underlying pain mechanisms, which can be nociceptive, neuropathic, sensitization and inflammatory, with often multiple mechanisms at play. Regardless of the mechanisms, the severity and impact of symptoms can be modified by various psychological and social factors. It is important to understand and, when possible, identify these processes because they have relevant effects on response to different interventions and can imply the need for different management approaches.

REFERENCES

1. IASP Task Force on Taxonomy. Classification of chronic pain. 2nd ed. Seattle, USA: IASP Press; 1994.
2. Prescott SA, Ma Q, De Koninck Y. Normal and abnormal coding of somatosensory stimuli causing pain. Nat Neurosci 2004; 17:183–91.
3. Roditi D, Robinson ME. The role of psychological interventions in the management of patients with chronic pain. Psychol Res Behav Manag 2011;4:41–9.
4. Williams AC, Craig KD. Updating the definition of pain. Pain 2016;157:2420–3.
5. Clovin L, Fallon M. ABC of pain. UK: John Wiley & Sons; 2002.
6. Torrance N, Elliott AM, Lee AJ, et al. Severe chronic pain is associated with increased 10 year mortality. A cohort record linkage study. Eur J Pain 2010;14:380–6.
7. Macfarlane GJ, Barnish MS, Jones GT. Persons with chronic widespread pain experience excess mortality: longitudinal results from UK Biobank and meta-analysis. Ann Rheum Dis 2017;76:1815–22.
8. Vardeh D, Mannion RJ, Woolf CJ. Toward a mechanism-based approach to pain diagnosis. J Pain 2016;17:T50–69.
9. Woolf CJ, Bennett GJ, Doherty M, et al. Towards a mechanism-based classification of pain? Pain 1998;77:227–79.
10. Wall & Melzack's textbook of pain. 6th ed. Philadelphia, USA: Elsevier; 2013.
11. Julius D, Basbaum AI. Molecular mechanism of nociception. Nature 2001;413:203–10.
12. Basbaum A, Bautista DM, Scherrer G, et al. Cellular and molecular mechanisms of pain. Cell 2009;139:267–84.
13. Basbaum A, Bushnell MC. Science of pain. USA: Academic Press; 2008.
14. Dubin AE, Patapoutian A. Nociceptors: the sensors of the pain pathway. J Clin Invest 2010;120:3760–72.
15. Arcourt A, Lechner SG. Peripheral and spinal circuits involved in mechanical allodynia. Pain 2015;156:220–1.
16. Kuner R, Flor H. Structural plasticity and reorganisation in chronic pain. Nat Rev Neurosci 2016;18:20–30.
17. Keefe FJ, Rumble ME, Scipio CD, et al. Psychological aspects of persistent pain: current state of the science. J Pain 2004;5:195–211.
18. Ossipov MH, Morimura K, Porreca F. Descending pain modulation and chronification of pain. Curr Opin Support Palliat Care 2014;8:143–51.
19. Ossipov MH, Dussor GO, Porreca F. Central modulation of pain. J Clin Invest 2010;120:3779–87.
20. Wiech K. Deconstructing the sensation of pain: the influence of cognitive processes on pain perception. Science 2016;354:584–7.
21. Eippert F, Bingel U, Schoell ED, et al. Activation of the opioidergic descending pain control system underlies placebo analgesia. Neuron 2009;63:533–43.
22. Benedetti F, Amanzio M, Rosato R, et al. Nonopioid placebo analgesia is mediated by CB1 cannabinoid receptors. Nat Med 2011;17:1228–30.
23. Pecina M, Zubieta JK. Molecular mechanisms of placebo responses in humans. Mol Psychiatry 2015;20:416–23.
24. Manchikanti L, Singh V, Rivera J, et al. Prevalence of cervical facet joint pain in chronic neck pain. Pain Physician 2002;5:243–9.
25. Uhrenholt L, Grunnet-Nilsson N, Hartvigsen J. Cervical spine lesions after road traffic accidents: a systematic review. Spine 2002;27:1934–41.
26. Jonsson H, Bring G, Rauschning W, et al. Hidden cervical spine injuries in traffic accident victims with skull fractures. J Spinal Disord 1991;4:251–63.
27. Taylor J, Taylor M. Cervical spinal injuries: an autopsy study of 109 blunt injuries. J Musculoskel Pain 1996;4:61–79.
28. Farrell SF, Osmotherly PG, Cornwall J, et al. Morphology of cervical spine meniscoids in individuals with chronic whiplash-associated disorder: a case-control study. J Orthop Sports Phys Ther 2016;46:902–10.
29. Stemper BD, Yoganandan N, Pintar FA. Gender and region-dependent local facet joint kinematics in rear impact: implications in whiplash injury. Spine 2004;29:764–71.
30. Bogduk N, Yoganandan N. Biomechanics of the cervical spine. Part 3: minor injuries. Clin Biomech (Bristol, Avon) 2001; 16:267–75.
31. Cavanaugh JM, Lu Y, Chen C, et al. Pain generation in lumbar and cervical facet joints. J Bone Joint Surg Am 2006;88:63–7.
32. McLain RF. Mechanoreceptor endings in human cervical facet joints. Spine 1994;19:495–501.
33. Cooper G, Bailey B, Bogduk N. Cervical zygapophysial joint pain maps. Pain Med 2007;8:344–53.
34. Dwyer A, Aprill C, Bogduk N. Cervical zygapophysial joint pain patterns I: a study in normal volunteers. Spine 1990;15:453–7.
35. Slipman CW, Plastaras C, Patel R, et al. Provocative cervical discography symptom mapping. Spine J 2005;5:381–8.
36. Bogduk N. Diagnostic nerve blocks in chronic pain. Best Pract Res Clin Anaesthesiol 2002;16:565–78.

37. Manchikanti L, Hirsch JA, Kaye AD, et al. Cervical zygapophysial (facet) joint pain: effectiveness of interventional management strategies. Postgrad Med 2016;128:54–68.

38. Gibson T, Bogduk N, Macpherson J, et al. Crash characteristics of whiplash associated chronic neck pain. J Musculoskelet Pain 2000;8:87–95.

39. Smith AD, Jull G, Schneider G, et al. Cervical radiofrequency neurotomy reduces central hyperexcitability and improves neck movement in individuals with chronic whiplash. Pain Med 2014;15:128–41.

40. Smith AD, Jull G, Schneider GM, et al. Modulation of cervical facet joint nociception and pain attenuates physical and psychological features of chronic whiplash: a prospective study. PM R 2015;7:913–21.

41. Colloca L, Ludman T, Bouhassira D, et al. Neuropathic pain. Nat Rev Dis Primers 2017;3:17002.

42. Finnerup NB, Jensen TS. Nerve damage and its relationship to neuropathic pain. In: Holdcraft A, Jagger S, editors. Core topics in pain. UK: Cambridge University Press; 2005.

43. Jensen TS, Finnerup NB. Allodynia and hyperalgesia in neuropathic pain: clinical manifestations and mechanisms. Lancet Neurol 2014;13:924–35.

44. Hatem S, Attal N, Willer JC, et al. Psychophysical study of the effects of topical application of menthol in healthy volunteers. Pain 2006;122:190–6.

45. Bennett G. Can we distinguish between inflammatory and neuropathic pain? Pain Res Manag 2006;11:11–15.

46. Attal NB, Bouhassira D. Can pain be more or less neuropathic? Pain 2004;112:223–4.

47. Tampin B, Slater H, Briffa NK. Neuropathic pain components are common in patients with painful cervical radiculopathy, but not in patients with nonspecific neck-arm pain. Clin J Pain 2013;29:846–56.

48. Sterling M, Jull G, Vicenzino B, et al. Sensory hypersensitivity occurs soon after whiplash injury and is associated with poor recovery. Pain 2003;104:509–17.

49. Chien A, Eliav E, Sterling M. Hypoesthesia occurs with sensory hypersensitivity in chronic whiplash-further evidence of a neuropathic condition. Man Ther 2009;14:138–46.

50. Tampin B, Slater H, Hall T, et al. Quantitative sensory testing somatosensory profiles in patients with cervical radiculopathy are distinct from those in patients with nonspecific neck-arm pain. Pain 2012;153:2403–12.

51. Chien A, Eliav E, Sterling M. Whiplash (grade II) and cervical radiculopathy share a similar sensory presentation: an investigation using quantitative sensory testing. Clin J Pain 2008; 24:595–603.

52. Sterling M, Treleaven J, Jull G. Responses to a clinical test of mechanical provocation of nerve tissue in whiplash associated disorders. Man Ther 2002;7:89–94.

53. Ide M, Ide J, Yamaga M, et al. Symptoms and signs of irritation of the brachial plexus in whiplash injuries. J Bone Joint Surg 2001;83:226–9.

54. Bennett M, Smith BH, Torrance N, et al. The S-LANSS score for identifying pain of predominantly neuropathic origin: validation for use in clinical and postal research. J Pain 2005;6:149–58.

55. Sterling M, Pedler A. A neuropathic pain component is common in acute whiplash and associated with a more complex clinical presentation. Man Ther 2009;14:173–9.

56. Freynhagen R, Baron R, Gockel U, et al. painDETECT: a new screening questionnaire to identify neuropathic components in patients with back pain. Curr Med Res Opin 2006;22: 1911–20.

57. Cappelleri JC, Koduru V, Bienen EJ, et al. A cross-sectional study examining the psychometric properties of the painDETECT measure in neuropathic pain. J Pain Res 2015;8:159–67.

58. Beith ID, Kemp A, Kenyon J, et al. Identifying neuropathic back and leg pain: a cross-sectional study. Pain 2011;152: 1511–16.

59. Morsø L, Kent PM, Albert HB. Are self-reported pain characteristics, classified using the PainDETECT questionnaire, predictive of outcome in people with low back pain and associated leg pain? Clin J Pain 2011;27:535–41.

60. Ji RR, Xu ZZ, Gao YJ. Emerging targets in neuroinflammation-driven chronic pain. Nat Rev Drug Discov 2014;13:533–48.

61. Zhang JM, An J. Cytokines, inflammation, and pain. Int Anesthesiol Clin 2007;45:27–37.

62. Schaible HG, Schmidt RF. Activation of groups III and IV sensory units in medial articular nerve by local mechanical stimulation of knee joint. J Neurophysiol 1983;49:35–44.

63. Schaible HG, Schmidt RF. Effects of an experimental arthritis on the sensory properties of fine articular afferent units. J Neurophysiol 1985;54:1109–22.

64. Ren K, Dubner R. Interactions between the immune and nervous systems in pain. Nat Med 2010;16:1267–76.

65. Latremoliere A, Woolf CJ. Central sensitisation: a generator of pain hypersensitivity by central neural plasticity. J Pain 2009;10:895–926.

66. Lund Håheim L, Nafstad P, Olsen I, et al. C-reactive protein variations for different chronic somatic disorders. Scand J Public Health 2009;37:640–6.

67. Stürmer T, Raum E, Buchner M, et al. Pain and high sensitivity C reactive protein in patients with chronic low back pain and acute sciatic pain. Ann Rheum Dis 2005;64:921–5.

68. Sterling M, Elliott JM, Cabot PJ. The course of serum inflammatory biomarkers following whiplash injury and their relationship to sensory and muscle measures: a longitudinal cohort study. PLoS ONE 2013;8:e77903.

69. Kivioja J, Ozenci V, Rinaldi L, et al. Systemic immune response in whiplash injury and ankle sprain: elevated IL-6 and IL-10. Clin Immunol 2001;101:106–12.

70. Pepys MB, Hirschfield GM. C-reactive protein: a critical update. J Clin Invest 2003;111:1805–12.

71. Pritchett JW. C-reactive protein levels determine the severity of soft-tissue injuries. Am J Orthop 1996;25:759–61.

72. Davis CG. Mechanisms of chronic pain from whiplash injury. J Forensic Leg Med 2013;20:74–85.

73. Bolay H, Moskowitz MA. Mechanisms of pain modulation in chronic syndromes. Neurology 2002;59:S2–7.

74. Koelbaek Johansen M, Graven-Nielsen T, Schou Olesen A, et al. Generalised muscular hyperalgesia in chronic whiplash syndrome. Pain 1999;83:229–34.

75. Yarnitsky D, Arendt-Nielsen L, Bouhassira D, et al. Recommendations on terminology and practice of psychophysical DNIC testing. Eur J Pain 2010;14:339.

76. Staud R, Robinson ME, Price DD. Temporal summation of second pain and its maintenance are useful for characterizing widespread central sensitisation of fibromyalgia patients. J Pain 2007;8:893–901.

77. Chien A, Sterling M. Sensory hypoesthesia is a feature of chronic whiplash but not chronic idiopathic neck pain. Man Ther 2010;15:48–53.

78. Scott D, Jull G, Sterling M. Widespread sensory hypersensitivity is a feature of chronic whiplash-associated disorder but not chronic idiopathic neck pain. Clin J Pain 2005;21:175–81.

79. Herren-Gerber R, Weiss S, Arendt-Nielsen L, et al. Modulation of central hypersensitivity by nociceptive input in chronic pain after whiplash injury. Pain Med 2004;5:366–76.

80. Bovim G. Cervicogenic headache, migraine, and tension-type headache. Pressure-pain threshold measurements. Pain 1992;51: 169–73.

81. Assapun J, Uthaikhup S. Localized pain hypersensitivity in older women with cervicogenic headache: a quantitative sensory testing study. J Oral Facial Pain Headache 2017;31:80–6.

82. Banic B, Petersen-Felix S, Andersen OK, et al. Evidence for spinal cord hypersensitivity in chronic pain after whiplash injury and in fibromyalgia. Pain 2004;107:7–15.

83. Johnston V, Jimmieson NL, Jull G, et al. Quantitative sensory measures distinguish office workers with varying levels of neck pain and disability. Pain 2008;137:257–65.

84. Raak R, Wallin M. Thermal thresholds and catastrophizing in individuals with chronic pain after whiplash injury. Biol Res Nurs 2006;8:138–46.

85. Sterling M, Hendrikz J, Kenardy J. Similar factors predict disability and posttraumatic stress disorder trajectories after whiplash injury. Pain 2011;152:1272–8.

86. Sterling M, Hodkinson E, Pettiford C, et al. Psychologic factors are related to some sensory pain thresholds but not nociceptive flexion reflex threshold in chronic whiplash. Clin J Pain 2008;24:124–30.

87. Stone AM, Vicenzino B, Lim EC, et al. Measures of central hyperexcitability in chronic whiplash associated disorder–a systematic review and meta-analysis. Man Ther 2013;18: 111–17.

88. Malfliet A, Kregel J, Cagnie B, et al. Lack of evidence for central sensitisation in idiopathic, non-traumatic neck pain: a systematic review. Pain Physician 2015;18:223–36.

89. Sterling M, Jull G, Vicenzino B, et al. Physical and psychological factors predict outcome following whiplash injury. Pain 2005;114:141–8.

90. Sterling M, Kenardy J, Jull G, et al. The development of psychological changes following whiplash injury. Pain 2003;106: 481–9.

91. Wager TD, Atlas LY, Lindquist MA, et al. An fMRI-based neurologic signature of physical pain. N Engl J Med 2013;368: 1388–97.

92. Robinson MJ, Edwards SE, Iyengar S, et al. Depression and pain. Front Biosci 2009;14:5031–51.

93. Vachon-Presseau E, Martel MO, Roy M, et al. Acute stress contributes to individual differences in pain and pain-related brain activity in healthy and chronic pain patients. J Neurosci 2013;33:6826–33.

94. McGaugh JL. Significance and remembrance: the role of neuromodulatory systems. Psychol Sci 1990;1:15–25.

95. Pitman RK. Post-traumatic stress disorder, hormones, and memory. Biol Psychiatry 1989;26:221–3.

96. McEwen BS. Stress, adaptation, and disease: allostasis and allostatic load. Ann N Y Acad Sci 1998;840:33–44.

97. Li X, Hu L. The role of stress regulation on neural plasticity in pain chronification. Neural Plast 2016;6402942.

98. McLean SA. The potential contribution of stress systems to the transition to chronic whiplash-associated disorders. Spine 2011;36:S226–32.

99. Sterling M, Jull G, Vicenzino B, et al. Characterization of acute whiplash-associated disorders. Spine 2004;29:182–8.

100. Gaab J, Baumann S, Budnoik A, et al. Reduced reactivity and enhanced negative feedback sensitivity of the hypothalamus-pituitary-adrenal axis in chronic whiplash-associated disorder. Pain 2005;119:219–24.

101. Griep EN, Boersma JW, Lentjes EG, et al. Function of the hypothalamic-pituitary-adrenal axis in patients with fibromyalgia and low back pain. J Rheumatol 1998;25:1374–81.

102. Muhtz C, Rodriguez-Raecke R, Hinkelmann K, et al. Cortisol response to experimental pain in patients with chronic low back pain and patients with major depression. Pain Med 2013;14:498–503.

103. McEwen BS, Kalia M. The role of corticosteroids and stress in chronic pain conditions. Metabolism 2010;59:S9 15.

104. Riva R, Mork PJ, Westgaard RH, et al. Comparison of the cortisol awakening response in women with shoulder and neck pain and women with fibromyalgia. Psychoneuroendocrinology 2012;37:299–306.

105. Zimmer C, Basler HD, Vedder H, et al. Sex differences in cortisol response to noxious stress. Clin J Pain 2003;19:233–9.

106. McLean SA, Clauw DJ, Abelson JL, et al. The development of persistent pain and psychological morbidity after motor vehicle collision: integrating the potential role of stress response systems into a biopsychosocial model. Psychosom Med 2005;67:783–90.

107. McLean SA, Diatchenko L, Lee YM, et al. Catechol O-methyltransferase haplotype predicts immediate musculoskeletal neck pain and psychological symptoms after motor vehicle collision. J Pain 2011;12:101–7.

108. Diatchenko L, Slade GD, Nackley AG, et al. Genetic basis for individual variations in pain perception and the development of a chronic pain condition. Hum Mol Genet 2005;14:135–43.

109. Zubieta JK, Heitzeg MM, Smith YR, et al. COMT val158met genotype affects mu-opioid neurotransmitter responses to a pain stressor. Science 2003;299:1240–3.

110. Vargas-Alarcon G, Fragoso JM, Cruz-Robles D, et al. Catechol-O-methyltransferase gene haplotypes in Mexican and Spanish patients with fibromyalgia. Arthritis Res Ther 2007;9:R110.

111. Wells RE, Kaptchuk TJ. To tell the truth, the whole truth, may do patients harm: the problem of the nocebo effect for informed consent. Am J Bioeth 2012;12:22–9.

112. Sawamoto N, Honda M, Okada T, et al. Expectation of pain enhances responses to non-painful somatosensory stimulation in the anterior cingulate cortex and parietal operculum/posterior insula: an event-related functional magnetic resonance imaging study. J Neurosci 2000;20:7438–45.

113. Price DD. Psychological and neural mechanisms of the affective dimension of pain. Science 2000;288:1769–72.

114. Carroll LJ. Beliefs and expectations for recovery, coping, and depression in whiplash-associated disorders: lessening the transition to chronicity. Spine 2011;36:S250–6.

115. Carroll LJ, Holm LW, Ferrari R, et al. Recovery in whiplash-associated disorders: do you get what you expect? J Rheumatol 2009;36:1063–70.

116. Holm LW, Carroll LJ, Cassidy JD, et al. Expectations for recovery important in the prognosis of whiplash injuries. PLoS Med 2008;5:e105.

117. Kessner S, Forkmann K, Ritter C, et al. The effect of treatment history on therapeutic outcome: psychological and neurobiological underpinnings. PLoS ONE 2014;9:e109014.

118. Crombez G, Vlaeyen JW, Heuts PH, et al. Pain-related fear is more disabling than pain itself: evidence on the role of pain-related fear in chronic back pain disability. Pain 1999;80:329–39.

119. McCracken LM, Gross RT, Sorg PJ, et al. Prediction of pain in patients with chronic low back pain: effects of inaccurate prediction and pain-related anxiety. Behav Res Ther 1993;31:647–52.

120. Vlaeyen JW, Linton SJ. Fear-avoidance and its consequences in chronic musculoskeletal pain: a state of the art. Pain 2000;85:317–32.

121. Sullivan MJ, Adams H, Martel MO, et al. Catastrophizing and perceived injustice: risk factors for the transition to chronicity after whiplash injury. Spine 2011;36:S244–9.

122. Ritchie C, Sterling M. Recovery Pathways and Prognosis After Whiplash Injury. J Orthop Sports Phys Ther 2016;46:851–61.

123. Carroll LJ, Cassidy JD, Côté P. The role of pain coping strategies in prognosis after whiplash injury: passive coping predicts slowed recovery. Pain 2006;124:18–26.

124. Mercado AC, Carroll LJ, Cassidy JD, et al. Coping with neck and low back pain in the general population. Health Psychol 2000;19:333–8.

125. Falla D, Peolsson A, Peterson G, et al. Perceived pain extent is associated with disability, depression and self-efficacy in individuals with whiplash-associated disorders. Eur J Pain 2016;20:1490–501.

126. Falla D, Peolsson A, Heneghan N, et al. Widespread pain is associated with greater perceived pain and disability, but not with psychological features in patients with cervical radiculopathy. Congress of the World Confederation for Physical Therapy 2017;2–4. July; Cape Town, South Africa.

127. Fitzcharles MA, Rampakakis E, Ste-Marie PA, et al. The association of socioeconomic status and symptom severity in persons with fibromyalgia. J Rheumatol 2014;41:1398–404.

128. Ariëns GA, van Mechelen W, Bongers PM, et al. Psychosocial risk factors for neck pain: a systematic review. Am J Ind Med 2001;39:180–93.

129. Ariëns GA, Bongers PM, Hoogendoorn WE, et al. High quantitative job demands and low coworker support as risk factors for neck pain: results of a prospective cohort study. Spine 2001;26:1896–901.

130. Johnston V, Jimmieson NL, Souvlis T, et al. Interaction of psychosocial risk factors explain increased neck problems among female office workers. Pain 2007;129:311–20.

131. Butler RJ, Johnson WG, Côté P. It pays to be nice: employer-worker relationships and the management of back pain claims. J Occup Environ Med 2007;49:214–25.

132. Montoya P, Larbig W, Braun C, et al. Influence of social support and emotional context on pain processing and magnetic brain responses in fibromyalgia. Arthritis Rheum 2004;50:4035–44.

3

MOVEMENT AND POSTURE IN NECK PAIN DISORDERS

T he cervical spine is an intriguing and complex structure. Both sophisticated mobility and stability are demanded concurrently; mobility to subserve vision and hearing, stability to support the weight of the head and in large part, the load of the upper limbs. The cervical spine is also an important sensory organ. It provides knowledge of head position in relation to the body and makes an important contribution to balance and coordination of eye and head movement. This chapter overviews posture and movement of the cervical region, as well as the interactions with adjacent regions in the healthy state. Impairments in posture and movement in neck pain disorders are then explored to inform clinical reasoning in patient assessment. Control of posture and movement and impairments in neuromuscular and sensorimotor control in neck pain disorders are discussed in Chapters 5 and 6.

CERVICAL POSTURE

A common aim of rehabilitation of people with neck pain is to train patients to function in an upright neutral posture, based on the premise that neck pain is often associated with prolonged postures, which expose the cervical spine to excessive mechanical load at or near end ranges (e.g., a forward head posture). A neutral cervical posture is one where load is distributed evenly through the anterior (vertebral bodies and discs) and posterior (articular processes and facet joints) elements of the cervical segments,[1,2] the joints are in a mid-position and there is minimal muscle activity to support the position. The shape of the "ideal" cervical lordosis

permits optimal sharing of loads between anterior and posterior elements. In contrast, a flattened cervical lordosis increases compressive forces on anterior vertebral elements and tensile forces on posterior vertebral elements. An increased lordosis increases compressive forces on the posterior elements and tensile forces on the anterior vertebral elements.[3] Altered load distribution may irritate pain-sensitive structures. Certain sitting postures (e.g., a slumped posture) place motion segments towards the limit of their range with potential for adverse load.[4]

The position of the head and the angle of the cervical lordosis at any moment in time is largely dependent on the orientation of the cervicothoracic junction and head orientation for vision. The cervical spine has a strong biomechanical relationship with the thorax and the lumbopelvic region.[5] The sagittal orientation of the cervicothoracic junction largely dictates the angle of the cervical lordosis.[6,7] Because the angle of the thoracic kyphosis changes with age, the shape of the cervical lordosis changes.[8] Thus the orientation of the thoracic spine, combined with the need to maintain forward vision, potentially dictates the loading mechanisms of the cervical spine.

MOVEMENT OF THE CERVICAL SPINE

From a movement perspective, the functional cervical spine extends from the occiput to the upper thoracic region. There are three functional divisions; the craniocervical (C0–2), cervical (C2–7) and cervicothoracic regions. C2–3 and C7–T1 are transitional segments.[9,10]

The craniocervical and cervical regions have distinct motion characteristics. Motion of these areas is independent or interdependent depending on the task. There is also an intimate relationship between cervical movement and function of the thorax, the upper limbs and the craniomandibular region.

Movements of the craniocervical region

The craniocervical region comprises the atlanto–occipital and atlanto–axial articulations. The craniocervical segments overall provide approximately one-third of the flexion and extension excursion of the head and one-half of the axial rotation of the cervical region.[11] The shape of the atlanto–occipital (C0–1) articulation permits a generous range of motion in the sagittal plane, but minimal motion in lateral flexion and axial rotation because of the steepness of the lateral walls of the atlas sockets and the tension of the joint capsules.[12] The atlanto–axial (C1–2) articulation consists of four joints: two biconvex joints laterally and two joints medially, between the odontoid process and the ring of the atlas and the transverse ligament. C1–2 can be regarded as a pivot joint. It permits a large excursion of axial rotation, and some flexion and extension. This freedom of head motion facilitates great visual excursion. With this mobility, specific craniocervical ligaments, such as the alar and transverse ligaments as well as the tectorial membrane, enhance the stability of the region.[11,13,14]

Movements at the C0–1 and C1–2 segments are coupled, such that rotation is accompanied by contralateral lateral flexion at each segment.[15–17] Any coupled flexion-extension motion with these movements is negligible.[15] Translational movements occur with the angular movements in the craniocervical joints, but likewise, the excursions are minimal.[11]

Functionally, nodding and shaking the head in the act of saying yes and no are predominantly craniocervical motion. Of clinical interest, C1–2 axial rotation can be accurately localized from axial rotation of the cervical region by fully flexing the cervical region before performing head rotation,[18] the basis for the flexion-rotation test (Fig. 3.1).[19]

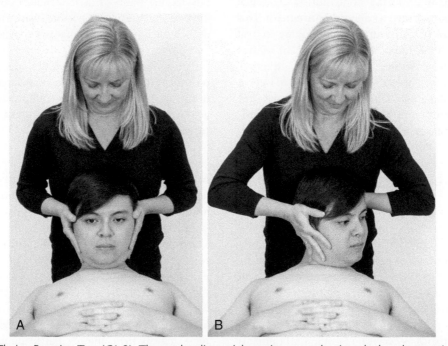

Fig. 3.1 ■ The Flexion Rotation Test (C1-2). The test localizes axial rotation to predominantly the atlanto–axial joints. (A) The patient is asked to lift their head to look at their feet to assist the clinician to gain full cervical flexion. (B) The head is rotated to encounter a solid end feel. Cut-off values for the test are less than 30-degrees head rotation or an asymmetry between sides of more than10 degrees.[105]

Movements of the cervical region (C2–7)

The movements of the C2–7 segments reflect some of the unique features of the cervical motion segment. The adult cervical motion segment is characterized by the formation and presence of uncovertebral joints and the transverse fissure dividing the posterior aspect of the intervertebral disc.[20,21] Fissuring of the disc is a normal response to the formation of the uncinate processes and the repeated translational and torsional strain imposed by large excursions of cervical movement. By the age of 40 years, adjacent vertebral bodies are bound together only by the anterior annulus and the two longitudinal ligaments.[20]

Movements in the C2–7 cervical segments are guided by the orientation of the facet joints and uncinate processes. Flexion and extension at each segment consist of an angular and a translational displacement. The angular excursion is highest in the middle segments (largest at C5–6) and least at C2–3 and C7–T1. Accompanying translational displacements are highest at C2–3 and progressively decline down the spine.[22] Translational displacements are small. An in vivo study using kinetic magnetic resonance imaging (MRI) documented 0.85 ± 1.22 mm translation at C2–3, declining to 0.16 ± 0.86 mm at C6–7.[22] All segments contribute to axial rotation with the middle segments (C3–C6) making the greatest contribution.[16,17] Likewise, all segments contribute to lateral flexion, with a progressively increasing contribution from C2–3 to C6–7.[15] However, rotation and lateral flexion are separated artificially because in vivo, there is a strong ipsilateral coupling of these movements.[15,16,22] The exception is the transitional C2–3 segment, where contralateral coupling is frequent.[23] When rotation is performed, it is associated with extension at the C2–5 levels, and flexion at the C5–7 segments.[16,17]

Movements of the cervicothoracic region (C7-T4)

The cervicothoracic region acts functionally with the cervical spine,[24] although it is far stiffer compared with adjacent cervical segments.[10] This reflects the presence of the ribs and their attachments to the manubrium. Motion in this region, although lesser ranges, has the same characteristics as cervical segments. Coupling of axial rotation and lateral flexion is usually ipsilateral.[25,26] Upper thoracic motion occurs with head excursions in all directions in the magnitudes of roughly 10 degrees

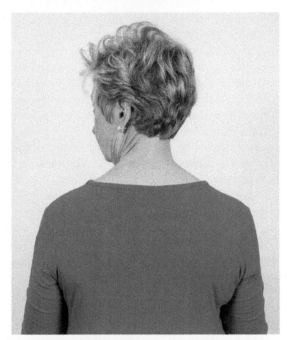

Fig. 3.2 ■ Full head rotation is a sum of movement at the craniocervical, cervical and cervicothoracic regions. In the person depicted, the reduced excursion of motion is mainly emanating from the lower cervical and cervicothoracic regions.

for each of flexion and extension, 8 degrees for axial rotation and 5 degrees for lateral flexion in each direction.[24,27] From a clinical viewpoint, this means that full head excursions cannot occur without a contribution from the cervicothoracic region (Fig. 3.2).

Integrated segmental motion

An intriguing aspect of coupled axial rotation and lateral flexion in the cervical spine is its contralateral nature in the craniocervical segments and ipsilateral nature in the cervical segments. This is a good example of the integrated nature of segmental motion. Opposite coupling between the two regions allows the head to maintain vertical alignment during axial rotation.[28]

Radiological studies have been undertaken to analyze the dynamics (movement amplitude and timing) of individual cervical motion segments during active cervical movements in each plane.[12] Some basic patterns emerge. Flexion may be initiated and terminated predominantly in lower cervical segments (C4–7), with middle cervical (C2–4) and craniocervical (C0–2) segments contributing mostly during the middle phase of motion. The C0–2 segments tend to move towards extension at end range flexion because of passive insufficiency of the nuchal ligament. Clinically, this means that the examination of flexion should be undertaken separately for the craniocervical segments because their capacity for flexion will not be adequately examined during flexion of the entire neck (Fig. 3.3 A and B). A similar pattern of motion is observed during extension although C0–2 reaches its maximum extension during the final phase of movement.[29,30] Segmental contributions can vary through range. Some display greatest motion during a movement rather than at the end range, emphasizing the flaws of analyzing movement at the end of range only.[29] Likewise, when the segments move depends on the movement task. If the task is a nodding movement of the head, movement will be initiated and mainly confined to the craniocervical segments. Protraction/retraction movements result in another pattern. Protraction places the lower segments near their end range of flexion and the upper levels in progressively greater extension, replicating the orientation of the neck

in a forward head posture. Retraction positions the lower segments in a mid-extension range with each superior level demonstrating more flexion, with C0–1 and C1–2 achieving full flexion.[31] These variations have underpinned the clinical practice of examining different movement tasks and movement sequences as in, for example, combined movement examination protocols[32,33] and may in part explain differences in symptomatic responses.

RELATIONSHIPS TO ADJACENT REGIONS

The cervical region has functional relationships with the upper limbs and craniomandibular region in postures and movement.

The cervical spine and upper limb

The shoulder girdle and upper limb have a close relationship to the cervical region via the axioscapular muscles, which suspend the scapula, clavicle and upper limb. This important relationship in function and dysfunction is

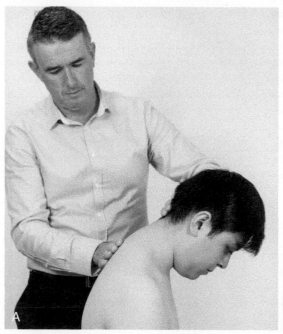 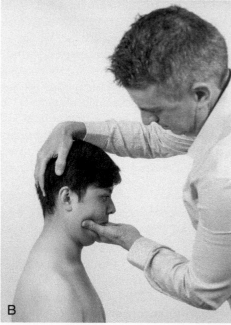

Fig. 3.3 ▪ (A) The examination of cervical flexion (cervical and cervicothoracic) is undertaken with the craniocervical region remaining relaxed. If the craniocervical region is flexed, insufficiency in the ligamentum nuchae prevents full flexion of the cervical and cervicothoracic regions. (B) Craniocervical flexion is assessed with the cervical region in a more neutral position.

discussed in Chapter 5. Although we often think in terms of loads transmitted to the cervical spine as a result of upper limb function,[34] here the focus is on spinal movement associated with upper limb function.

The thoracic spine moves during arm elevation.[35–38] To achieve full arm elevation bilaterally requires around 10 degrees of thoracic extension. All thoracic segments move, although the segmental contribution is more in the mid-lower thoracic region than the cervicothoracic region (T1–6). There is a strong correlation between the angle of thoracic kyphosis and arm elevation.[37] Not surprisingly, the presence of a slumped posture will prevent full shoulder elevation.[38] Single arm elevation also induces movement in the thoracic region. Extension again occurs, but in the upper thoracic region (T1–6), the movement is predominantly rotation, coupled with lateral flexion. The coupling is usually ipsilateral, but there is variability.[39,40] These are important relationships to consider in assessment and management from both neck and shoulder perspectives (Fig. 3.4).

The cervical segments also move with arm abduction under light load.[41] Although passive abduction essentially elicits no movement of cervical segments, it has been shown that the addition of a 2-kg resistance at the 0-degrees position and at each of four abduction angles between 30 to 120 degrees, induced cervical segmental rotation at each cervical segment (C1–T1) (Fig. 3.5). Displacement of C6 was greatest and most marked at the lower angles of right arm abduction, notably ranges where most functional activities might take place. Rotation of most segments was to the left, which could reflect the angle of muscle pull. This segmental movement, which is a normal occurrence with load, is a likely mechanism by which the cervical spine absorbs and distributes the load of upper limb function.

The cervical spine and the craniomandibular region

The craniomandibular complex is in close anatomical relationship with the cervical spine, and from a neurophysiological perspective, both regions in common, access the trigeminocervical nucleus. With these close anatomical and neurophysiological links, some interdependent relationships can be expected, such as an overlap in pain distributions. From a movement and posture perspective, the orientation of the mandible

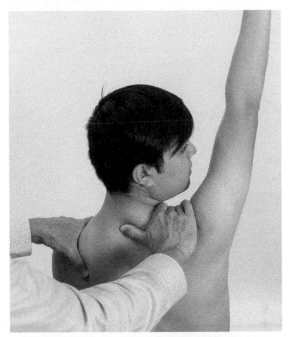

Fig. 3.4 ■ Movement in the cervicothoracic region is necessary to achieve full arm elevation. Arm movement can be used to assess cervicothoracic movement. The patient performs single arm elevation while the clinician palpates for displacement of the thoracic spinous processes at each thoracic segment (C7–T1 to T3–4 or T4–5). This examination technique can be used as a treatment technique. In treatment, the clinician performs a passive transverse glide through the spinous process of the hypomobile thoracic segments to augment the rotation occurring as the patient performs single arm elevation.

can be influenced by head and neck posture.[42] For example, the mandible pursues a more posterior path of opening in a forward head postural position.[42] The neck and the mandible also exhibit coordinated movement with wide opening and closing of the mouth. These movements are associated with craniocervical extension and flexion respectively.[43,44] Full extension of the cervical spine is dependent on mouth opening, particularly in the presence of reduced extensibility of the hyoid muscles. Coexistent osseous changes have been found in the temporomandibular joint and upper cervical joints. Sonnesen et al.[45] contend that these coexisting changes might either reflect a biomechanical relationship or at least a shared general disposition between the upper cervical spine and temporomandibular joint for degenerative osseous changes. In line

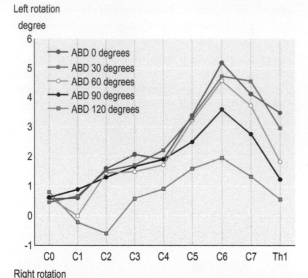

Left rotation
degree

Fig. 3.5 ■ The motion induced in each cervical segmental with right shoulder abduction under a 2-kg load assessed by magnetic resonance imaging. *ABD,* Abduction. (From Takasaki H, Hall T, Kaneko S, et al. Cervical segmental motion induced by shoulder abduction assessed by magnetic resonance imaging. Spine 2009;34:E122–126.)

with this contention, intraarticular interventions for temporomandibular joint osteoarthritis have been shown to improve neck pain and range of movement.[46]

There is a popular belief that head and neck posture is often related to temporomandibular joint dysfunction and pain, yet the evidence is inconclusive.[47] Historically, studies have been at odds in their findings and the situation continues. Current studies range from finding no relationship between head and neck posture and temporomandibular pain disorders, to others claiming close links between changes in craniocervical postures and disc displacement in the temporomandibular joint.[48–51] At this time, clinicians cannot automatically presume or dismiss a relationship. Each patient must be examined individually to determine the presence or not of any relationship between cervical posture and their presenting craniomandibular disorder.

CERVICAL POSTURE AND NECK PAIN DISORDERS

There has been a long-standing interest in the relationship between cervical posture and neck pain. In particular, most interest has been in the forward head posture because it places joints more towards their end of range.[4]

The head assumes a more forward posture as a factor of age.[52,53] Not surprisingly, and historically, there have been disparate findings regarding the relationship between the static forward head posture and the presence or magnitude of neck pain. This is apparent when the measurements of the cervical lordosis are made either radiographically[53–55] or measured using external landmarks and measurement techniques.[56–60] Quite simply, whereas some studies find that neck pain is associated with a forward head posture, others do not. This probably reflects large individual variations in spinal and even segmental curvatures[55] as well as age effects, which challenge interpretations of clinical significance. There is some evidence that the posture of the cervicothoracic region might better predict neck pain than the forward head position.[57] A traditional interpretation that a flattened cervical curve on x-ray is associated with neck pain is also questionable because a flattened cervical curve occurs with similar frequency in asymptomatic populations.[55,61] It is possible that the cervical curve on x-ray might need to be kyphotic rather than flattened to be of any clinical significance.[55,61] Once more, clinicians cannot automatically presume or dismiss a relationship between the static forward head position and neck pain, and any relationship must be decided on an individual patient basis.

External measurements of posture or the radiological measure of lordosis in the static upright posture might not be the critical measure. The posture adopted by the patient in function may be more relevant. This was illustrated in studies showing that measurements of the static posture at the start of a computer task did not differ between neck pain and control groups, but persons with neck pain drifted into a more forward head posture as they worked on the computer.[62,63] In addition to changes in posture, increases occur in cervical flexor and extensor muscle activity in persons with neck pain during such tasks, which can increase load on cervical structures.[64–66] Cervical extensor activity is 40% higher in the slouched posture.[67] The current high use of smartphones and tablets by the very young to the elderly has escalated the adoption of prolonged head flexion postures. Note that the mechanical demand on extensor muscles increases 3 to 5 times with the head flexed using a tablet versus sitting in a neutral posture.[68] Thus the functional posture adopted by the patient during work may be of greatest importance. Importantly, a poor habitual posture is modifiable by rehabilitation. It is more difficult to change a static postural shape.

Cervical movement disturbances in neck pain disorders

Movement disturbances are pathognomonic of cervical musculoskeletal disorders. The disturbances present in several ways, ranging from changes in the nature and extent of neck motion at the segmental and regional levels to how movement is performed and controlled.

Range of motion

Loss of cervical motion is characteristic of both mechanical neck pain and pain of traumatic origin (e.g., whiplash associated disorders) and distinguishes between healthy persons and those with cervical disorders.[69] Both primary plane movements and associated conjunct motions are reduced.[70,71] In accord, segmental movement is usually reduced.[72] Several processes might underlie the loss of cervical motion including; changes in articular or other soft tissues as a result of injury; the degenerative or ageing process; local segmental or regional muscle spasm as a response to pain; increased muscle activity as part of a change in neuromuscular or sensorimotor control associated with a neck pain disorder; and possibly fear of movement.

It is often difficult to identify an injury or relevant pathology with current imaging methods and guidelines. Yet lesions and pathological changes do occur in both the cervical discs and zygapophysial joints and the pathophysiological processes together with attendant nociception can be responsible for the abnormal motion in the acute or chronic states.[73–79] Structural changes as a result of injury or disease will affect motion but the nature of abnormal segmental motion may vary depending on the type or stage of the disorder. For example, capsular and joint changes associated with osteoarthritis of the zygapophysial joints restrict motion, whereas in early to moderate stages of disc degeneration, translatory motion increases slightly before it declines in advanced disc degeneration.[80]

The craniocervical region has the potential for instability as a result of trauma (e.g., whiplash, sports injury), inflammatory arthropathies as rheumatoid arthritis[81] or a genetic disorder such as Down syndrome. Loss of transverse ligament integrity permits anterior and posterior migration of the atlas from the dens during sagittal plane motion. A loss of alar ligament integrity influences stability of both C0–1 and C1–2 motion segments in multiple motion planes, but especially rotary stability.[82] The challenge is to identify ligament injuries. Debate continues about the relevance of MRI signal changes of alar and transverse ligaments to a whiplash induced lesion and symptoms[83,84] and the value of clinical tests is uncertain.[85] Another example of excessive abnormal movement in the craniocervical complex is manifest in the neck tongue syndrome, which is a relatively rare presentation, more common in children or adolescents. In this condition, the excessive movement is associated with a temporary, abnormal subluxation of C1–2 with sudden turning of the head which impinges the C2 ventral ramus against bone, producing the neck and tongue symptoms.[86] At the other extreme, and again more common in children, is atlanto–axial rotatory fixation, presenting as an acute wry neck.[87]

One of the major causes of restricted segmental and regional motion is muscle spasm as a reaction to pain or pathology. The muscle spasm may be "regional" as seen in an acute wry neck or in cases of severe pain. More frequently, the muscle spasm is more "segmental" and clinicians are very familiar with the "hardness" perceived when palpating over symptomatic cervical zygapophysial joints. Increased muscle activity as feature of a change in neuromuscular control associated with a neck pain disorder may also limit motion. This might occur when there is excessive co-contraction of the cervical flexors and extensors[65] or when muscles display a loss of direction specificity.[88]

Movement performance

Historically in manipulative therapy practice, interest in movement has been largely around range of movement and pain response. In recent years, more attention is being given to what might be called *movement performance*. These movement or kinematic disturbances are explored fully in Chapter 6. Poor movement performance is an expression of altered sensorimotor function.[89,90] It is included here to encourage expansion in observations and interpretation of the movement examination. Poor movement performance points to the need for other specific tests (e.g., proprioception).

Reduced acceleration and velocity of neck movement are commonly documented in the presence of neck pain.[70,89,91,92] It is proposed that reduced velocity is an impairment of greater consequence functionally than some loss of range of movement. Picture the rapid head movement required to check that it is safe to change lanes while driving. Furthermore, altered neck movement velocity, more so than range of motion, appears to be a particularly sensitive and specific measure of neck pain.[91] Variability in acceleration, commonly termed *reduced smoothness of movement* has also been found during cervical rotation in individuals with neck pain.[70,89,91] Other movement disturbances include unsteady or irregular head movements in prescribed tasks.[93–95]

Disturbances are also apparent in more general activities, not only in specific neck movements. For example, abnormal helical axes (instantaneous axes of motion) have been observed when patients perform functional tasks with their upper limbs.[96] It has also been observed that people with chronic neck pain walk with reduced trunk rotation.[97] Consideration of the elements of movement performance is a necessary part of the clinical examination of the neck pain patient.

Psychological considerations

Range and performance of movement may be restricted by unhelpful beliefs such as fear of movement,[98,99] although there are often many interacting factors.[100] It is understandable that a person in acute pain may be guarding their neck and be reluctant to move because it hurts. As witnessed in the clinic as well as in clinical trials, this guarding in many cases resolves as pain subsides and range of movement returns. This is observed in both acute and chronic pain states.[101,102] Nevertheless a fear of movement (kinesiophobia) with the belief that pain is harmful and threatening is counterproductive to recovery.[103] The effect of psychosocial features is considered further in Chapter 7. However, characteristics such as kinesiophobia reinforce the need to consider patients in both biological and psychological contexts so all features contributing to abnormal movement are considered in developing a multimodal management program.

Nevertheless, presumptions should not be made that kinesiophobia is an automatic occurrence. A study of factors associated with movement performance and

sensorimotor features in patients with neck pain determined that range and velocity of motion were not related to fear of motion but rather to visual disturbances, pain and balance.[90] In another recent study which examined factors associated with reduced range of active neck movements in persons with chronic whiplash associated disorders ($n = 216$), only age and measures of perceived pain and disability correlated with range of motion, whereas fear of movement, pain catastrophizing, anxiety and depression were not related to reduced motion.[104]

CONCLUSION

Posture, especially work postures or postures adopted when using various electronic devices or during other recreational activities, can overload cervical structures and contribute or precipitate a pain state. Movement is a critical function of the multisegmented cervical region. Both the range and how movement is performed and controlled can be affected by pain, injury, degenerative disease and ageing. Understanding the complexities of posture and movement from the segmental to the regional level in the healthy and pain states forms the basis for a relevant examination of the patient with a cervical disorder to inform diagnosis and management.

REFERENCES

1. Kumaresan S, Yoganandan N, Pintar F. Posterior complex contribution on compression and distraction cervical spine behavior: a finite element model. J Musculoskelet Res 1998;2:257–65.
2. Pal G, Routal R. A study of weight transmission through the cervical and upper thoracic regions of the vertebral column in man. J Anat 1986;148:245–61.
3. Harrison D, Harrison D, Janik T, et al. Comparison of axial and flexural stresses in lordosis and three buckled configurations of the cervical spine. Clin Biomech 2001;16:276–84.
4. Harms-Ringdahl K, Ekholm J, Schuldt K, et al. Load moments and myoelectric activity when the cervical spine is held in full flexion and extension. Ergonomics 1986;29:1539–52.
5. Caneiro J, O'Sullivan P, Burnett A, et al. The influence of different sitting postures on head/neck posture and muscle activity. Man Ther 2010;15:54–60.
6. Hardacker JW, Shuford RF, Capicotto P, et al. Radiographic standing cervical segmental alignment in adult volunteers without neck symptoms. Spine 1997;22:1472–3.
7. Loder R. The sagittal profile of the cervical and lumbosacral spine in Scheuermann thoracic kyphosis. J Spinal Disord 2001;14:226–31.

8. Boyle J, Milne N, Singer K. Influence of age on cervicothoracic spinal curvature: an ex vivo radiographic survey. Clin Biomech (Bristol, Avon) 2002;17:361–7.

9. Mestdagh H. Morphological aspects and biomechanical properties of the vertebroaxial joint (C_2-C_3). Acta Morphol Neerl Scand 1976;14:19–30.

10. Simon S, Davis M, Odhner D, et al. CT imaging techniques for describing motions of the cervicothoracic junction and cervical spine during flexion, extension, and cervical traction. Spine 2006;31:44–50.

11. Lopez A, Scheer J, Leibl K, et al. Anatomy and biomechanics of the craniovertebral junction. Neurosurg Focus 2015; 38:E2.

12. Bogduk N, Mercer S. Biomechanics of the cervical spine. I: normal kinematics. Clin Biomech 2000;15:633–48.

13. Osmotherly P, Rivett D, Mercer S. Revisiting the clinical anatomy of the alar ligaments. Eur Spine J 2013;22:60–4.

14. Osmotherly P, Rivett D, Rowe L. The anterior shear and distraction tests for craniocervical instability. An evaluation using magnetic resonance imaging. Man Ther 2012;17:416–21.

15. Ishii T, Mukai Y, Hosono N, et al. Kinematics of the cervical spine in lateral bending: in vivo three-dimensional analysis. Spine 2006;31:155–60.

16. Salem W, Lenders C, Mathieu J, et al. In vivo three-dimensional kinematics of the cervical spine during maximal axial rotation. Man Ther 2013;18:339–44.

17. Zhao X, Wu Z, Han B, et al. Three-dimensional analysis of cervical spine segmental motion in rotation. Arch Med Sci 2013;9:515–20.

18. Takasaki H, Hall T, Oshiro S, et al. Normal kinematics of the upper cervical spine during the flexion-rotation test - In vivo measurements using magnetic resonance imaging. Man Ther 2011;16:167–71.

19. Hall T, Robinson K, Fujinawa O, et al. Inter-tester reliability and diagnostic validity of the cervical flexion-rotation test. J Manipulative Physiol Ther 2008;31:293–300.

20. Mercer S, Bogduk N. The ligaments and annulus fibrosus of human adult cervical intervertebral discs. Spine 1999;24:619–26.

21. Tondury G. The behaviour of the cervical discs during life. In: Hirsch C, Zotterman Y, editors. Cervical pain. Oxford: Pergamon Press; 1972.

22. Xiong C, Suzuki A, Daubs M, et al. The evaluation of cervical spine mobility without significant spondylosis by kMRI. Eur Spine J 2015;24:2799–806.

23. Mimura M, Moriya H, Watanabe T, et al. Three-dimensional motion analysis of the cervical spine and special reference to the axial rotation. Spine 1989;14:1135–9.

24. Fiebert I, Spyropoulos T, Peterman D, et al. Thoracic segmental flexion during cervical forward bending. J Back Musculoskelet Rehabil 1993;3:80–5.

25. Penning L, Wilmink J. Rotation of the cervical spine: a CT study in normal subjects. Spine 1987;12:732–9.

26. Willems J, Jull G, Ng J. An in vivo study of the primary and coupled rotations of the thoracic spine. Clin Biomech 1996;11:311–16.

27. Tsang S, Szeto G, Lee R. Normal kinematics of the neck: the interplay between the cervical and thoracic spines. Man Ther 2013;18:431–7.

28. White AA, Panjabi M. Clinical biomechanics of the spine. 2nd ed. Philadelphia: J.B. Lippincott; 1990.

29. Anderst W, Donaldson W, Lee J, et al. Cervical motion segment contributions to head motion during flexion\extension, lateral bending, and axial rotation. Spine J 2015;15:2538–43.

30. Mameren HV, Drukker J, Sanches H, et al. Cervical spine motion in the sagittal plane (I) range of motion of actually performed movements, an X-ray cinematographic study. Eur J Morphol 1990;28:47–68.

31. Ordway N, Seymour R, Donelson R, et al. Cervical flexion, extension, protrusion, and retraction. Spine 1999;24:240–7.

32. Edwards BC. Manual of combined movements. 2nd ed. Edinburgh: Churchill Livingstone; 1999.

33. McCarthy C. Combined movement theory. UK: Churchill Livingstone, Elsevier; 2010.

34. Behrsin JF, Maguire K. Levator scapulae action during shoulder movement. A possible mechanism of shoulder pain of cervical origin. Aust J Physiother 1986;32:101–6.

35. Crawford H, Jull G. The influence of thoracic posture and movement on range of arm elevation. Physiother Theory Prac 1993;9:143–8.

36. Crosbie J, Kilbreath S, Hollmann L, et al. Scapulohumeral rhythm and associated spinal motion. Clin Biomech 2008;23:184–92.

37. Edmonston S, Ferguson A, Ippersiel P, et al. Clinical and radiological investigation of thoracic spine extension motion during bilateral arm elevation. J Orthop Sports Phys Ther 2012;42:861–9.

38. Malmström EM, Olsson J, Baldetorp J, et al. A slouched body posture decreases arm mobility and changes muscle recruitment in the neck and shoulder region. Eur J Appl Physiol 2015;115:2491–503.

39. Stewart S, Jull G, Willems J, et al. An initial analysis of thoracic spine motion with unilateral arm elevation in the scapular plane. J Man Manipulative Ther 1995;3:15–21.

40. Theodoridis D, Ruston S. The effect of shoulder movements on thoracic spine 3D motion. Clin Biomech 2002;17:418–21.

41. Takasaki H, Hall T, Kaneko S, et al. Cervical segmental motion induced by shoulder abduction assessed by magnetic resonance imaging. Spine 2009;34:E122–6.

42. Visscher C, Slater JH, Lobbezoo F, et al. Kinematics of the human mandible for different head postures. J Oral Rehabil 2000;27:299–305.

43. Eriksson P, Häggman-Henrikson B, Nordh E, et al. Co-ordinated mandibular and head-neck movements during rhythmic jaw activities in man. J Dent Res 2000;79:1378–84.

44. Zafar H, Nordh E, Eriksson P. Temporal coordination between mandibular and head-neck movements during jaw opening-closing tasks in man. Arch Oral Biol 2000;45:675–82.

45. Sonnesen L, Petersson A, Wiese M, et al. Osseous osteoarthritic-like changes and joint mobility of the temporomandibular joints and upper cervical spine: is there a relation? Oral Surg Oral Med Oral Pathol Oral Radiol 2017;123:273–9.

46. Guarda-Nardini L, Cadorin C, Frizziero A, et al. Interrelationship between temporomandibular joint osteoarthritis (OA) and cervical spine pain: effects of intra-articular injection with hyaluronic acid. Cranio 2017;35:276–82.

47. Manfredini D, Castroflorio T, Perinetti G, et al. Dental occlusion, body posture and temporomandibular disorders: where we are now and where we are heading for. J Oral Rehabil 2012;39:463–71.

48. An J, Jeon D, Jung W, et al. Influence of temporomandibular joint disc displacement on craniocervical posture and hyoid bone position. Am J Orthod Dentofacial Orthop 2015;147:72–9.

49. Câmara-Souza M, Figueredo O, Maia P, et al. Cervical posture analysis in dental students and its correlation with temporomandibular disorder. Cranio 2018;36:85–90.

50. Faulin E, Guedes C, Feltrin P, et al. Association between temporomandibular disorders and abnormal head postures. Braz Oral Res 2015;29:pii: S1806.

51. López-de-Uralde-Villanueva I, Beltran-Alacreu H, Paris-Alemany A, et al. Relationships between craniocervical posture and pain-related disability in patients with cervico-craniofacial pain. J Pain Res 2015;30:449–58.

52. Quek J, Pua Y-H, Clark R, et al. Effects of thoracic kyphosis and forward head posture on cervical range of motion in older adults. Man Ther 2013;18:65–71.

53. Sun A, Yeo H, Kim T, et al. Radiologic assessment of forward head posture and its relation to myofascial pain syndrome. Ann Rehabil Med 2014;38:821–6.

54. Farmer P, Snodgrass S, Buxton A, et al. An investigation of cervical spinal posture in cervicogenic headache. Phys Ther 2015;95:212–22.

55. Grob D, Frauenfelder H, Mannion AF. The association between cervical spine curvature and neck pain. Eur Spine J 2007;16:669–78.

56. Kim E-K, Kim J. Correlation between rounded shoulder posture, neck disability indices, and degree of forward head posture. J Phys Ther Sci 2016;28:2929–32.

57. Lau K, Cheung K, Chan K, et al. Relationships between sagittal postures of thoracic and cervical spine, presence of neck pain, neck pain severity and disability. Man Ther 2010;15:457–62.

58. Oliveira A, Silva A. Neck muscle endurance and head posture: a comparison between adolescents with and without neck pain. Man Ther 2016;22:62–7.

59. Richards K, Beales D, Smith A, et al. Neck posture clusters and their association with biopsychosocial factors and neck pain in Australian adolescents. Phys Ther 2016;96:1576–87.

60. Yip C, Chiu T, Poon A. The relationship between head posture and severity and disability of patients with neck pain. Man Ther 2008;13:148–54.

61. Johansson M, Liane MB, Bendix T, et al. Does cervical kyphosis relate to symptoms following whiplash injury? Man Ther 2011;16:378–83.

62. Falla D, Jull G, Russell T, et al. Effect of neck exercise on sitting posture in patients with chronic neck pain. Phys Ther 2007;87:408–17.

63. Szeto G, Straker L, Raine S. A field comparison of neck and shoulder postures in symptomatic and asymptomatic office workers. Appl Erg 2002;33:75–84.

64. Falla D, Bilenkij G, Jull G. Patients with chronic neck pain demonstrate altered patterns of muscle activation during performance of a functional upper limb task. Spine 2004;29: 1436–40.

65. Johnston V, Jull G, Souvlis T, et al. Neck movement and muscle activity characteristics in office workers with neck pain. Spine 2008;33:555–63.

66. Szeto G, Straker L, O'Sullivan P. EMG median frequency changes in the neck-shoulder stabilizers of symptomatic office workers when challenged by different physical stressors. J Electromyogr Kinesiol 2005;15:544–55.

67. Edmondston S, Sharp M, Symes A, et al. Changes in mechanical load and extensor muscle activity in the cervico-thoracic spine induced by sitting posture modification. Ergonomics 2011;54:179–86.

68. Vasavada A, Nevins D, Monda S, et al. Gravitational demand on the neck musculature during tablet computer use. Ergonomics 2015;58:990–1004.

69. Stenneberg M, Rood M, Bie RD, et al. To what degree does active cervical range of motion differ between patients with neck pain, patients with whiplash, and those without neck pain? A systematic review and meta-analysis. Arch Phys Med Rehabil 2017;98:1407–34.

70. Röijezon U, Djupsjöbacka M, Björklund M, et al. Kinematics of fast cervical rotations in persons with chronic neck pain: a cross-sectional and reliability study. BMC Musculoskelet Disord 2010;11:222.

71. Woodhouse A, Vasseljen O. Altered motor control patterns in whiplash and chronic neck pain. BMC Musculoskelet Disord 2008;9:90.

72. Dvorak J, Froehlich D, Penning L, et al. Functional radiographic diagnosis of the cervical spine. Flexion/extension. Spine 1988;13:748–55.

73. Betsch M, Blizzard S, Shinseki M, et al. Prevalence of degenerative changes of the atlanto-axial joints. Spine J 2015;15:275–80.

74. Engel A, Rappard G, King W, et al. The effectiveness and risks of fluoroscopically-guided cervical medial branch thermal radiofrequency neurotomy: a systematic review with comprehensive analysis of the published data. Pain Med 2016;17:658–69.

75. Farrell S, Osmotherly P, Cornwall J, et al. Morphology of cervical spine meniscoids in individuals with chronic whiplash-associated disorder: a case-control study. J Orthop Sports Phys Ther 2016;46:902–10.

76. Farrell S, Osmotherly P, Cornwall J, et al. Cervical spine meniscoids: an update on their morphological characteristics and potential clinical significance. Eur Spine J 2017;26:939–47.

77. Manchikanti L, Cash K, Pampati V, et al. Two-year follow-up results of fluoroscopic cervical epidural injections in chronic axial or discogenic neck pain: a randomized, double-blind, controlled trial. Int J Med Sci 2014;11:309–20.

78. Russo V, Duits A, Dhawan R, et al. Joint arthropathy at the cranio-vertebral junction. Scintigraphic patterns on bone SPECT/CT. Br J Neurosurg 2017;31:45–9.

79. Taylor J. The Cervical Spine. An atlas of normal anatomy and the morbid anatomy of ageing and injuries. Australia: Elsevier; 2017.

80. Miyazaki M, Hong S, Yoon S, et al. Kinematic analysis of the relationship between the grade of disc degeneration and motion unit of the cervical spine. Spine 2008;33:187–93.

81. Joaquim A, Ghizoni E, Tedeschi H, et al. Radiological evaluation of cervical spine involvement in rheumatoid arthritis. Neurosurg Focus 2015;38:E4.

82. Panjabi M, Dvorak J, Crisco J, et al. Effects of alar ligament transection on upper cervical spine rotation. J Orthop Res 1991;9:584–93.

83. Li Q, Shen H, Li M. Magnetic resonance imaging signal changes of alar and transverse ligaments not correlated with whiplash-associated disorders: a meta-analysis of case-control studies. Eur Spine J 2013;22:14–20.

84. Myran R, Zwart J, Kvistad K, et al. Clinical characteristics, pain, and disability in relation to alar ligament MRI findings. Spine 2011;36:E862–7.

85. Hutting N, Scholten-Peeters G, Vijverman V, et al. Diagnostic accuracy of upper cervical spine instability tests: a systematic review. Phys Ther 2013;93:1686–95.

86. Gelfand A, Johnson H, Lenaerts M, et al. Neck-tongue syndrome: a systematic review. Cephalalgia 2018;38:374–82.

87. Roche C, O'Malley M, Dorgan J, et al. A pictorial review of atlanto-axial rotatory fixation: key points for the radiologist. Clin Radiol 2001;56:947–58.

88. Lindstrøm R, Schomacher J, Farina D, et al. Association between neck muscle coactivation, pain, and strength in women with neck pain. Man Ther 2011;16:80–6.

89. Sjölander P, Michaelson P, Jaricb S, et al. Sensorimotor disturbances in chronic neck pain-Range of motion, peak velocity, smoothness of movement, and repositioning acuity. Man Ther 2008;13:122–31.

90. Treleaven J, Chen X, Bahat HS. Factors associated with cervical kinematic impairments in patients with neck pain. Man Ther 2016;22:109–15.

91. Bahat HS, Chen X, Reznik D, et al. Interactive cervical motion kinematics: sensitivity, specificity and clinically significant values for identifying kinematic impairments in patients with chronic neck pain. Man Ther 2015;20:295–302.

92. Tsang S, Szeto G, Lee R. Relationship between neck acceleration and muscle activation in people with chronic neck pain: implications for functional disability. Clin Biomech 2016;35:27–36.

93. Baydal-Bertomeu J, Page Á, Belda-Lois J, et al. Neck motion patterns in whiplash-associated disorders: quantifying variability and spontaneity of movement. Clin Biomech 2011;26:29–34.

94. Kristjansson E, Oddsdottir G. "The Fly": a new clinical assessment and treatment method for deficits of movement control in the cervical spine: reliability and validity. Spine 2010;35:E1298–305.

95. Woodhouse A, Stavdahl O, Vasseljen O. Irregular head movement patterns in whiplash patients during a trajectory task. Exp Brain Res 2010;201:261–70.

96. Grip H, Sundelin G, Gerdle B, et al. Cervical helical axis characteristics and its center of rotation during active head and upper arm movements-comparisons of whiplash-associated disorders, non-specific neck pain and asymptomatic individuals. J Biomech 2008;41:2799–805.

97. Falla D, Gizzi L, Parsa H, et al. People with chronic neck pain walk with a stiffer spine. J Orthop Sports Phys Ther 2017;47:268–77.

98. Bahat HS, Weiss P, Sprecher E, et al. Do neck kinematics correlate with pain intensity, neck disability or with fear of motion? Man Ther 2014;19:252–8.

99. Pool J, Ostelo R, Knol D, et al. Are psychological factors prognostic indicators of outcome in patients with sub-acute neck pain? Man Ther 2010;15:111–16.

100. Pedler A, Kamper S, Sterling M. Addition of posttraumatic stress and sensory hypersensitivity more accurately estimates disability and pain than fear avoidance measures alone after whiplash injury. Pain 2016;157:1645–54.

101. Jull G, Kenardy J, Hendrikz J, et al. Management of acute whiplash: a randomized controlled trial of multidisciplinary stratified treatments. Pain 2013;154:1798–806.

102. Smith A, Jull G, Schneider G, et al. Cervical radiofrequency neurotomy reduces central hyperexcitability and improves neck movement in individuals with chronic whiplash. Pain Med 2014;15:128–41.

103. Feeus A, Dalen TV, Bierma-Zeinstra1 S, et al. Kinesiophobia in patients with non-traumatic arm, neck and shoulder complaints: a prospective cohort study in general practice. BMC Musculoskelet Disord 2007;8:117.

104. Falla D New insights into motor adaptations in low back pain and neck pain: implications for sports medicine and rehabilitation. European College of Sports Science; 2017 Essen, Germany 5-8th July.

105. Hall T, Briffa K, Hopper D, et al. Long-term stability and minimal detectable change of the cervical flexion-rotation test. J Orthop Sports Phys Ther 2010;40:225–9.

4 NEURAL TISSUE IN NECK PAIN DISORDERS

■ ■

Neck pain disorders may include injury to, or pathology of, neural structures. Identifying involvement of these tissues is essential because it may signal the need for a change in management strategy, and in more serious cases, a potential safety concern for the patient requiring immediate medical referral. This chapter discusses the potential mechanisms underlying the direct involvement of nerve tissue in neck pain disorders, their clinical manifestations and common conditions.

NERVE INJURY AND NECK PAIN DISORDERS

Specific structural characteristics and pathologies of the cervical spine and upper limb may render the spinal cord and peripheral nerves susceptible to injury. The term *neuropathy* describes abnormal states of the peripheral nerves that may involve numerous pathological and functional changes in the nervous system. Myelopathy is the relevant term for similar states of the spinal cord and these terms will be used in this chapter.

Neuropathy may be a manifestation of many health-related or hereditary disorders such as chronic alcoholism, multiple sclerosis, diabetes mellitus,[1] cancer (e.g., Pancoast tumour),[2] metabolic disturbances and nutritional deficits.[3,4] Such conditions may result in polyneuropathies presenting as muscle weakness, atrophy and sensory deficits, but they may also present in less severe forms mimicking features commonly related to musculoskeletal conditions. Although it is beyond the scope of this chapter to describe such conditions in detail, clinicians should be aware of their potential presentation (refer to Azhary et al.[1] for a discussion on differential diagnosis). The focus of this chapter is on conditions involving neural tissue associated with musculoskeletal conditions of the cervical spine.

PATHOPHYSIOLOGICAL MECHANISMS OF NERVE INJURY—THE BASIS FOR CLINICAL PRESENTATION AND EXAMINATION PROCEDURES

This section considers the pathophysiological basis of neuropathy and myelopathy related to neck pain disorders and the subsequent clinical presentations. Some clinical presentations have relatively clear indications of nerve involvement, yet others may be difficult to differentially diagnose. An understanding of pathophysiological processes and subsequent clinical manifestation may assist the clinical reasoning process. Specific details regarding examination procedures of nerve tissue are discussed in Chapter 9.

Pathophysiological mechanisms of neuropathy in neck pain disorders

Neuropathy of variable severity may be secondary to injury or pathology of interfacing musculoskeletal structures. It may be associated with perineural inflammation and/or nerve entrapment and compression. Alternately, neuropathy may also arise from direct trauma to the nerve.

41

Musculoskeletal injury and perineural inflammation

Injury or pathology of musculoskeletal structures that interface nerves may result in the release of inflammatory mediators and the development of perineural inflammation. For example, the release of inflammatory mediators is a feature of cervical disc lesions and is thought to contribute to the development of cervical radiculopathy.[5–7] Animal studies have shown that perineural inflammation along a nerve trunk can induce pain in the organ innervated by the nerve[8–11] within a few hours of nerve exposure.[9,12,13] Nerve-related pain can result from the presence of chronic mild inflammation even without evidence of nerve damage, or from a more severe inflammatory process that does result in nerve damage.[11,13,14] Perineural inflammation may induce spontaneous neurophysiological activity and mechanosensitivity in the affected nerve.[15–18]

Nerve entrapment and compression

Nerves may be directly entrapped in the cervical spine (e.g., cervical myelopathy, cervical radiculopathy),[19,20] or neck pain disorders may be associated with nerve entrapment in the upper limb (e.g., cubital tunnel syndrome,[21] carpal tunnel syndrome[22]) in a double crush scenario.[23,24] Degenerative or injured musculoskeletal interfaces within the spine and periphery may reduce the space containing the nerve, resulting in nerve compression that may affect nerve tissue both local and remote to the site of compression.

Local compression of peripheral nerves has been shown in animal studies to impair neural circulation. This may result in: intraneural ischaemia, disturbance of the blood-nerve-barrier, neuroinflammation and intraneural oedema,[25–29] Schwann cell reaction and demyelination[30] and changes in nodal structure.[31] Furthermore, there may be reduced thresholds for firing and ectopic impulse generation from nociceptive fibres and nerve fibres that have become mechanosensitive.[32–35] Nerve compression may affect both myelinated and unmyelinated fibres.[31,36] Animal studies show that even mild compression can cause degeneration of small diameter axons and demyelination of larger diameter fibres.[36]

Changes have also been observed remotely following peripheral nerve injury with the release of inflammatory mediators[36–38] and ectopic activity[36,39] of the dorsal root ganglion. With the close proximity of cell bodies from different peripheral nerves within the dorsal root ganglion, adjacent intact neurones may also be affected by the neuroinflammatory process within the dorsal root ganglion, which may alter their firing threshold.[40] These changes in the dorsal root ganglion, together with reported changes within the spinal cord[41] and brain,[42,43] are proposed to explain a patient's spread of symptoms, which are sometimes well beyond the normal distribution of the injured peripheral nerve.[40] For detailed information regarding pathophysiological processes underlying nerve compression and the association with neuropathic pain, the reader is directed to very comprehensive reviews on this topic by Schmid et al.[40,44]

Injury to a peripheral nerve may occur at more than one site. The term *double crush syndrome* was used to explain how injury at one site of a nerve made that nerve more susceptible to injury at another location.[23] In the upper limb, this association has been often drawn between carpal tunnel syndrome and cervical radiculopathy.[45,46] It was reasoned that compression at one location on a nerve's axon would predispose that same axon to injury elsewhere because of disrupted bidirectional transport of essential nutrients along the axon. The nerve would then be prone to undergoing morphological and functional changes.[23] Although this mechanism has been supported,[47] there is still speculation as to other potential mechanisms underlying the double crush syndrome.[48] It has also been suggested that the term double crush syndrome be replaced with the term *multifocal neuropathy* to reflect that nerve injury may occur at more than two sites and can occur because of stretch and not just compression.[24] The term also incorporates the potential impact that systemic conditions such as diabetes may have on the clinical sequelae.[24]

Traumatic nerve injury

Nerve trauma may be catastrophic (such as cervical spinal cord injury), or less severe (such as brachial neuropraxia). Brachial neuropraxia (stinger) describes a transient episode of neural symptoms (shooting, electric pain or paraesthesia) and weakness[49] in an upper extremity following a significant blow to the head and/or shoulder, which commonly occurs in contact sports.[50,51] It is thought to mostly reflect a cervical extension-compression injury,[52] usually involving the

C5 to C6 nerve roots or the upper trunk of the brachial plexus.[50,53] Brachial neuropraxia may occur recurrently.[54]

Stretch-induced neuropathies range from a single traumatic tensile strain to the brachial plexus (e.g., abrupt stop in a bus when the person is standing and holding a handle) to severe conditions such as a brachial plexus avulsion in a motor bike accident. Prolonged tensile strain may result in stretch-induced neuropathy such as that reported during surgical procedures involving sustained upper limb elevation.[55,56] Animal studies have shown that prolonged stretch to a nerve will impair blood flow,[57] axonal transport[47] and conduction.[58] Nerve injury may also occur during surgical procedures, such as accessory nerve injury during neck dissection surgery for head and neck cancer with resultant effects on trapezius function.[59] Similarly, trauma to the long thoracic nerve and associated palsy of the serratus anterior muscle is well documented and may have significant implications for shoulder girdle function and recovery.[60]

Clinical manifestations of neuropathy and relationship to examination findings

The consequences of injury to a nerve and the resultant clinical manifestations (patient-reported and physical examination findings) are commonly referred to in terms of a gain (e.g., mechanosensitivity) or loss (e.g., nerve conduction deficit) of nerve function.[40]

FOCUS POINT

A patient's pain may not always be associated with nerve compression. Structures such as the dorsal root ganglion may be involved or the pain may be associated with the presence of perineural inflammation and the development of nerve mechanosensitivity.

Patient reported symptoms

Patient reported symptoms may be pathognomic of nerve involvement. A loss of nerve function indicates reduced impulse generation, resulting in numbness (anaesthesia) or weakness. In contrast, a gain in function reflects reduced inhibition or abnormal excitability, presenting as paraesthesia, spontaneous pain, hyperalgesia and allodynia.[4] Pain may not always be associated with nerve compression and may be dependent on involvement of certain nerve structures, such as the dorsal root ganglion,[61,62] or the presence of perineural inflammation and the development of nerve mechanosensitivity. There are characteristic symptoms of nerve-related pain that are distinctive to those associated with somatic referred pain. Symptoms described as burning, electric shocks, cold pain in conjunction with paraesthesia, anaesthesia, tingling and itching, may improve identification of nerve involvement.[63] However, caution needs to be taken because considerable overlap in symptoms has been shown in individuals reporting conditions with and without nerve involvement.[64] This overlap may partly be caused by changes at various levels of the nervous system which explains the experience of symptoms beyond the normal distribution of the injured peripheral nerve (e.g., non-dermatomal distribution).[40] Differentiation of neuropathic pain may be assisted by the use of specific questionnaires such as the self-report version of the Leeds Assessment of Neuropathic Symptoms and Signs[65] and the Neuropathic Pain Questionnaire.[66]

Nerve conduction integrity

A traditional clinical neurological examination (lower tract: spinal reflexes, strength, sensation; upper tract: Hoffmann's sign, Babinski, clonus) may detect compromise of nerve conduction, signalling a loss of nerve function. Similar but more quantitative evaluation of the integrity of nerve conduction may be undertaken with electrodiagnostic testing methods.[67] Although these forms of evaluation are still warranted in patients with referred upper limb pain or other reported symptoms (e.g., paraesthesia, anaesthesia, weakness), their capacity

---

FOCUS POINT

Adjacent intact neurones may be affected by neuroinflammatory processes within the dorsal root ganglion which alters their firing threshold. Together with changes in the spinal cord and brain, the consequences of neuroinflammation may explain the spread of symptoms beyond the distribution of the injured peripheral nerve.

to detect the presence of conduction deficits has limitations.[40] For example, electrodiagnostic tests only evaluate large myelinated motor neurons and Aβ fibres, but not the small diameter fibres (Aδ and C fibres).[68] Yet the evidence suggests that these smaller diameter fibres are affected in entrapment neuropathies, sometimes before the larger myelinated fibres.[36] Because these traditional methods of assessment have limitations, their findings may correlate poorly with the patients' symptoms and disability level.[69,70] Elements of Quantitative Sensory Testing may assist the identification of a loss of nerve function, such as a deterioration in thermal and mechanical detection thresholds.[40,71] Specifically, a loss of function may implicate dysfunction in specific nerve fibres: elevated vibration detection thresholds implicates Aβ fibres; altered cold detection threshold implicates Aδ fibres; altered warm detection threshold implicates C-fibres.[71] It should be noted that this is separate to the use of Quantitative Sensory Testing to detect a gain in nerve function such as allodynia and temporal summation, which may indicate central mediated pain mechanisms, especially if widespread[71–74] (Chapter 2).

Nerve mechanosensitivity

The nervous system slides relative to its interfacing structures during movement of the body and is subjected to compressive and stretch forces.[75–78] As discussed previously, processes resulting from perineural inflammation or nerve compression from injury to interfacing musculoskeletal structures may predispose the nerve to mechanosensitivity. Although healthy nerves can tolerate compressive and stretch forces associated with movement, animal studies indicate that irritated, inflamed or injured nerves may have increased mechanical sensitivity, resulting in ectopic impulses in response to movement and compression.[16,17] Elements of the physical examination, such as neurodynamic tests, active and passive movement examination and nerve palpation,[79–81] may identify nerve mechanosensitivity. Specifically, neurodynamic tests aim to identify the presence of nerve mechanosensitivity by causing nerve gliding in relationship to interfacing structures[76,82–85] and nerve elongation potentially affecting intraneural pressure.[86] Ectopic impulse generation may occur in response to very small amounts of nerve elongation or applied pressure on inflamed nerves.[17] This may reproduce

> **FOCUS POINT**
>
> Examination of the neural system attempts to identify altered nerve function such as nerve conduction deficits (a loss of function) or neural mechanosensitivity (a gain of function) that is relevant to the neck pain disorder.

symptoms and aberrant protective muscle responses during a test and reduce excursion of joint motion.[87] Interpretation of neurodynamic test responses needs to be made with some caution as sensory[88] and protective muscle responses[89] during neurodynamic tests are also present in asymptomatic individuals. Criteria for clinical testing and interpretation of tests of neuromechanosensitivity are described in Chapter 9.

CERVICAL SPINE-RELATED NERVE CONDITIONS

The aetiology of nerve-related conditions of the upper body may have a direct relationship with the cervical spine (e.g., cervical myelopathy, cervical radiculopathy), or conditions of the cervical spine may potentially contribute to other nerve-related upper limb conditions. Symptoms and signs of either carpal tunnel or cubital tunnel syndrome may extend beyond normal territories of the nerves involved if associated with a double crush mechanism particularly at the cervical spine,[45,46] or with neuronal changes in the dorsal root ganglion and central nervous system[41–43] as occurs in some cases of peripheral nerve injury.[40] This section will focus on nerve conditions with a direct relationship to the cervical spine.

Degenerative cervical myelopathy

Degenerative cervical myelopathy describes a collection of pathological conditions which, individually, or in combination, cause compression of the cervical spinal cord.[19] Degenerative cervical myelopathy incorporates conditions such as cervical spondylotic myelopathy.[90] These non-traumatic degenerative forms of cervical myelopathy are the most common cause of spinal cord impairment in the elderly.[91] Their incidence and prevalence in North America is estimated at a minimum of 41 and 605 per million people, respectively.[92]

The cervical cord is somewhat vulnerable to degenerative change because the width of the spinal canal reduces from C1 to C6 whereas the width of the cord area increases[93] placing the lower cervical cord at increased risk of stenosis and subsequent compression.[94] Canal stenosis and subsequent compression may be congenital, the result of trauma or acquired as a result of cervical spondylosis or neoplasms. Degenerative cervical myelopathy may result from spondylosis/degenerative osteoarthritic processes (e.g., facet joint degeneration, degenerative disc disease), non-osteoarthritic ligament degeneration (hypertrophy, ossification, calcification) or cervical hypermobility (e.g., Ehlers-Danlos syndrome). Individuals with congenital conditions such as Down syndrome and Klippel-Feil syndrome are predisposed to cervical myelopathy.[92] In any stenotic state, further canal narrowing during physiological or pathological motion (particularly during cervical extension), may exacerbate spinal cord compression.[90,95–98]

Similar to changes in peripheral nerves, compression of the spinal cord may disrupt blood supply leading to cord ischaemia.[96] It has been demonstrated in animal models that chronic compression of the cervical spinal cord results in spinal cord ischaemia, blood-spinal cord barrier disruption, neuroinflammation and apoptotic signalling activation.[99] Pathological processes within the cord may include grey and white matter degeneration, anterior horn cell loss, cystic cavitation, Wallerian degeneration and degeneration of the corticospinal tract.[99–101] Reviews by Wilson et al.[90] and Nouri et al.[92] provide a more detailed evaluation of the pathological processes associated with degenerative cervical myelopathy.

Clinical signs associated with cervical myelopathy are varied because of the extensive and variable changes to the spinal cord. No one clinical finding is pathognomonic, but cervical myelopathy is typified by gait imbalance, loss of hand dexterity and sphincter dysfunction.[19] Symptoms may also include numbness or paraesthesia of the arms and hands, weakness of the legs, Lhermitte's sign (electrical sensation up or down the spine ± limbs usually with neck flexion). Signs include corticospinal distribution motor deficits, atrophy of intrinsic hand muscles, hyperreflexia, positive Hoffman sign, up going plantar responses and lower limb spasticity.[102] Cord signal change on MRI may not correlate well with upper extremity reflex examination findings.[103]

Natural progression of the condition is highly variable. Some patients remain clinically stable in the long term, but a large proportion experience clinical deterioration if left untreated.[90] Current evidence suggests that in patients with cervical canal stenosis and cord compression secondary to spondylosis, but without clinical evidence of myelopathy, approximately 8% will develop clinical evidence of myelopathy at 1-year follow-up and 23% at a median of 44-months follow-up.[104] Furthermore 20% to 60% of patients will deteriorate neurologically over time without surgical intervention.[95]

Management of the condition is still uncertain. Evidence supports the efficacy of surgical treatment for symptomatic patients with degenerative cervical myelopathy;[90] however non-surgical management may still be an option for those patients who have radiological evidence of canal stenosis and cord compression but may not be myelopathic or have only minimal symptoms. Nevertheless, clinicians need to be aware of the potential for neurological decline in this patient group that requires immediate medical care. Continual re-evaluation of clinical presentation including regular neurological evaluation is indicated for these patients.

Cervicobrachial disorders and cervical radiculopathy

Nerves may be affected by musculoskeletal injury or pathology as they course through and exit the cervical spine. Cervical nerves exit through the intervertebral foramen, which is bordered by the pedicles superiorly and inferiorly, by the facet joint and capsule dorsally, and by the posterolateral disc, uncovertebral joint and vertebral artery ventrally. Pathology in any of the interfacing musculoskeletal structures may potentially affect the local nerve structures or, in the presence of stenosis, compress nerves. Coexisting neck and arm pain is associated with greater levels of self-reported disability than neck pain alone.[105] Clinically, there is a spectrum of cervicobrachial conditions. Some present as somatic referral of arm pain with no apparent nerve involvement, whereas some present with varying degrees and mix of physical signs of altered nerve conduction and mechanosensitivity.

Cervical radiculopathy is characterized by objective signs of nerve conduction loss including some combination of sensory loss, motor loss or impaired reflexes in a segmental distribution.[7] The lower cervical nerve roots

(C6, C7) are most vulnerable. This is consistent with the mismatch in size between the intervertebral foramen and spinal nerves and the prevalent degenerative changes at the C5-6 and C6-7 motion segments.[106–108] Encroachment of cervical nerve roots as they exit the intervertebral foramen is from spondylosis in approximately 70% to 75% of cases (reduced disc height, degenerative zygapophyseal or uncovertebral joints), disc lesions in approximately 20% to 25% of cases or nerve root sleeve fibrosis.[107,109,110] Injury to the nerve underlying cervical radicular pain may be caused by compression of the nerve and/or the presence of perineural inflammation.[5–7]

Cervical radiculopathy has a prevalence of 0.10% to 0.35% for the entire population but mostly affects individuals between 40 and 65 years of age.[111,112] Pain may or may not be present and may be non-dermatomal.[113] As discussed, compression of the peripheral nerve alone may not provoke pain but instead pain may be reliant on factors such as the presence of perineural inflammation, or the development of intraneural inflammation or the involvement of the dorsal root ganglion.[61] There is also some evidence for altered central pain processing mechanisms in cervical radiculopathies.[72]

Occipital neuralgia

Occipital neuralgia is an uncommon cause of occipital pain and headache caused by irritation of the greater, lesser or third occipital nerves and may be characterized by paroxysmal lancinating pain.[114] It is proposed that irritation and entrapment of the greater occipital nerve may occur at various locations along its anatomic course including where it branches from C2 between the axis and atlas, or where it courses between the inferior oblique and semispinalis muscles or where it pierces the belly of the semispinalis muscle or aponeurosis of the trapezius.[115,116] Although many pathoanatomic aetiologies of occipital neuralgias have been proposed (trauma, fibrositis, myositis, C1–2 and C2–3 pathology, neural malformations),[117] their aetiology is largely unknown and most presentations are considered idiopathic.[114] For a discussion of potential aetiologies underlying occipital neuralgias, comprehensive reviews on this topic are provided by Dougherty[114] and Cesmebasi et al.[117] Although the exact aetiology may be difficult to identify, from the clinician's perspective the distribution and nature of headache symptoms associated with occipital neuralgia justifies a thorough

examination of the cervical spine, including a detailed examination of the nervous system incorporating tests of nerve conduction and mechanosensitivity.

Thoracic outlet syndrome

Thoracic outlet syndrome still remains a controversial condition.[118] It is a blanket term encapsulating many different clinical entities.[119] The syndrome is characterized by pain, paraesthesia, weakness and discomfort in the upper limb, which is aggravated by elevation of the arms or by exaggerated movements of the head and neck.[120] The thoracic outlet refers to an area from the supraclavicular fossa to the axilla, through which course the brachial plexus (C5 to T1 nerve fibres), as well as the subclavian and axillary arteries and veins.[119] Therefore thoracic outlet syndrome may involve compromise of neural tissues, vascular tissues, or both. Three classifications have been described; (1) neurologic thoracic outlet syndrome, (2) vascular thoracic outlet syndrome (arterial and venous) and (3) neurovascular/combined. Vascular thoracic outlet syndrome is rare (< 5% of cases) with neurologic thoracic outlet syndrome the main contributor.[118,121,122] Stewman et al.[119] provide a full description of the subcategories and prevalence of subcategories of thoracic outlet syndrome.

Potential sites of neurovascular compromise include the interscalene triangle, costoclavicular space and subcoracoid space,[123–125] but there may be significant anatomic variation in these regions between individuals. There is the potential for compromise as the brachial plexus and subclavian artery exit through the anterior and middle scalene muscles that, together with the first rib, form the scalene triangle. The C5 or C6 ventral rami may penetrate the anterior scalene muscle,[126] but most commonly they penetrate the middle scalene along with the dorsal scapular nerve.[127] Atrophy, spasm or the common presence of the additional scalenus minimus muscle may compromise travel of neurovascular structures through the scalene triangle.[126,128,129] The double crush syndrome may be a relevant factor for thoracic outlet syndrome with respect to compression of the brachial plexus and distal sites of nerve compression.[130] Overall, there is still uncertainty about the underlying mechanisms of thoracic outlet. Its diverse presentations underpin recommendations that diagnoses rely on a thorough examination because there is currently no gold standard test for its diagnosis.[119]

CONCLUSION

Neck pain disorders commonly involve injury or pathology of nerve tissue. The cervical spine may be directly implicated in some neural conditions such as cervical radiculopathy or myelopathy. Cervical conditions may also be implicated in some upper limb neuropathies such as carpal tunnel syndrome. The identification of the presence and nature of neuropathy in neck pain disorders depends on a judicious structural differential examination. In particular, determining the relative presence of nerve conduction and nerve mechanosensitivity features will guide the most appropriate and safe course of management for these sometimes-complex neck pain presentations.

REFERENCES

1. Azhary H, Farooq MU, Bhanushali M, et al. Peripheral neuropathy: differential diagnosis and management. Am Fam Physician 2010;81:887–92.
2. Thampy E, Cherian SV. An unusual but classic cause of hand numbness: pancoast tumour. Postgrad Med J 2017;93:779.
3. Woolf CJ, Mannion RJ. Neuropathic pain: aetiology, symptoms, mechanisms, and management. Lancet 1999;353:1959–64.
4. Woolf CJ. Dissecting out mechanisms responsible for peripheral neuropathic pain: implications for diagnosis and therapy. Life Sci 2004;74:2605–10.
5. Kang JD, Georgescu HI, McIntyre-Larkin L, et al. Herniated cervical intervertebral discs spontaneously produce matrix metalloproteinases, nitric oxide, interleukin-6, and prostaglandin E2. Spine 1995;20:2373–8.
6. Furusawa N, Baba H, Miyoshi N, et al. Herniation of cervical intervertebral disc: immunohistochemical examination and measurement of nitric oxide production. Spine 2001;26:1110–16.
7. Bogduk N. The anatomy and pathophysiology of neck pain. Phys Med Rehabil Clin N Am 2011;22:367–82.
8. Benoliel R, Wilensky A, Tal M, et al. Application of a pro-inflammatory agent to the orbital portion of the rat infraorbital nerve induces changes indicative of ongoing trigeminal pain. Pain 2002;99:567–78.
9. Eliav E, Herzberg U, Ruda MA, et al. Neuropathic pain from an experimental neuritis of the rat sciatic nerve. Pain 1999;83:169–82.
10. Chacur M, Milligan ED, Gazda LS, et al. A new model of sciatic inflammatory neuritis (SIN): induction of unilateral and bilateral mechanical allodynia following acute unilateral peri-sciatic immune activation in rats. Pain 2001;94:231–44.
11. Gazda LS, Milligan ED, Hansen MK, et al. Sciatic inflammatory neuritis (SIN): behavioral allodynia is paralleled by peri-sciatic proinflammatory cytokine and superoxide production. J Peripher Nerv Syst 2001;6:111–29.
12. Eliav E, Gracely RH. Sensory changes in the territory of the lingual and inferior alveolar nerves following lower third molar extraction. Pain 1998;77:191–9.
13. Milligan ED, Maier SF, Watkins LR. Sciatic inflammatory neuropathy in the rat: surgical procedures, induction of inflammation, and behavioral testing. Methods Mol Med 2004;99:67–89.
14. Eliav E, Tal M, Benoliel R. Experimental malignancy in the rat induces early hypersensitivity indicative of neuritis. Pain 2004;110:727–37.
15. Eliav E, Benoliel R, Tal M. Inflammation with no axonal damage of the rat saphenous nerve trunk induces ectopic discharge and mechanosensitivity in myelinated axons. Neurosci Lett 2001;311:49–52.
16. Bove GM, Ransil BJ, Lin HC, et al. Inflammation induces ectopic mechanical sensitivity in axons of nociceptors innervating deep tissues. J Neurophysiol 2003;90:1949–55.
17. Dilley A, Lynn B, Pang SJ. Pressure and stretch mechanosensitivity of peripheral nerve fibres following local inflammation of the nerve trunk. Pain 2005;117:462–72.
18. Eliav E, Benoliel R, Herzberg U, et al. The role of IL-6 and IL-1beta in painful perineural inflammatory neuritis. Brain Behav Immun 2009;23:474–84.
19. Tetreault L, Goldstein CL, Arnold P, et al. Degenerative cervical myelopathy: a spectrum of related disorders affecting the aging spine. Neurosurgery 2015;77(Suppl. 4):S51–67.
20. Shedid D, Benzel EC. Cervical spondylosis anatomy: pathophysiology and biomechanics. Neurosurgery 2007;60(1 Suppl 1):S7–13.
21. Assmus H, Antoniadis G, Bischoff C, et al. Cubital tunnel syndrome - a review and management guidelines. Cent Eur Neurosurg 2011;72:90–8.
22. Bland JD. Carpal tunnel syndrome. Curr Opin Neurol 2005;18:581–5.
23. Upton AR, McComas AJ. The double crush in nerve entrapment syndromes. Lancet 1973;2:359–62.
24. Cohen BH, Gaspar MP, Daniels AH, et al. Multifocal neuropathy: expanding the scope of double crush syndrome. J Hand Surg Am 2016;41:1171–5.
25. Rydevik B, Lundborg G, Bagge U. Effects of graded compression on intraneural blood blow. An in vivo study on rabbit tibial nerve. J Hand Surg Am 1981;6:3–12.
26. Rydevik B, Lundborg G. Permeability of intraneural microvessels and perineurium following acute, graded experimental nerve compression. Scand J Plast Reconstr Surg 1977;11:179–87.
27. Mueller M, Leonhard C, Wacker K, et al. Macrophage response to peripheral nerve injury: the quantitative contribution of resident and hematogenous macrophages. Lab Invest 2003;83:175–85.
28. Moalem G, Tracey DJ. Immune and inflammatory mechanisms in neuropathic pain. Brain Res Rev 2006;51:240–64.
29. Moalem G, Xu K, Yu L. T lymphocytes play a role in neuropathic pain following peripheral nerve injury in rats. Neuroscience 2004;129:767–77.
30. Mackinnon SE. Pathophysiology of nerve compression. Hand Clin 2002;18:231–41.

31. Schmid AB, Bland JD, Bhat MA, et al. The relationship of nerve fibre pathology to sensory function in entrapment neuropathy. Brain 2014;137(Pt 12):3186–99.

32. Devor M. Sodium channels and mechanisms of neuropathic pain. J Pain 2006;7(1 Suppl. 1):S3–12.

33. Moalem G, Grafe P, Tracey DJ. Chemical mediators enhance the excitability of unmyelinated sensory axons in normal and injured peripheral nerve of the rat. Neuroscience 2005;134: 1399–411.

34. Sorkin LS, Xiao WH, Wagner R, et al. Tumour necrosis factor-alpha induces ectopic activity in nociceptive primary afferent fibres. Neuroscience 1997;81:255–62.

35. Grossmann L, Gorodetskaya N, Baron R, et al. Enhancement of ectopic discharge in regenerating A- and C-fibers by inflammatory mediators. J Neurophysiol 2009;101:2762–74.

36. Schmid AB, Coppieters MW, Ruitenberg MJ, et al. Local and remote immune-mediated inflammation after mild peripheral nerve compression in rats. J Neuropathol Exp Neurol 2013;72:662–80.

37. Hu P, Bembrick AL, Keay KA, et al. Immune cell involvement in dorsal root ganglia and spinal cord after chronic constriction or transection of the rat sciatic nerve. Brain Behav Immun 2007;21:599–616.

38. Hu P, McLachlan EM. Macrophage and lymphocyte invasion of dorsal root ganglia after peripheral nerve lesions in the rat. Neuroscience 2002;112:23–38.

39. Schafers M, Sommer C, Geis C, et al. Selective stimulation of either tumor necrosis factor receptor differentially induces pain behavior in vivo and ectopic activity in sensory neurons in vitro. Neuroscience 2008;157:414–23.

40. Schmid AB, Nee RJ, Coppieters MW. Reappraising entrapment neuropathies–mechanisms, diagnosis and management. Man Ther 2013;18:449–57.

41. Watkins LR, Maier SF. Beyond neurons: evidence that immune and glial cells contribute to pathological pain states. Physiol Rev 2002;82:981–1011.

42. Mor D, Bembrick AL, Austin PJ, et al. Anatomically specific patterns of glial activation in the periaqueductal gray of the sub-population of rats showing pain and disability following chronic constriction injury of the sciatic nerve. Neuroscience 2010;166:1167–84.

43. LeBlanc BW, Zerah ML, Kadasi LM, et al. Minocycline injection in the ventral posterolateral thalamus reverses microglial reactivity and thermal hyperalgesia secondary to sciatic neuropathy. Neurosci Lett 2011;498:138–42.

44. Schmid AB. The peripheral nervous system and its compromise in entrapment neuropathies. In: Jull G, Moore A, Falla D, et al, editors. Grieve's modern musculoskeletal physiotherapy. 4th ed. Edinburgh: Elsevier; 2015. p. 78–92.

45. Hurst LC, Weissberg D, Carroll RE. The relationship of the double crush to carpal tunnel syndrome (an analysis of 1,000 cases of carpal tunnel syndrome). J Hand Surg [Br] 1985;10: 202–4.

46. Morgan G, Wilbourn AJ. Cervical radiculopathy and coexisting distal entrapment neuropathies: double-crush syndromes? Neurology 1998;50:78–83.

47. Dahlin LB, McLean WG. Effects of graded experimental compression on slow and fast axonal transport in rabbit vagus nerve. J Neurol Sci 1986;72:19–30.

48. Schmid AB, Coppieters MW. The double crush syndrome revisited–a Delphi study to reveal current expert views on mechanisms underlying dual nerve disorders. Man Ther 2011;16:557–62.

49. Shannon B, Klimkiewicz JJ. Cervical burners in the athlete. Clin Sports Med 2002;21:29–35.

50. Standaert CJ, Herring SA. Expert opinion and controversies in musculoskeletal and sports medicine: stingers. Arch Phys Med Rehabil 2009;90:402–6.

51. Castro FP Jr. Stingers, cervical cord neurapraxia, and stenosis. Clin Sports Med 2003;22:483–92.

52. Meyer SA, Schulte KR, Callaghan JJ, et al. Cervical spinal stenosis and stingers in collegiate football players. Am J Sports Med 1994;22:158–66.

53. Krivickas LS, Wilbourn AJ. The pathomechanics of chronic, recurrent cervical nerve root neurapraxia: the chronic burner syndrome. Am J Sports Med 1998;26:603–4.

54. Green J, Zuckerman SL, Dalton SL, et al. A 6-year surveillance study of "stingers" in NCAA American Football. Res Sports Med 2017;25:26–36.

55. Coppieters MW. Shoulder restraints as a potential cause for stretch neuropathies: biomechanical support for the impact of shoulder girdle depression and arm abduction on nerve strain. Anesthesiology 2006;104:1351–2.

56. Coppieters MW, Van de Velde M, Stappaerts KH. Positioning in anesthesiology: toward a better understanding of stretch-induced perioperative neuropathies. Anesthesiology 2002;97: 75–81.

57. Lundborg G, Rydevik B. Effects of stretching the tibial nerve of the rabbit. A preliminary study of the intraneural circulation and the barrier function of the perineurium. J Bone Joint Surg Br 1973;55:390–401.

58. Wall EJ, Massie JB, Kwan MK, et al. Experimental stretch neuropathy. Changes in nerve conduction under tension. J Bone Joint Surg Br 1992;74:126–9.

59. Goldstein DP, Ringash J, Bissada E, et al. Scoping review of the literature on shoulder impairments and disability after neck dissection. Head Neck 2014;36:299–308.

60. Vastamaki M, Ristolainen L, Vastamaki H, et al. Isolated serratus palsy etiology influences its long-term outcome. J Shoulder Elbow Surg 2017;26:1964–9.

61. Howe JF, Loeser JD, Calvin WH. Mechanosensitivity of dorsal root ganglia and chronically injured axons: a physiological basis for the radicular pain of nerve root compression. Pain 1977;3: 25–41.

62. Song XJ, Hu SJ, Greenquist KW, et al. Mechanical and thermal hyperalgesia and ectopic neuronal discharge after chronic compression of dorsal root ganglia. J Neurophysiol 1999;82: 3347–58.

63. Bouhissera D, Attal N. Novel strategies for neuropathic pain. In: Villannueva L, Dickensen A, Ollat H, editors. The pain system in normal and pathological states. Seattle: IASP press; 2004.

64. Rasmussen P, Sindrup S, Jensen T, et al. Symptoms and signs in patients with suspected neuropathic pain. Pain 2004;110:461–9.

65. Bennett MI, Smith BH, Torrance N, et al. The S-LANSS score for identifying pain of predominantly neuropathic origin: validation for use in clinical and postal research. J Pain 2005;6:149–58.

66. Krause SJ, Backonja MM. Development of a neuropathic pain questionnaire. Clin J Pain 2003;19:306–14.

67. Lee DH, Claussen GC, Oh S. Clinical nerve conduction and needle electromyography studies. J Am Acad Orthop Surg 2004;12:276–87.

68. Mallik A, Weir AI. Nerve conduction studies: essentials and pitfalls in practice. J Neurol Neurosurg Psychiatry 2005;76(Suppl. 2):ii23–31.

69. Mondelli M, Reale F, Sicurelli F, et al. Relationship between the self-administered Boston questionnaire and electrophysiological findings in follow-up of surgically-treated carpal tunnel syndrome. J Hand Surg [Br] 2000;25:128–34.

70. Longstaff L, Milner RH, O'Sullivan S, et al. Carpal tunnel syndrome: the correlation between outcome, symptoms and nerve conduction study findings. J Hand Surg [Br] 2001;26:475–80.

71. Rolke R, Baron R, Maier C, et al. Quantitative sensory testing in the German Research Network on Neuropathic Pain (DFNS): standardized protocol and reference values. Pain 2006;123:231–43.

72. Chien A, Eliav E, Sterling M. Whiplash (grade II) and cervical radiculopathy share a similar sensory presentation: an investigation using quantitative sensory testing. Clin J Pain 2008;24:595–603.

73. Schmid AB, Soon BT, Wasner G, et al. Can widespread hypersensitivity in carpal tunnel syndrome be substantiated if neck and arm pain are absent? Eur J Pain 2012;16:217–28.

74. Treede RD, Handwerker HO, Baumgärtner U, et al. Hyperalgesia and allodynia: taxonomy, assessment, and mechanisms. In: Brune K, Handwerker HO, editors. Hyperalgesia: molecular mechanisms and clinical implications. Seattle: IASP Press; 2004. p. 1e15.

75. McLellan DL, Swash M. Longitudinal sliding of the median nerve during movements of the upper limb. J Neurol Neurosurg Psychiatry 1976;39:566–70.

76. Coppieters MW, Alshami AM, Babri AS, et al. Strain and excursion of the sciatic, tibial, and plantar nerves during a modified straight leg raising test. J Orthop Res 2006;24:1883–9.

77. Gelberman RH, Hergenroeder PT, Hargens AR, et al. The carpal tunnel syndrome. A study of carpal canal pressures. J Bone Joint Surg Am 1981;63:380–3.

78. Coppieters MW, Butler DS. Do 'sliders' slide and 'tensioners' tension? An analysis of neurodynamic techniques and considerations regarding their application. Man Ther 2008;13:213–21.

79. Baselgia LT, Bennett DL, Silbiger RM, et al. Negative neurodynamic tests do not exclude neural dysfunction in patients with entrapment neuropathies. Arch Phys Med Rehabil 2017;98:480–6.

80. Elvey RL. Physical evaluation of the peripheral nervous system in disorders of pain and dysfunction. J Hand Ther 1997;10:122–9.

81. Hall TM, Elvey RL. Nerve trunk pain: physical diagnosis and treatment. Man Ther 1999;4:63–73.

82. Byl C, Puttlitz C, Byl N, et al. Strain in the median and ulnar nerves during upper-extremity positioning. J Hand Surg Am 2002;27:1032–40.

83. Dilley A, Lynn B, Greening J, et al. Quantitative in vivo studies of median nerve sliding in response to wrist, elbow, shoulder and neck movements. Clin Biomech (Bristol, Avon) 2003;18:899–907.

84. Wilgis EF, Murphy R. The significance of longitudinal excursion in peripheral nerves. Hand Clin 1986;2:761–6.

85. Wright TW, Glowczewskie F Jr, Cowin D, et al. Radial nerve excursion and strain at the elbow and wrist associated with upper-extremity motion. J Hand Surg Am 2005;30:990–6.

86. Millesi H, Zoch G, Reihsner R. Mechanical properties of peripheral nerves. Clin Orthop Relat Res 1995;314:76–83.

87. Coppieters MW, Stappaerts KH, Wouters LL, et al. Aberrant protective force generation during neural provocation testing and the effect of treatment in patients with neurogenic cervicobrachial pain. J Manipulative Physiol Ther 2003;26:99–106.

88. Coppieters MW, Stappaerts KH, Everaert DG, et al. Addition of test components during neurodynamic testing: effect on range of motion and sensory responses. J Orthop Sports Phys Ther 2001;31:226–35.

89. Coppieters MW, Stappaerts KH, Staes FF, et al. Shoulder girdle elevation during neurodynamic testing: an assessable sign? Man Ther 2001;6:88–96.

90. Wilson JR, Tetreault LA, Kim J, et al. State of the art in degenerative cervical myelopathy: an update on current clinical evidence. Neurosurgery 2017;80:S33–45.

91. Kalsi-Ryan S, Karadimas SK, Fehlings MG. Cervical spondylotic myelopathy: the clinical phenomenon and the current pathobiology of an increasingly prevalent and devastating disorder. Neuroscientist 2013;19:409–21.

92. Nouri A, Tetreault L, Singh A, et al. Degenerative cervical myelopathy: epidemiology, genetics, and pathogenesis. Spine 2015;40:E675–93.

93. Ulbrich EJ, Schraner C, Boesch C, et al. Normative MR cervical spinal canal dimensions. Radiology 2014;271:172–82.

94. Morishita Y, Naito M, Wang JC. Cervical spinal canal stenosis: the differences between stenosis at the lower cervical and multiple segment levels. Int Orthop 2011;35:1517–22.

95. Karadimas SK, Erwin WM, Ely CG, et al. Pathophysiology and natural history of cervical spondylotic myelopathy. Spine 2013;38:S21–36.

96. Baptiste DC, Fehlings MG. Pathophysiology of cervical myelopathy. Spine J 2006;6:190S–197S.

97. Lestini WF, Wiesel SW. The pathogenesis of cervical spondylosis. Clin Orthop Relat Res 1989;239:69–93.

98. Rao R. Neck pain, cervical radiculopathy, and cervical myelopathy: pathophysiology, natural history, and clinical evaluation. J Bone Joint Surg Am 2002;84-A:1872–81.

99. Karadimas SK, Moon ES, Yu WR, et al. A novel experimental model of cervical spondylotic myelopathy (CSM) to facilitate translational research. Neurobiol Dis 2013;54:43–58.

100. Karadimas SK, Laliberte AM, Tetreault L, et al. Riluzole blocks perioperative ischemia-reperfusion injury and enhances

postdecompression outcomes in cervical spondylotic myelopathy. Sci Transl Med 2015;7(316):316ra194.

101. Karadimas SK, Moon E, Fehlings M. The sodium channel/glutamate blocker riluzole is complementary to decompression in a preclinical experimental model of cervical spondylotic myelopathy: implications for translational clinical application. Neurosurgery 2012;71:E543.

102. Fortin M, Dobrescu O, Courtemanche M, et al. Association between paraspinal muscle morphology, clinical symptoms, and functional status in patients with degenerative cervical myelopathy. Spine 2017;42:232–9.

103. Nemani VM, Kim HJ, Piyaskulkaew C, et al. Correlation of cord signal change with physical examination findings in patients with cervical myelopathy. Spine 2014;40:6–10.

104. Wilson JR, Barry S, Fischer DJ, et al. Frequency, timing, and predictors of neurological dysfunction in the non-myelopathic patient with cervical spinal cord compression, canal stenosis, and/or ossification of the posterior longitudinal ligament. Spine 2013;38:S37–54.

105. Daffner SD, Hilibrand AS, Hanscom BS, et al. Impact of neck and arm pain on overall health status. Spine 2003;28:2030–5.

106. Osborn A. Diagnostic neuroradiology. St. Louis: CV Mosby; 1994.

107. Shedid D, Benzel EC. Cervical spondylosis anatomy: pathophysiology and biomechanics. Neurosurgery 2007;60:S7–13.

108. Harrop JS, Hanna A, Silva MT, et al. Neurological manifestations of cervical spondylosis: an overview of signs, symptoms, and pathophysiology. Neurosurgery 2007;60:S14–20.

109. Epstein J, Epstein B, Lavine L, et al. Cervical myelo-radiculopathy caused by arthrotic hypertrophy of the posterior facets and laminae. J Neurosurgery 1978;49:387–92.

110. Carette S, Fehlings MG. Clinical practice. Cervical radiculopathy. N Engl J Med 2005;353:392–9.

111. Radhakrishnan K, Litchy WJ, O'Fallon WM, et al. Epidemiology of cervical radiculopathy. A population-based study from Rochester, Minnesota, 1976 through 1990. Brain 1994;117(Pt 2):325–35.

112. Salemi G, Savettieri G, Meneghini F, et al. Prevalence of cervical spondylotic radiculopathy: a door-to-door survey in a Sicilian municipality. Acta Neurol Scand 1996;93:184–8.

113. Murphy DR, Hurwitz EL, McGovern EE. A nonsurgical approach to the management of patients with lumbar radiculopathy secondary to herniated disk: a prospective observational cohort study with follow-up. J Manipulative Physiol Ther 2009;32:723–33.

114. Dougherty C. Occipital neuralgia. Curr Pain Headache Rep 2014;18:411.

115. Loukas M, El-Sedfy A, Tubbs RS, et al. Identification of greater occipital nerve landmarks for the treatment of occipital neuralgia. Folia Morphol 2006;65:337–42.

116. Narouze S. Occipital neuralgia diagnosis and treatment: the role of ultrasound. Headache 2016;56:801–7.

117. Cesmebasi A, Muhleman MA, Hulsberg P, et al. Occipital neuralgia: anatomic considerations. Clin Anat 2015;28:101–8.

118. Sanders RJ, Hammond SL, Rao NM. Thoracic outlet syndrome: a review. Neurologist 2008;14:365–73.

119. Stewman C, Vitanzo PC Jr, Harwood MI. Neurologic thoracic outlet syndrome: summarizing a complex history and evolution. Curr Sports Med Rep 2014;13:100–6.

120. Lindgren KA, Oksala I. Long-term outcome of surgery for thoracic outlet syndrome. Am J Surg 1995;169:358–60.

121. Ferrante MA. The thoracic outlet syndromes. Muscle Nerve 2012;45:780–95.

122. Sanders RJ, Hammond SL, Rao NM. Diagnosis of thoracic outlet syndrome. J Vasc Surg 2007;46:601–4.

123. Nichols AW. Diagnosis and management of thoracic outlet syndrome. Curr Sports Med Rep 2009;8:240–9.

124. Wilbourn AJ. Thoracic outlet syndromes. Neurol Clin 1999;17:477–97.

125. Dahlstrom KA, Olinger AB. Descriptive anatomy of the interscalene triangle and the costoclavicular space and their relationship to thoracic outlet syndrome: a study of 60 cadavers. J Manipulative Physiol Ther 2012;35:396–401.

126. Harry WG, Bennett JD, Guha SC. Scalene muscles and the brachial plexus: anatomical variations and their clinical significance. Clin Anat 1997;10:250–2.

127. Wiater JM, Flatow EL. Long thoracic nerve injury. Clin Orthop 1999;368:17–27.

128. Rusnak-Smith S, Moffat M, Rosen E. Anatomical variations of the scalene triangle: dissection of 10 cadavers. J Orthop Sports Phys Ther 2001;31:70–80.

129. Makhoul RG, Machleder HI. Developmental anomalies at the thoracic outlet: an analysis of 200 consecutive cases. J Vasc Surg 1992;16:534–42.

130. Mackinnon SE, Novak CB. Thoracic outlet syndrome. Curr Probl Surg 2002;39:1070–145.

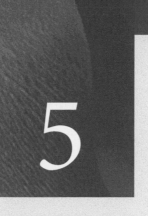

5

NEUROMUSCULAR DISTURBANCES IN NECK PAIN DISORDERS

The cervical region is equipped with elaborate musculature and the coordinated activity of all muscles influences the orientation of the cervical spine and head position. The intricate neural control of the cervical spine dictates that nociception can have a profound influence on the control of head movement and stability.

A number of theories have been proposed over the years to account for the neuromuscular adaptations accompanying pain. This includes classic models such as the pain adaptation model[1] and the vicious circle model[2] which both predict very stereotypical changes in the presence of pain. Although a number of experimental findings supported each model, neither model is able to explain the complexity and diversity of neuromuscular adaptations seen in people with musculoskeletal pain, including the diverse neuromuscular adaptations accompanying neck pain. As a result, contemporary theories have been proposed to better explain motor adaptations to injury/pain, which encompass the greater diversity of motor adaptations seen in clinical cases.[3,4] Some of the key principles of contemporary theory indicate that;[3–5] (1) pain-related neuromuscular adaptations involve a diversity of changes ranging from subtle redistribution of activity within a muscle to complete avoidance of movement; (2) despite common features, individuals will present with their own unique mix of neuromuscular adaptations; (3) pain-related neuromuscular adaptations have a common aim initially to protect the painful/threatened body region from real or anticipated further pain/injury; (4) neuromuscular adaptations can be initiated in the presence of pain/injury but may also be the initial trigger for the development of pain; and (5) if maintained, neuromuscular adaptations can lead to secondary adaptations and/or long-term consequences. Such contemporary theory is underpinned by a wealth of data from experimental and clinical studies including those in people with neck pain disorders.

The various features of this contemporary understanding of neuromuscular adaptations to pain will be reviewed in this chapter as it applies to neck pain disorders. Following a brief overview of anatomic considerations of the cervical musculature, a number of studies will be considered, which describe varying neuromuscular adaptations in individuals with neck pain. These changes range from more general modifications such as decreased neck muscle strength, through to subtle variations in the distribution of activity within and between neck muscles. There is convincing evidence that nociception/injury is the initial trigger for such adaptations[6–13] although, continued or maladaptive changes in neuromuscular control can contribute to the chronicity, maintenance and recurrence of neck pain.[14] That is, altered muscle coordination which involves less efficient combinations of muscle synergies may alter loading on cervical structures including the muscles themselves and increase the vulnerability of the cervical region to strain resulting in the maintenance or initiation of nociception.[5,6,15] Moreover, neck pain has been associated with a number of peripheral adaptations within muscle including changes in muscle cross-sectional area, fatty infiltration of muscle tissue and specific modifications of muscle fibres, which may in part be driven by ongoing alterations of muscle behaviour. These adaptations will also be reviewed within this chapter.

ANATOMICAL CONSIDERATIONS

There are 44 muscles in the neck which collectively work to control and stabilize head movement in three-dimensional space while simultaneously executing voluntary movements. Neck muscles are topographically arranged, with some acting solely over the upper cervical region, others acting only over the mid and lower cervical region and others spanning the entire cervical spine. The neck muscles can be further considered according to their functional roles. Generally speaking, the larger superficial muscles (e.g., splenius capitis, sternocleido-mastoid) have larger lever arms and cross-sectional areas and a greater capacity to exert torque than deeper muscles (e.g., multifidus, longus colli and longus capitis).[16] In contrast, the deeper muscles are typically segmentally arranged with direct attachments to the cervical vertebrae and have larger spindle densities.[17,18] The suboccipital (e.g., rectus capitis posterior major and minor) and deep cervical muscles (e.g., multifidus and longus colli) have the highest density of muscle spindles of all muscles in the body.[17,18] Moreover, the deep muscles are characterized by a greater proportion of low-threshold slow twitch muscle fibres relative to the superficial muscles reflecting their contribution to postural support of the cervical spine.[17,18] Accordingly, a model of the cervical spine demonstrated regions of local segmental instability when only the large superficial muscles of the neck were simulated to produce movement in the absence of deep muscle activation[19] confirming the relevance of the deep muscle layer in contributing to general postural support. Our recent work using shear wave elastography revealed that the deep muscle layer has greater passive and active stiffness compared with the superficial neck muscles.[20] These findings are supported by observations of high passive stiffness of the multifidus muscle, which was demonstrated on muscle fibre bundle examinations.[21] Similar to all deep muscles, the cervical multifidus is predominantly composed of low-threshold, slow-twitch muscle fibres,[17,18] which are stiffer[22,23] than fast-twitch fibres.

The sternocleidomastoid, anterior scalene and hyoid muscles form the superficial layer of the neck muscles anterolaterally. Bilateral contraction of the sternocleido-mastoid induces extension at the upper cervical region and flexion of the lower cervical region. Bilateral contraction of the anterior scalene will also contribute to flexion of the neck whereas ipsilateral contraction induces ipsilateral lateral flexion. During neck extension (when the neck flexor muscles act eccentrically), it is estimated that the flexor moment arms of both the sternocleido-mastoid and the anterior scalene muscles reduce as extension progresses such that in extreme extension, their moment arms are less than 25% of their value in a neutral upright position.[16] Thus as extension progresses, the deeper muscles progressively contribute more to control the position of the head.

The deepest layer of the flexor group consists of the longus capitis, longus colli and rectus capitis anterior. These muscles act to counter the accentuation of the cervical lordosis induced by extensor muscle contraction and head weight.[19,24,25] The longus capitis muscle overlaps the superior portion of longus colli and has attachments from the transverse processes of the third, fourth, fifth and sixth cervical vertebrae to insert on the inferior surface of the basilar part of the occipital bone. The longus colli has direct attachment to the anterior surface of the cervical vertebrae and spans from the atlas to the third thoracic vertebra. An increase in electromyographic (EMG) activity is evident in these deep cervical flexor muscles either when load is applied to the top of the head, that is, a load which accentuate the lordosis, or when the lordosis is actively straightened during postural realignment tasks.[26,27]

The neck extensor muscles are organized in four layers. Levator scapulae and upper trapezius constitute the superficial layer and, although they have attachments to the cranium and cervical spine, they are primarily considered muscles of the shoulder girdle responsible for bearing the load and absorbing the forces induced on the cervical segments during upper limb function.[28] This implies that the upper trapezius and levator scapulae muscles may induce compressive loading on cervical motion segments because of their attachments. Compared with the levator scapulae, the mechanical effects of upper trapezius are less owing to its relatively small cross sectional area and attachments primarily to the ligamentum nuchae.[29–31] However, the vertical orientation of the levator scapulae fibres and direct attachments to the upper four cervical vertebrae may induce compressive forces on the cervical spine.[32] Understandably, forces imposed on the cervical spine from excessive or aberrant axioscapular muscle activity may be potentially adverse and contribute to the development of neck pain during static work postures and/or tasks imposing repetitive arm movements.[28,32]

Splenius capitis forms the second layer and acts on the head to produce extension, ipsilateral rotation and ipsilateral lateral flexion of the neck.[33] The semispinalis capitis forms the third layer, and semispinalis cervicis, multifidus and rotatores muscles form the deepest layer together with the suboccipital muscle group. The rotatores are small and short muscles lying close to the vertebral arch and spinous process and act to rotate the vertebra to the opposite side. Multifidus has direct attachments to the cervical vertebrae and similarly the fibres of semispinalis cervicis originate from the transverse processes of T1 to T5–T6 inserting on to the spinous processes of C2 to C5 respectively down to C7. Collectively, the multifidus, rotatores and semispinalis cervicis form the transversospinalis muscle which produces extension, ipsilateral lateral flexion and contralateral rotation of the neck.

The suboccipital muscle group includes the rectus capitis posterior major and minor, and the obliquus capitis superior and inferior. These muscles contribute to the fine control of head movement in addition to providing support for the upper cervical segments, which is accredited to their relatively small moment arms, direct attachments to the cervical vertebrae, high proportion of slow-twitch fibres and high density of muscle spindles.[34–39]

The knowledge on the differing functional roles of the neck muscles is relevant because studies in people with neck pain disorders support a differential effect of pain on the deeper postural muscles of the neck versus the larger torque producing muscles. These differential effects are reviewed in this chapter.

CHANGES IN MOTOR OUTPUT IN PEOPLE WITH NECK PAIN

Several biomechanical disturbances are noted in people with neck pain including reduced range of motion,[40–42] reduced concurrent motions in the associated planes,[43] slower movement speed[44,45] and reduced smoothness of movement[44,42] as reviewed in Chapters 3. In addition

to these biomechanical disturbances, people with neck pain commonly display other impairments in motor output including reduced neck muscle strength, endurance and force steadiness.

Decreased neck strength is a common physical feature in people with neck pain regardless of the aetiology of their symptoms, and is typically diminished around all axes.[46] The extent to which neck strength is affected in people with neck pain varies widely with reports ranging from a 13% to 90% reduction compared with asymptomatic people.[47,48] Neck muscle endurance is also commonly affected and multiple studies have confirmed poor endurance of the neck flexors, extensors and craniocervical flexor muscles in people with neck pain across a range of contraction intensities.[49–52] Similar to observations for neck strength, reduced endurance appears to be independent of the aetiology of the patient's symptoms and has been documented for people with different neck pain disorders including cervicogenic headache,[51] cervical radiculopathy,[53] and idiopathic neck pain.[50,54] A loss of endurance in the craniocervical flexor muscles has also been observed indirectly as a reduced ability to maintain an upright sitting posture.[55] That is, compared with asymptomatic people, those with neck pain drift into a more forward head position during prolonged sitting.[55]

An impaired ability to maintain a steady force output around a target force value during isometric contractions is a further indicator of disturbed motor output in people with neck pain.[50,56,57] As an example, note the larger fluctuations in force illustrated in Fig. 5.1 when the patient with chronic neck pain attempts to control a force at 15 N while performing a circular contraction of their head and neck as compared with the representative example from an asymptomatic person.[56] Reduced ability to maintain a steady force output has been documented for people with neck pain across a range of contraction intensities.[50,56,57]

Some of the variability in neck muscle functional performance seen in people with neck pain can be explained by the presence of psychological features. For instance, approximately 13% of the variability in neck muscle strength in a group of patients with chronic neck pain could be explained by their level of fear avoidance.[46] Nevertheless, when their current pain during the neck muscle strength testing was taken into account, current pain and fear avoidance explained around 27% of the variance in neck muscle strength.[46] A recent study

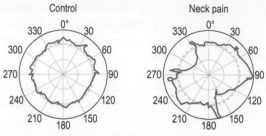

Fig. 5.1 ■ Representative force traces obtained for a control subject and a patient performing a circular contraction at 15 N. Note that the patient presents with less accuracy in producing the circular contraction compared with the control subject, which is reflected in a greater coefficient of variation of force for the patient compared with the control subject. In this example, the coefficient of variation of force is 7.4% and 17.5% for the control and patient respectively. (From Schomacher J, Farina D, Lindstroem R, et al. Chronic trauma-induced neck pain impairs the neural control of the deep semispinalis cervicis muscle. Clin Neurophysiol 2012;123:1403–1408.)

also showed that most of the variability in performance on physical tests of neck muscle function in people with whiplash-associated disorders could be best explained by their level of pain intensity and disability rather than their scores on various psychological questionnaires.[58]

Underlying these general changes in motor output, there may be numerous modifications in muscle behaviour including altered coordination both between and within muscles as now explored.

CHANGES IN THE COORDINATION BETWEEN MUSCLES

As indicated, there are 44 muscles in the neck which collectively facilitate the control and support of the cervical spine while simultaneously executing voluntary movements. Our central nervous system (CNS) copes with the anatomic complexity and redundancy of the neck muscles by developing consistent muscle synergies to generate multidirectional patterns of force.[6,59–61] Normally, the neck muscles show well-defined preferred directions of activation, which are in accordance with their anatomic position relative to the spine.[30,56,61,62] The recruitment of neck muscles for a given movement or task is therefore optimized and dependent on the task requirements. This changes when pain or anticipated pain is present.

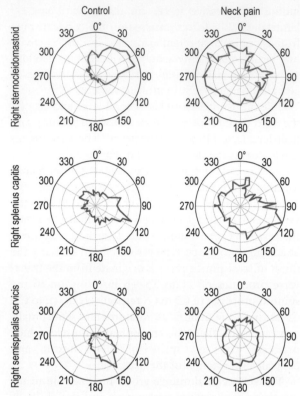

Fig. 5.2 ■ Representative directional activation curves obtained from the sternocleidomastoid, splenius capitis and semispinalis cervicis muscles during a circular contraction performed at 15 N presented for a control subject and a patient with chronic neck pain. Note the defined activation of the sternocleidomastoid, splenius capitis and semispinalis cervicis for the control subject with minimal activity during the antagonist phase of the task. Conversely, the directional activation curves for the patient indicate more even activation levels of each muscle for all directions. (From Falla D, Lindstrom R, Rechter L, et al. Effect of pain on the modulation in discharge rate of sterno-cleidomastoid motor units with force direction. Clin Neurophysiol 2010;121:744–753; Schomacher J, Farina D, Lindstroem R, et al. Chronic trauma-induced neck pain impairs the neural control of the deep semispinalis cervicis muscle. Clin Neurophysiol 2012;123:1403–1408; Lindstrom R, Schomacher J, Farina D, et al. Association between neck muscle co-activation, pain, and strength in women with neck pain. Man Ther 2011;16:80–86.)

Studies have shown that people with neck pain display distinct changes in neck muscle coordination including reduced specificity of neck muscle activity with respect to asymptomatic individuals[56,63,64] (Fig. 5.2). This includes people with chronic whiplash-associated disorders in addition to those with idiopathic neck pain. The reduced specificity of neck muscle activity is associated with a reduced modulation in the discharge rate of individual motor units with force direction.[56] Notably, reduced specificity of neck muscle activity also implies an increase in neck flexor and extensor coactivation as seen in Fig. 5.2, because a high level of antagonistic neck muscle activity is present in association with neck pain. Greater coactivation of the superficial cervical flexor and extensor muscles has also been observed in people with chronic neck pain and headache during isometric neck contractions[64,65] and in office workers with neck pain during a typing task.[66] Increased coactivation of the neck flexor and extensor muscles is inversely correlated with total neck strength and positively correlated with levels of pain and perceived disability.[64]

Higher levels of neck muscle coactivation may serve to initially protect a painful neck, that is, increased neck muscle coactivation may reflect an attempt to voluntarily increase the stability of the head/neck for the fear of performing potentially painful movements. This fits with the contemporary theory that motor adaptation to pain has a general aim (at least in the short term) to protect the painful/threatened body part from real or anticipated further pain/injury.[3] However, if maintained, this may ultimately lead to excessive loading on cervical structures further perpetuating neck symptoms and may act to facilitate ongoing nociception.

A number of additional studies support the observation of heightened activity of the superficial neck muscles in people with neck pain disorders. In particular, increased activation of the sternocleidomastoid and anterior scalene muscles is commonly observed during performance of the craniocervical flexion test; an observation that has been made in a number of studies evaluating different patient populations including cervicogenic headache,[67,68] idiopathic neck pain,[69,70] whiplash-induced neck pain[70–72] and occupationally-induced neck pain[73,74] (Fig. 5.3). The heightened activity of the superficial flexors was thought to reflect a compensatory strategy for weakness or inhibition of the longus colli and longus capitis reflecting a reorganization of the motor strategy to perform the task. Reduced activation of the deep cervical flexors was subsequently confirmed via direct measures of the EMG amplitude of longus colli and longus capitis during performance of this test in people with chronic neck

pain.[69] Recent work confirmed the interpretation that higher activity of the superficial flexor muscles during performance of this test, is an indicator of reduced activity of the deep cervical flexors.[75] That is, a moderate negative correlation was identified between the average EMG amplitude of the deep cervical flexors and sternocleidomastoid across all stages of the craniocervical flexion test.

Increased activation of the superficial neck flexors is not unique to the task of craniocervical flexion. Indeed, several studies have reported augmented activation of these muscles as people with neck pain perform other tasks including repeated upper limb movements[66,76] and isometric neck contractions.[56,77] Moreover, a recent study which examined the behaviour of sternocleidomastoid motor units, found that the people with mechanical neck pain showed significantly higher initial and mean firing rates during isometric cervical flexion contractions,[78] which supports earlier observations from surface EMG studies of greater sternocleidomastoid muscle activity in people with neck pain disorders. Additional findings of reduced modulation of the discharge rates of sternocleidomastoid motor units[56] (Fig. 5.4) and decreased sternocleidomastoid motor unit short-term synchronization[78] further support an altered neuromuscular control strategy in people with chronic neck pain. Interestingly, a recent study using real-time, ultrasound measurements of muscle deformation showed reduced variability in the interplay between different neck flexor muscles in people with whiplash-associated disorders during repeated arm elevation.[79]

Consistent with the observation of reduced activation of the deep cervical flexor muscles, studies have also demonstrated that people with neck pain commonly present with reduced activation of the deep extensors, semispinalis cervicis and multifidus. This has been demonstrated in several studies applying different methodologies including functional magnetic resonance imaging[80] and intramuscular EMG.[63,81] In contrast, higher activity of the superficial extensors (e.g., splenius capitis) is frequently seen in people with neck pain and this has been demonstrated in a number of tasks including typing on a keyboard,[82] isometric neck extension and lateral flexion,[83] repetitive upper limb movement[66] and isometric circular contractions in the horizontal plane.[64]

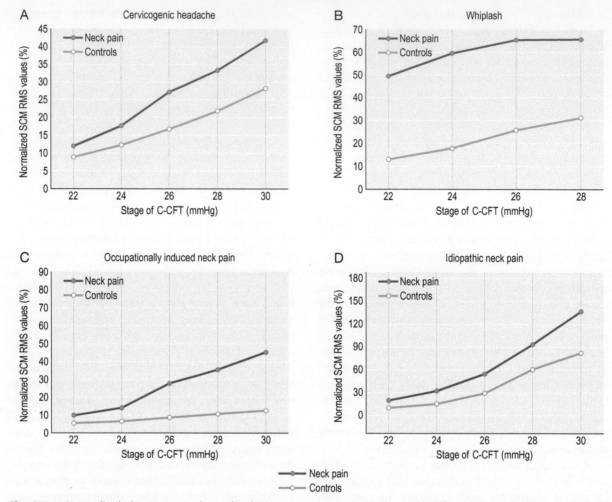

Fig. 5.3 ■ Normalized electromyograph amplitude (root mean square, RMS) recorded for the sternocleidomastoid muscle (SCM) during performance of the craniocervical flexion test (C-CFT) in people with neck pain (*dark blue*) versus healthy controls (*light blue*). Note the higher activity of the sternocleidomastoid muscle for the patients regardless of the aetiology of their neck pain. (A) cervicogenic headache,[67] (B) whiplash-induced neck pain,[72] (C) occupationally-induced neck pain[73] and (D) idiopathic neck pain.[69]

These seemingly contrasting effects on deep and superficial muscle activity suggests that more deeply and superficially situated muscles may be affected differentially by either central or peripheral mechanisms.[15] Another explanation could be that the CNS prioritizes a solution of increased stiffness/protection by coactivating the larger, superficial muscles[84] yet this comes at the expense of loss of control of the deeper postural muscles. Similar hypotheses have been proposed to explain trunk muscle adaptations in people with low-back pain.[84]

Besides changes in neck muscle activation, altered axioscapular muscle activation may be present in people with neck pain despite the absence of shoulder or arm pain[76,85–88] and can be induced experimentally with injection of hypertonic saline into neck muscles.[89,90] For instance, changes in upper trapezius muscle activity have been observed in patients with neck pain of both traumatic and non-traumatic origin[66,76,86] during repetitive movements of the upper limb. Likewise, altered masticatory muscle activation has been observed in

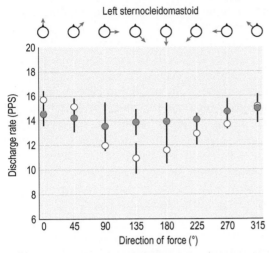
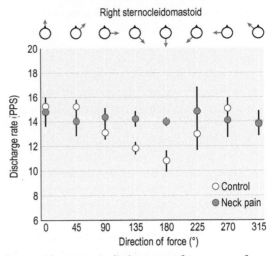

Fig. 5.4 ■ Mean and standard deviation of left and right sternocleidomastoid motor unit discharge rate for a group of control subjects and patients with chronic neck pain during 10-second contractions performed at 15 N of force in eight directions (45-degree intervals from 0–360 degrees) in the horizontal plane. The symbols at the top of the image illustrate the directions of force. The asymptomatic subjects display a modulation in discharge of motor units depending on the direction of force. In contrast, the patient group displayed the same neural drive to the sternocleidomastoid muscle for all force directions. *PPS*, Pulses per second. (From Falla D, Lindstrom R, Rechter L, et al. Effect of pain on the modulation in discharge rate of sternocleidomastoid motor units with force direction. Clin Neurophysiol 2010;121:744–753.)

people with persistent neck pain despite the absence of orofacial pain or temporomandibular disorders.[91,92]

SUBTLE VARIATIONS IN THE DISTRIBUTION OF ACTIVITY WITHIN MUSCLES

High density, two-dimensional surface EMG provides a measure of the electrical potential distribution over a large surface area during muscle contraction and unlike classic bipolar surface EMG applications, provides a topographic representation of EMG amplitude.[93] This method can be used to evaluate the distribution of activity within a muscle and can identify relative adaptations in the intensity of activity within regions of a muscle during both static and dynamic contractions.

One of the most relevant findings revealed by high-density EMG over the last decade is spatial heterogeneity of muscle activity and how it changes during sustained constant-force contractions,[94,95] contractions of increasing load,[95,96] and dynamic contractions.[10,97] These findings likely indicate a nonuniform distribution of motor units or spatial dependency in the control of motor units.[98,99] Importantly, studies in healthy individuals have

shown that this spatial reorganization of muscle activity during contractions has the physiological significance of minimizing muscle fatigue, that is, prolonging endurance, and is potentially relevant to avoid overload of the same muscle fibres during prolonged activation.[94] For example, a progressive shift of activity occurs towards the cranial region of the upper trapezius muscle when healthy individuals perform sustained shoulder abduction[9,94,100,101] resulting in a total shift of the centre of activity within the muscle. This response reflects a greater progressive recruitment of motor units within the cranial region of the upper trapezius muscle[99,102] and likely reflects an optimization of the neural strategy with fatigue. Variability is an important neural strategy because variation effectively shares the load so that one tissue or structure is not repeatedly loaded.

In the presence of either experimentally induced muscle pain[9,10,101,103] or clinical pain,[91,92,97,100] there is less redistribution of activity to different muscle regions during sustained and/or dynamic contractions. Thus when pain is present, muscle contractions are performed by increasing the activation of a region within the muscle over the duration of the task, that is, without the normal variability of muscle activity characteristic for asymptomatic subjects. These findings suggest that nociception interferes with the normal adaptation of activity within a muscle, which may ultimately induce overuse of similar muscle compartments with fatigue. Our recent work also revealed that neck muscle pain induces a shift of the spatial distribution of upper trapezius muscle activity during a repetitive task, which may help to explain the perpetuation of pain with repetitive activity. The study identified that regions of the trapezius muscle, which would not normally be as active, became active in the painful condition and that regions, which would normally be active (based on their anatomical action), became less active. This new motor strategy may be seen as an effective mechanism to "protect" the painful region. However, this "new" pattern of trapezius muscle activation in the painful condition can be seen as an inefficient motor strategy and would likely be relevant for perpetuation of symptoms.

CHANGES IN THE TEMPORAL CHARACTERISTICS OF NECK MUSCLE ACTIVITY

Besides changes in the extent of neck muscle activation, alterations in the timing of neck muscle activity may occur in association with neck pain. Alterations in the temporal aspects of neck muscle activation have been explored by evaluating both the onset of muscle activity, typically via perturbations, and the offset of muscle activity, typically as time to relaxation following voluntary contractions.

Delayed onset of neck muscle activity

The onset of neck muscle activation has been tested during both internal and external perturbations. Internal perturbations, such as a rapid movement of the arm, produce reactive forces, which are of equal magnitude and opposite direction to the forces produced by the arm movement.[104] These forces are transferred to body segments eliciting a series of postural adjustments to maintain equilibrium. One strategy of the nervous system, which is detectable by EMG during internal perturbations, is feed-forward muscle activation. This mechanism helps to maintain or regain stability in the presence of external forces, or when a body part is required to act as a steady base for movement to occur. When asymptomatic people perform rapid arm movements in standing, both the deep and superficial neck muscles are activated in a feed-forward manner.[105,106] In contrast, the onset of neck muscle activity is delayed in people with neck pain.[106] Notably, the delay in onset exceeds the criteria for feed-forward contraction. Moreover, unlike observations in asymptomatic people, the activation of the deep cervical flexors adopts a direction specific response suggesting that the change is not simply a delay that could be explained by factors such as decreased motor neuron excitability, but instead is consistent with the change in the strategy used by the CNS to control the cervical spine.[106]

More recent work has shown that when people with neck pain are exposed to rapid, full-body postural perturbations, they demonstrate delayed activation of the sternocleidomastoid and splenius capitis muscles with respect to asymptomatic people[107] (Fig. 5.5). The reduced ability to activate neck muscles in response to an unexpected event, such as a trip, slip or jolt, may leave the neck vulnerable to further injury.

Delayed offset of muscle activity

Delayed muscle relaxation has been documented after neck[108] and upper limb contractions[109] in people with neck pain. For instance, a significant reduction in the ability to relax the upper trapezius and infraspinatus muscles was observed in people with chronic whiplash-associated disorders as they performed repetitive shoulder flexion.[110] Lower relative rest times have also been observed for people with occupationally-induced neck pain during the performance of standardized short-term computer work.[111] A number of other studies have confirmed that people with neck pain may have difficulty relaxing the upper trapezius both between and following repetitive arm movements.[76,112] It has also shown that this muscle is generally susceptible to increased activity during tasks involving mental demand.[113] Similarly, there is some evidence to suggest that people with neck pain may have difficulty relaxing their anterior scalene and sternocleidomastoid muscles following activation.[76]

In a recent study examining the flexion-relaxation phenomenon and flexion-relaxation ratios of the cervical extensor muscles using surface EMG in computer workers with and without chronic neck pain, a lower flexion-relaxation ratio was observed for the

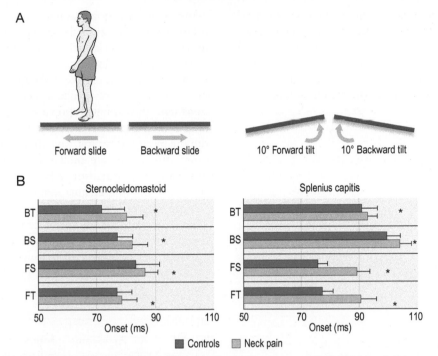

Fig. 5.5 ■ Patients with chronic neck pain and healthy controls stood on a moveable platform and were exposed to randomized full body postural perturbations (8-cm forward slides [*FS*], 8-cm backward slides [*BS*], 10-degrees forward tilts [*FT*], and 10-degrees backward tilts [*BT*]). (B) Mean and standard deviation of the onset of the sternocleidomastoid and splenius capitis muscles in response to the perturbations. Note the significantly (*$P < 0.05$) delayed onset time of the neck muscles for the patients with neck pain regardless of the perturbation direction. (From Boudreau S, Farina D, Kongstad L, et al. The relative timing of trunk muscle activation is retained in response to unanticipated postural-perturbations during acute low back pain. Exp Brain Res 2011;210:259–267.)

semispinalis capitis muscle in the symptomatic group. This change was attributed to pain-induced overactivity of the semispinalis capitis muscle.[114] In another study, the flexion-relaxation phenomenon for the cervical extensors was observed in around 85% of the asymptomatic subjects whereas it was only present in around 36% of the participants with chronic neck pain.[115] Moreover, for the patients who did show the phenomenon, the period between onset and offset was reduced. A lower cervical flexion-relaxation ratio has also been documented in people with subclinical neck pain.[116]

INDIVIDUAL VARIABILITY IN MOTOR ADAPTATIONS TO PAIN

The earlier sections of this chapter have outlined common features of neuromuscular impairment in people with neck pain, yet it must be noted that there is considerable variability between individuals. This is typically evident when considering the large standard deviation of EMG data reported for people with neck pain relative to healthy control groups. Not every person with neck pain will present with such changes in neuromuscular control and certainly not to the same extent. There is some evidence suggesting that the variability existing between individuals with neck pain is partially related to the magnitude of their pain and perceived disability.[76,117,118] For instance, the level of activity of the sternocleidomastoid and anterior scalene muscles during a repeated upper limb task was shown to be greatest for those reporting higher levels of perceived pain and disability as reflected by their Neck Disability Index score.[76] Higher levels of pain intensity were also associated with slower onset of the deep cervical flexors during rapid flexion shoulder and lower activation of these muscles during the craniocervical flexion test.[118] Besides the relation to symptom severity, the variability between individuals likely also relates to the presence and magnitude of attendant stress reactions and may even relate to different functional histories, experiences with pain, or habitual postures/movement patterns.

Supporting the variability observed in clinical studies, there is convincing evidence from experimental pain studies that nociception will trigger individual specific neuromuscular adaptations.[6,119,120] For instance, in a study which examined the effects of experimentally induced neck muscle pain on multi-muscle control of neck movements during an aiming task,[6] each subject in the study adopted an individual control strategy to cope with the painful stimulus. This allowed each subject to perform the task in the painful condition without altering their neck kinematics but rather taking advantage of the redundancy of neck muscle activation and changing their control strategy (Fig. 5.6). Interestingly, on average across the group, the sternocleidomastoid muscle displayed increased activity in the painful condition. Yet inspection of the individual data presented in Fig. 5.6

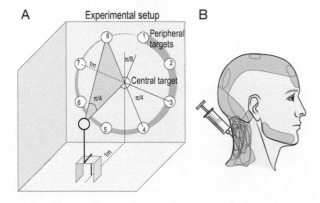

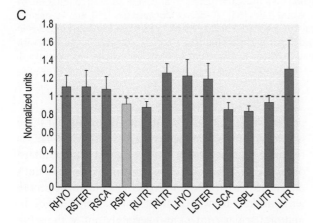

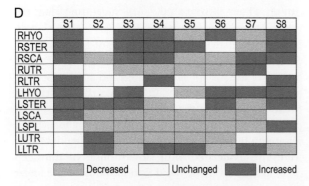

Fig. 5.6 ■ (A) Participants performed multidirectional, multiplanar aiming movements of the head. Nine circular targets (one "central target" plus eight "peripheral targets") were placed on a whitewall following a circular trajectory. Participants wore a helmet mounted with laser pointers and the task consisted of moving their head and neck to aim laser pointers from the central target to each peripheral target following the tempo provided by a metronome. Electromyography (EMG) was recorded from multiple neck muscles. (B) The task was completed at baseline (no pain) and immediately following the injection of hypertonic saline into the right splenius capitis muscle (painful condition). (C) Mean and standard deviation of the EMG amplitude recorded for each muscle in the painful condition normalized relative to the baseline condition. The blue dotted line indicates the level of activity which would be comparable between conditions. The injected muscle, the right splenius capitis, is highlighted in grey; note the overall decreased activity of this muscle. Other muscles showed either an increase or decrease of activity when averaged across all subjects. (D) Individual data for each of the eight subjects showing the direction of change in EMG amplitude of each muscle between the baseline and painful condition. Dark blue indicates an increase of EMG amplitude in the painful condition compared with baseline, grey indicates decreased EMG amplitude and white indicates no change. Note the individual specific patterns of modulation of muscle activity. No two subjects showed the same strategy. *HYO*, Sternohyoid; *L*, left; *LTR*, lower trapezius; *R*, Right; *LTR*, lower trapezius; *SCA*, anterior scalene; *SPL*, splenius capitis; *STER*, sternocleidomastoid; *UTR*, upper trapezius). (From Gizzi L, Muceli S, Petzke F, et al. Experimental muscle pain impairs the synergistic modular control of neck muscles. PLoS One 2015;18:e0137844.)

shows that for some people, their "new" motor strategy involved reduced activation of the sternocleidomastoid. Thus even though at a group level it was a common strategy to increase the activation of the sternocleidomastoid, this was not universal for all subjects. This example supports the contemporary theory of a heterogeneous adaptation of motor control in response to pain despite common changes on average[3,121] and clearly has important implications for management.

CHANGES IN PERIPHERAL PROPERTIES OF NECK MUSCLES

Besides changes in neck muscle behaviour, a number of biochemical, histological and morphological muscle adaptations have been observed in people with chronic neck pain. Biochemical alterations include increased interstitial levels of glutamate detected in the upper division of the trapezius muscle in people with trapezius myalgia[122] and higher interstitial interleukin and serotonin in those with chronic whiplash-associated disorders.[123] Additional observations in people with trapezius myalgia include morphological signs of disturbed mitochondrial function (ragged red and cytochrome-c oxidase negative fibres),[124–126] and increased cross-sectional area of type I muscle fibres despite a lower capillary to fibre area ratio.[127–129]

Further specific changes to muscle fibres include a significant increase in the proportion of type IIC fibres in both the neck flexors and extensors of people with chronic neck pain, suggesting preferential atrophy of slow-twitch oxidative type I fibres.[130] Interestingly, this observation was found to be independent from the type of neck pathology[130] and may partially explain the greater myoelectrical manifestations of fatigue detected for the cervical and axioscapular muscles in people with neck pain during both static and dynamic conditions.[53,131–133]

Elevated fatty infiltration of neck muscles has been observed in people with neck pain following a whiplash trauma.[134–137] This has been most notable in muscles known to possess a larger proportion of type I fibres and a higher density of muscle spindles, that is, the deep sleeve of cervical muscles including the rectus capitis minor and major, longus capitis, longus colli, semispinalis cervicis and multifidus.[134–137] This degeneration of muscle tissue has been noted particularly in people with persistent moderate to severe levels of pain

following the injury[135,137] and in contrast, is not a common finding in people with insidious-onset neck pain.[138] However, a recent study showed larger amounts of fat infiltrates in the rectus capitis posterior major and minor and splenius capitis muscles in elders with cervicogenic headache.[139] Of interest, the total amount of fat within the neck extensor muscles in people with chronic whiplash-associated disorders was shown to be correlated to sensory, physical, kinaesthetic and psychological features, with cold hyperalgesia showing the strongest correlation.[135] Elevated levels of neck muscle fatty infiltration has also been associated with poor functional recovery.[137] The mechanisms underlying the development of fat within the neck muscles following trauma is not fully understood and could be attributed to a number of factors ranging from generalized disuse of the muscles to chronic denervation of the muscle. Considering that these changes are not typically identified in people with idiopathic neck pain, it is likely that the actual trauma plays a role.

Atrophy has been noted for some muscles in people with chronic neck pain disorders and may be present in both deep (e.g., multifidus[139–141]) and superficial muscles (e.g., semispinalis capitis[142]). Some studies have reported the opposite, that is, a larger cross-sectional area of the multifidus muscles was documented in people with whiplash-induced neck pain[143] and a larger cross-sectional area was noted for the semispinalis cervicis and multifidus in fighter pilots with chronic neck pain.[144] In whiplash, the larger cross-sectional area probably represents muscle pseudohypertrophy because of the higher fat content of the muscles.[145] A measure of relative muscle cross-sectional area was introduced to account for the presence of fatty tissue infiltration and one study reported that for 93% of muscles examined, the relative muscle cross-sectional area was the same or even smaller for the patients compared with the control subjects.[145]

TIME COURSE FOR DEVELOPMENT OF NEUROMUSCULAR DYSFUNCTION

Muscle behaviour adapts very rapidly to the presence of nociception. This has been demonstrated experimentally in a number of studies[6–9,13,90,103] and the type of adaptations seen in people with chronic neck pain can be artificially induced through experimental pain models.[7,9,103] As an example, local excitation of nociceptive afferents in the upper trapezius muscle unilaterally, induced a significant decrease in longus colli and longus capitis activation;[7] a common finding in people with chronic neck pain disorders.[69] In addition to this experimental data, clinical observations in patients with acute neck pain also support the presence of early neuromuscular adaptations. For instance, increased activation of the sternocleidomastoid muscle has been observed in people with acute pain following a whiplash trauma when they perform the craniocervical flexion test.[72] As detailed earlier, increased activation of the sternocleidomastoid muscle on this test is a direct reflection of lower activation of the deep cervical flexors.[75] For these reasons, exercise is advocated as an essential component of management from the outset, as is discussed in Chapter 15.

In contrast, it appears that the peripheral adaptations do not occur immediately and may take several months, if not longer, to develop. An example is the presence of fatty tissue infiltration of the extensor muscle group which first becomes apparent three months after the injury in those suffering with moderate to severe pain.[137] Consider also the example presented in Fig. 5.7, which shows a greater relative increase in the proportion of type II fibres with increasing pain duration.[130,146] Although the mechanisms underlying the development of these peripheral changes are not entirely known, they may at least be, in part, considered secondary adaptations of disrupted muscle behaviour. This knowledge provides an even greater incentive to ensure early and effective exercise for people with acute neck pain with the aim of preventing these adaptations.

IMPLICATIONS FOR MANAGEMENT

Exercise is recommended for people with neck pain and is likely the most widely used conservative intervention.[147] Systematic reviews confirm its effectiveness in relieving neck pain [147-151] and also for the prevention of pain.[152] In addition, there is strong evidence that exercise is effective for restoring or enhancing neuromuscular function.[55,153-158] When considering the analgesic effect of exercise, multiple forms of exercise have been proposed to relieve neck pain including general strength and endurance training, exercises for flexibility and range of motion, graded activity, motor control, and aerobic exercise for general fitness. In terms of the effect on pain, then there is little evidence to support one type of exercise over another and the same holds true for low-back pain.[121] For example, higher-load resistance training for the neck flexor muscles provides the same degree of pain relief compared with low-load motor control exercises for the neck flexors.[153] It is suggested that the decision on the type of exercise to use should be dictated by clinician and patient preference.

Nevertheless, although various exercises may be effective for relief of chronic neck pain, some exercises have superior immediate analgesic effects and become particularly relevant and a greater priority for those with acute symptoms. For instance, one study[159] compared the immediate effects of a low-load craniocervical

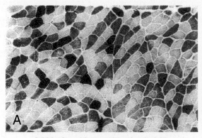 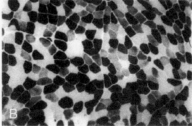

SCM **after 12 months** of pain with
6% of type-IIB fibres (dark)

SCM **after 36 months** of pain with
44% of type-IIB fibres (dark)

Fig. 5.7 ■ Biopsy taken from the sternocleidomastoid (*SCM*) muscle shows a greater relative increase in the proportion of type II fibres with increasing pain duration. (A) SCM after 12 months of pain with 6% of type-IIB fibres (*dark*). (B) SCM after 36 months of pain with 44% of type-IIB fibres (*dark*). (From Uhlig Y, Weber BR, Grob D, et al. Fiber composition and fiber transformations in neck muscles of patients with dysfunction of the cervical spine. J Orthop Res 1995;13:240–249.)

flexion exercise versus a head lift exercise on neck pain intensity at rest and during active cervical motion, and on pressure pain thresholds (PPT) and thermal pain thresholds measured over the cervical spine and at a remote site over the tibialis anterior muscle. Additional measures of sympathetic nervous system function were evaluated including blood flux, skin conductance, skin temperature, heart rate and blood pressure. The study revealed that the craniocervical exercise produced the most significant immediate hypoalgesic effect. This improvement was in the order of 14% to 21% of pre-exercise PPT levels measured over the neck as opposed to only a 3% to 7% change for the head lift exercise. Neither exercise influenced pressure pain sensitivity at the remote site. There was no indication of sympathetic nervous system excitation following exercise which would have been indicative of a systemic effect. There was a significant reduction in pain during active movement post-exercise following the craniocervical flexion exercise only. Other studies have confirmed an immediate reduction in neck pain intensity and increase in PPT over the neck region following craniocervical flexion exercise.[160] In addition, gentle active scapular retraction and depression has been shown to induce an immediate reduction in neck pain intensity and increase in PPT over the neck region.[161] Although these specific neck exercises did not induce immediate systemic pain modulating effects, the immediate localized hypoalgesia that can be gained from these exercises has important implications for exercise prescription.

Variability in symptomatic response to exercise

Although clinical trials confirm that standardized exercise programs are effective on average for people with neck pain, a review of individual responses often reveals that some patients have an excellent outcome with complete relief of their symptoms and others have only minimal or even no benefit.[162] Thus the often applied "one size fits all" exercise for neck pain is usually inadequate. There are a number of reasons for such variability in outcome. One, is the presence of central sensitization which may impede positive exercise outcomes.[163] Psychological factors have also been shown to impede a favourable outcome from neck exercise programs.[164]

A further important consideration is the type and degree of neuromuscular impairments present in the individual before the commencement of training, which can be an important determinant of symptom relief. As reviewed in this chapter, although there are common features of neuromuscular impairment in people with neck pain, there is considerable variability between individuals. Not every person with neck pain will present with the same changes in neuromuscular control and not to the same extent. Thus it is not surprising that standardized exercise programs provide varying results in people with neck pain given that some of the patients in a trial would display minimal impairment in the targeted neuromuscular function. The data presented in Fig. 5.8A and B supports this reasoning. It presents the results of a study[162] in which the physiological effects of a 6-week craniocervical flexion exercise program for people with chronic neck pain were examined. Participants, regardless of their baseline performance in the craniocervical flexion test, performed this exercise over a 6-week period and were instructed to perform their exercise twice daily, with supervized sessions with a physiotherapist once a week. Fig. 5.8A shows the relation between their baseline level of deep cervical flexor muscle activity versus the amount of improvement in deep cervical flexor muscle activity following the exercise intervention. As predicted, those with the least activation of their deep cervical flexor muscles before training were those who had the greatest increase in activation following training. Fig. 5.8B shows the relation between change in pain following the exercise intervention and the amount of improvement in the activation of their deep cervical flexor muscles post-intervention. Once again, a linear relation is observed. That is, the patients who showed the greatest improvement in the activation of their deep cervical flexor muscles were those who gained the greatest pain relief from training. Some patients had no change or only minimal change in pain despite participating in a 6-week exercise program. It is likely that those patients had other more relevant features that were not targeted by the exercise. Thus to optimize exercise prescription and outcome for people with neck pain, exercises must be assessment-driven and targeted to the patient's unique mix of presenting features for more effective management of neck pain.[121]

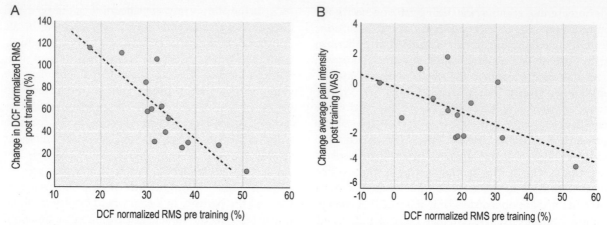

Fig. 5.8 ■ (A) Scatter plot of pre-training normalized deep cervical flexor (*DCF*) electromyography (EMG) amplitude and the percentage change in DCF EMG amplitude values after 6 weeks of craniocervical flexion training in a group of patients with chronic neck pain. (B) Scatter plot of post-training normalized DCF EMG amplitude and change in average neck pain intensity rated on a visual analogue scale (*VAS*) post-training. *RMS*, Root mean square. (From Falla D, O'Leary S, Farina D, et al. The change in deep cervical flexor activity after training is associated with the degree of pain reduction in patients with chronic neck pain. Clin J Pain 2012;28:628–634.)

A recent study further supported the benefit of tailored exercise interventions.[165] The only factor significantly associated with a reduction of both neck pain and neck-related disability at 3 and 12 months following different exercise interventions for chronic whiplash-associated disorders, was participation in a specific neck exercise program, based on a detailed assessment of the patient and tailored to each individual. Patients allocated to this group had up to 5.3 times higher odds of achieving disability reduction, and 3.9 times higher odds of achieving pain reduction compared with those who participated in general physical activity, even if both groups did have a significant benefit from exercise overall.[165] This data further supports the benefit of tailoring and targeting exercises according to detailed assessment of neuromuscular function to account for the variability in people with neck pain disorders.

Neuromuscular adaptations to exercise

Reductions in pain and disability are often the main outcome measures in randomized controlled trials for various types of exercise programs in patients with neck pain and as illustrated previously, various training approaches can relieve neck pain. Nevertheless, when managing people with neck pain, relief of pain is only one consideration. Equally important is the restoration

of function. This is particularly relevant considering that many people develop recurrent pain following their first episode of neck pain.[166] Thus the challenge with treatment is not only to resolve an acute episode of pain, which can be achieved relatively easily via a number of different techniques, but to prevent or limit its recurrence for future quality of life. In that respect, exercise to restore neuromuscular function plays a critical role in the long-term management of the neck pain disorder with aims to prevent or lessen recurrent episodes of pain. Its prescription and application have to be thought about in quite different terms compared with exercise for its analgesic effects.

There is convincing evidence that neuromuscular function of the neck can be enhanced by training. However, although multiple forms of exercise have been shown to relieve neck pain, there is evidence supporting the need for specificity in training when the aim is for rehabilitation of neuromuscular function. For example, low-load exercise to facilitate activation of the deep cervical flexor muscles is effective at increasing the activation of these muscles,[156] restoring the coordination between the deep and superficial flexors,[156,160] enhancing the speed of activation of the deep cervical flexor muscles when challenged by a postural perturbation[156] and improving the patient's ability to maintain an upright posture of the cervical spine during prolonged sitting.[55] These improvements of neuromuscular function were not obtained when people with chronic neck pain participated in a strength and endurance training program for their neck flexor muscles, despite comparable changes in pain and perceived disability.[55,156] In contrast, exercise programs using higher-load endurance and strength protocols for the neck flexors induce superior gains in neck muscle strength, endurance and resistance to fatigue compared with craniocervical exercises.[153,155] This is hardly surprising because the low-load nature of craniocervical flexion exercises would not be expected to substantially change strength and fatigability of the superficial cervical flexors especially when an aim of the exercise is to decrease the relative activity of these muscles during performance of the task. Thus the provision of a load to challenge the neck muscles is required to induce a change in higher-load function. These observations are in line with multiple studies examining neuromuscular adaptations to training which confirm that specific neuronal, muscle and functional changes in motor output in response to exercise are specific to the mode of exercise.[167–170] This knowledge further supports the need for assessment-driven targeted exercises for people with neck pain if neuromuscular function is to be improved.

CONCLUSION

Neuromuscular adaptations are a common and expected reaction to nociception. There is an abundance of literature describing such changes in people with various neck pain disorders and some of the common features are summarized in Fig. 5.9. Although these changes may have some short-term benefit by acting to protect a painful neck, in the longer term such adaptations become maladaptive and can contribute to persistence and recurrence of symptoms. This could occur, for example, if the adaptation to protect the neck results in increased load on cervical structures (e.g., greater coactivation of the neck muscles) or if there is an increased risk of further injury (e.g., delayed neck muscle activation during body perturbations). Potentially, changes in muscle behaviour may lead to altered muscle structure further contributing to ongoing symptoms and affecting functional recovery. Chapter 15 is devoted to the effective management of neuromuscular

Motor output
• Decreased strength
• Decreased endurance
• Decreased force steadiness
• Decreased range of motion
• Decreased speed of movement
• Reduced smoothness of movement

Muscle behaviour
• Increased muscle coactivation
• Reduced specificity of neck muscle activity
• Decreased activation of deep muscle activity
• Delayed muscle responses
• Reduced muscle relaxation
• Increased muscle fatigability

Muscle properties
• Muscle fatty tissue infiltrate
• Atrophy
• Reduced muscle microcirculation
• Muscle fibre transformations
• Biochemical alterations

Fig. 5.9 ■ Overview of common neuromuscular adaptations in people with neck pain disorders.

dysfunction, a critical component of rehabilitation for any neck pain disorder.

REFERENCES

1. Lund JP, Donga R, Widmer CG, et al. The pain-adaptation model: a discussion of the relationship between chronic musculoskeletal pain and motor activity. Can J Physiol Pharmacol 1991;69:683–94.
2. Johansson H, Sojka P. Pathophysiological mechanisms involved in genesis and spread of muscular tension in occupational muscle pain and in chronic musculoskeletal pain syndromes: a hypothesis. Med Hypotheses 1991;35:196–203.
3. Hodges PW, Tucker K. Moving differently in pain: a new theory to explain the adaptation to pain. Pain 2011;152:S90–8.
4. Murray GM, Peck CC. Orofacial pain and jaw muscle activity: a new model. J Orofac Pain 2007;21:263–78.
5. Hodges P, Falla D. Interaction between pain and sensorimotor control. In: Jull G, Moore A, Falla D, et al, editors. Grieve's modern musculoskeletal physiotherapy. UK: Elsevier; 2015.
6. Gizzi L, Muceli S, Petzke F, et al. Experimental muscle pain impairs the synergistic modular control of neck muscles. PLoS ONE 2015;18:e0137844.
7. Cagnie B, Dirks R, Schouten M, et al. Functional reorganization of cervical flexor activity because of induced muscle pain evaluated by muscle functional magnetic resonance imaging. Man Ther 2011;16:470–5.
8. Christensen SW, Hirata RP, Graven-Nielsen T. The effect of experimental neck pain on pressure pain sensitivity and axioscapular motor control. J Pain 2015;16:367–79.

9. Falla D, Arendt-Nielsen L, Farina D. Gender-specific adaptations of upper trapezius muscle activity to acute nociceptive stimulation. Pain 2008;138:217–25.

10. Falla D, Cescon C, Lindstroem R, et al. Muscle pain induces a shift of the spatial distribution of upper trapezius muscle activity during a repetitive task: a mechanism for perpetuation of pain with repetitive activity? Clin J Pain 2017;33:1006–13.

11. Falla D, Farina D, Graven-Nielsen T. Experimental muscle pain results in reorganization of coordination among trapezius muscle subdivisions during repetitive shoulder flexion. Exp Brain Res 2007;178:385–93.

12. Falla D, Farina D, Kanstrup Dahl M, et al. Pain-induced changes in cervical muscle activation do not affect muscle fatigability during sustained isometric contraction. J Electromyogr Kinesiol 2007;18:938–46.

13. Falla D, Farina D, Kanstrup Dahl M, et al. Muscle pain induces task-dependent changes in cervical agonist/antagonist activity. J Appl Physiol 2007;102:601–9.

14. Arendt-Nielsen L, Falla D. Motor control adjustments in musculoskeletal pain and the implications for pain recurrence. Pain 2009;142:171–2.

15. Hodges P, Schabrun S, Falla D. Reorganized motor-control at spinal and cortical level in neck and low back pain. In: Arendt-Nielsen L, Graven-Nielsen T, editors. Musculoskeletal pain - basic mechanisms and implications. Seattle: IASP Press; 2014.

16. Vasavada AN, Li S, Delp SL. Influence of muscle morphometry and moment arms on the moment-generating capacity of human neck muscles. Spine 1998;23:412–22.

17. Boyd Clark LC, Briggs CA, Galea MP. Comparative histochemical composition of muscle fibres in a pre- and a postvertebral muscle of the cervical spine. J Anat 2001;199:709–16.

18. Boyd Clark LC, Briggs CA, Galea MP. Muscle spindle distribution, morphology, and density in longus colli and multifidus muscles of the cervical spine. Spine 2002;27:694–701.

19. Winters JM, Peles JD. Neck muscle activity and 3D head kinematics during quasistatic and dynamic tracking movements. In: Winters JM, Woo SLY, editors. Multiple muscle systems: biomechanics and movement organisation. New York: Springer-Verlag; 1990. p. 461–80.

20. Dieterich AV, Andrade RJ, Le Sant G, et al. Shear wave elastography reveals different degrees of passive and active stiffness of the neck extensor muscles. Eur J Appl Physiol 2017;117: 17–18.

21. Ward SR, Tomiya A, Regev GJ, et al. The architectural design of the lumbar multifidus muscle supports its role as stabilizer. J Biomech 2009;42:1384–9.

22. Petit J, Filippi GM, Emonet-Denand F, et al. Changes in muscle stiffness produced by motor units of different types in peroneus longus muscle of cat. J Neurophysiol 1990;63:190–7.

23. Toursel T, Stevens L, Granzier H, et al. Passive tension of rat skeletal soleus muscle fibers: effects of unloading conditions. J Appl Physiol 2002;92:1465–72.

24. Panjabi MM, Cholewicki J, Nibu K, et al. Critical load of the human cervical spine: an in vitro experimental study. Clin Biomech (Bristol, Avon) 1998;13:11–17.

25. Mayoux-Benhamou MA, Revel M, Vallee C, et al. Longus colli has a postural function on cervical curvature. Surg Radiol Anat 1994;16:367–71.

26. Vitti M, Fujiwara M, Basmajian JV, et al. The integrated roles of longus colli and sternocleidomastoid muscles: an electromyographic study. Anat Rec 1973;177:471–84.

27. Falla D, O'Leary S, Fagan A, et al. Recruitment of the deep cervical flexor muscles during a postural-correction exercise performed in sitting. Man Ther 2007;12:139–43.

28. Takasaki H, Hall T, Kaneko S, et al. Cervical segmental motion induced by shoulder abduction assessed by magnetic resonance imaging. Spine 2009;34:E122–6.

29. Mayoux-Benhamou MA, Revel M, Vallee C. Selective electromyography of dorsal neck muscles in humans. Exp Brain Res 1997;113:353–60.

30. Vasavada AN, Peterson BW, Delp SL. Three-dimensional spatial tuning of neck muscle activation in humans. Exp Brain Res 2002;147:437–48.

31. Bull ML, Vitti M, De Freitas V. Electromyographic study of the trapezius (pars superior) and serratus anterior (pars inferior) muscles in free movements of the shoulder. Electromyogr Clin Neurophysiol 1989;29:119–25.

32. Behrsin JF, Maguire K. Levator scapulae action during shoulder movement. A possible mechanism of shoulder pain of cervical origin. Aust J Physiother 1986;32:101–6.

33. Sommerich CM, Joines SMB, Hermans V, et al. Use of surface electromyography to estimate neck muscle activity. J Electromyogr Kinesiol 2000;10:377–98.

34. Dutia MB. The muscles and joints of the neck: their specialisation and role in head movement. Prog Neurobiol 1991;37:165–78.

35. Abrahams VC, Richmond FJ. Specialization of sensorimotor organization in the neck muscle system. Prog Brain Res 1988;76:125–35.

36. Kamibayashi LK, Richmond FJ. Morphometry of human neck muscles. Spine 1998;23:1314–23.

37. Richmond F, Singh K, Corneil B. Marked non-uniformity of fiber-type composition in the primate suboccipital muscle obliquus capitis inferior. Exp Brain Res 1999;125:14–18.

38. Selbie WS, Thomson DB, Richmond FJ. Suboccipital muscles in the cat neck: morphometry and histochemistry of the rectus capitis muscle complex. J Morphol 1993;216:47–63.

39. Boyd-Clark LC, Briggs CA, Galea MP. Comparative histochemical composition of muscle fibres in a pre- and postvertebral muscle of the cervical spine. J Anat 2001;199:709–16.

40. Antonaci F, Bulgheroni M, Ghirmai S, et al. 3D kinematic analysis and clinical evaluation of neck movements in patients with whiplash injury. Cephalalgia 2002;22:533–42.

41. Dvir Z, Gal-Eshel N, Shamir B, et al. Cervical motion in patients with chronic disorders of the cervical spine: a reproducibility study. Spine 2006;31:E394–9.

42. Sjolander P, Michaelson P, Jaric S, et al. Sensorimotor disturbances in chronic neck pain-Range of motion, peak velocity, smoothness of movement, and repositioning acuity. Man Ther 2008;13:122–31.

43. Woodhouse A, Vasseljen O. Altered motor control patterns in whiplash and chronic neck pain. BMC Musculoskelet Disord 2008;9:90.

44. Grip H, Sundelin G, Gerdle B, et al. Cervical helical axis characteristics and its center of rotation during active head and upper arm movements-comparisons of whiplash-associated disorders, non-specific neck pain and asymptomatic individuals. J Biomech 2008;41:2799–805.

45. Ohberg F, Grip H, Wiklund U, et al. Chronic whiplash associated disorders and neck movement measurements: an instantaneous helical axis approach. IEEE Trans Inf Technol Biomed 2003;7:274–82.

46. Lindstrocm R, Graven-Nielsen T, Falla D. Current pain and fear of pain contribute to reduced maximum voluntary contraction of neck muscles in patients with chronic neck pain. Arch Phys Med Rehabil 2012;93:2042–8.

47. Chiu TT, Sing KL. Evaluation of cervical range of motion and isometric neck muscle strength: reliability and validity. Clin Rehabil 2002;16:851–8.

48. Prushansky T, Gepstein R, Gordon C, et al. Cervical muscles weakness in chronic whiplash patients. Clin Biomech (Bristol, Avon) 2005;20:794–8.

49. Edmondston S, Björnsdóttir G, Pálsson T, et al. Endurance and fatigue characteristics of the neck flexor and extensor muscles during isometric tests in patients with postural neck pain. Man Ther 2011;16:332–8.

50. O'Leary S, Jull G, Kim M, et al. Cranio-cervical flexor muscle impairment at maximal, moderate, and low loads is a feature of neck pain. Man Ther 2007;12:34–9.

51. Dumas JP, Arsenault AB, Boudreau G, et al. Physical impairments in cervicogenic headache: traumatic vs. non-traumatic onset. Cephalalgia 2001;21:884–93.

52. Watson DH, Trott PH. Cervical headache: an investigation of natural head posture and upper cervical flexor muscle performance. Cephalalgia 1993;13:272–84.

53. Halvorsen M, Abbott A, Peolsson A, et al. Endurance and fatigue characteristics in the neck muscles during sub-maximal isometric test in patients with cervical radiculopathy. Eur Spine J 2014;23:590–8.

54. Peolsson A, Kjellman G. Neck muscle endurance in nonspecific patients with neck pain and in patients after anterior cervical decompression and fusion. J Manipulative Physiol Ther 2007;30: 343–50.

55. Falla D, Jull G, Russell T, et al. Effect of neck exercise on sitting posture in patients with chronic neck pain. Phys Ther 2007;87:408–17.

56. Falla D, Lindstrom R, Rechter L, et al. Effect of pain on the modulation in discharge rate of sternocleidomastoid motor units with force direction. Clin Neurophysiol 2010;121:744–53.

57. Muceli S, Farina D, Kirkesola G, et al. Force steadiness in women with neck pain and the effect of short term vibration. J Electromyogr Kinesiol 2011;21:283–90.

58. New insights into motor adaptations in low back pain and neck pain: Implications for sports medicine and rehabilitation. European College of Sports Science; 2017 5-8th July; Essen, Germany.

59. Keshner EA, Campbell D, Katz RT, et al. Neck muscle activation patterns in humans during isometric head stabilization. Exp Brain Res 1989;75:335–44.

60. Keshner EA. Motor control of the cervical spine. In: Boyling JD, Jull G, editors. Grieve's modern manual therapy: the vertebral column. Edinburgh: Elsevier; 2004.

61. Keshner EA, Peterson BW. Motor control strategies underlying head stabilization and voluntary head movements in humans and cats. Prog Brain Res 1988;76:329–39.

62. Blouin JS, Siegmund GP, Carpenter MG, et al. Neural control of superficial and deep neck muscles in humans. J Neurophysiol 2007;98:920–8.

63. Schomacher J, Farina D, Lindstroem R, et al. Chronic trauma-induced neck pain impairs the neural control of the deep semispinalis cervicis muscle. Clin Neurophysiol 2012;123: 1403–8.

64. Lindstrom R, Schomacher J, Farina D, et al. Association between neck muscle co-activation, pain, and strength in women with neck pain. Man Ther 2011;16:80–6.

65. Fernandez-de-las-Penas C, Falla D, Arendt-Nielsen L, et al. Cervical muscle co-activation in isometric contractions is enhanced in chronic tension-type headache patients. Cephalalgia 2008;28:744–51.

66. Johnston V, Jull G, Souvlis T, et al. Alterations in cervical muscle activity in functional and stressful tasks in female office workers with neck pain. Eur J Appl Physiol 2008;103:253–64.

67. Jull G, Amiri M, Bullock-Saxton J, et al. Cervical musculoskeletal impairment in frequent intermittent headache. Part 1: subjects with single headaches. Cephalalgia 2007;27:793–802.

68. Jull G, Barrett C, Magee R, et al. Further clinical clarification of the muscle dysfunction in cervical headache. Cephalalgia 1999;19:179–85.

69. Falla D, Jull G, Hodges PW. Patients with neck pain demonstrate reduced electromyographic activity of the deep cervical flexor muscles during performance of the craniocervical flexion test. Spine 2004;29:2108–14.

70. Jull G, Kristjansson E, Dall'Alba P. Impairment in the cervical flexors: a comparison of whiplash and insidious onset neck pain patients. Man Ther 2004;9:89–94.

71. Jull GA. Deep cervical flexor muscle dysfunction in whiplash. J Musculoskel Pain 2000;8:143–54.

72. Sterling M, Jull G, Vicenzino B, et al. Development of motor dysfunction following whiplash injury. Pain 2003;103:65–73.

73. Johnston V, Jull G, Souvlis T, et al. Neck movement and muscle activity characteristics in female office workers with neck pain. Spine 2008;33:555–63.

74. Steinmetz A, Claus A, Hodges PW, et al. Neck muscle function in violinists/violists with and without neck pain. Clin Rheumatol 2016;35:1045–51.

75. Jull G, Falla D. Does increased superficial neck flexor activity in the craniocervical flexion test reflect reduced deep flexor activity in people with neck pain? Man Ther 2016;25:43–7.

76. Falla D, Bilenkij G, Jull G. Patients with chronic neck pain demonstrate altered patterns of muscle activation during performance of a functional upper limb task. Spine 2004;29: 1436–40.

77. Falla D, Jull G, Edwards S, et al. Neuromuscular efficiency of the sternocleidomastoid and anterior scalene muscles in patients with chronic neck pain. Disabil Rehabil 2004;26:712–17.

78. Yang CC, Su FC, Yang PC, et al. Characteristics of the motor units during sternocleidomastoid isometric flexion among patients with mechanical neck disorder and asymptomatic individuals. PLoS ONE 2016;11:e0167737.

79. Peterson G, Nilsson D, Trygg J, et al. Novel insights into neck muscle coordination in individuals with whiplash-associated disorders. Sci Rep 2015;5:15289.

80. O'Leary S, Cagnie B, Reeve A, et al. Is there altered activity of the extensor muscles in chronic mechanical neck pain? A functional magnetic resonance imaging study. Arch Phys Med Rehabil 2011;92:929–34.

81. Schomacher J, Boudreau S, Petzke F, et al. Localized pressure pain sensitivity is associated with lower activation of the semispinalis cervicis muscle in patients with chronic neck pain. Clin J Pain 2013;10:898–906.

82. Szeto GP, Straker LM, O'Sullivan PB. A comparison of symptomatic and asymptomatic office workers performing monotonous keyboard work 1: neck and shoulder muscle recruitment patterns. Man Ther 2005;10:270–80.

83. Kumar S, Narayan Y, Prasad N, et al. Cervical electromyogram profile differences between patients of neck pain and control. Spine 2007;32:E246–53.

84. Hodges P, Cholewicki J. Functional control of the spine. In: Vleeming A, Mooney V, Stoeckart R, editors. Movement, stability and lumbopelvic pain. Edinburgh: Elsevier; 2007.

85. Christensen SW, Hirata RP, Graven Nielsen T. Altered pain sensitivity and axioscapular muscle activity in neck pain patients compared with healthy controls. Eur J Pain 2017;21:1763–71.

86. Nederhand MJ, Ijzerman MJ, Hermens HJ, et al. Cervical muscle dysfunction in the chronic whiplash associated disorder grade II (WAD-II). Spine 2000;25:1938–43.

87. Zakharova-Luneva E, Jull G, Johnston V, et al. Altered trapezius muscle behavior in individuals with neck pain and clinical signs of scapular dysfunction. J Manipulative Physiol Ther 2012;35:346–53.

88. Helgadottir H, Kristjansson E, Einarsson E, et al. Altered activity of the serratus anterior during unilateral arm elevation in patients with cervical disorders. J Electromyogr Kinesiol 2011;21:947–53.

89. Christensen SW, Hirata RP, Graven-Nielsen T. The effect of experimental neck pain on pressure pain sensitivity and axioscapular motor control. J Pain 2015;16:367–79.

90. Christensen SW, Hirata RP, Graven Nielsen T. Bilateral experimental neck pain reorganize axioscapular muscle coordination and pain sensitivity. Eur J Pain 2017;21:681–91.

91. Testa M, Geri T, Gizzi L, et al. High-density EMG reveals novel evidence of altered masseter muscle activity during symmetrical and asymmetrical bilateral jaw clenching tasks in people with chronic nonspecific neck pain. Clin J Pain 2017;33:148–59.

92. Testa M, Geri T, Gizzi L, et al. Alterations in masticatory muscle activation in people with persistent neck pain despite the absence of orofacial pain or temporomandibular disorders. J Oral Facial Pain Headache 2015;29:340–8.

93. Falla D, Farina D. Advances in Electromyography. In: Jull G, Moore A, Falla D, et al, editors. Grieve's modern musculoskeletal physiotherapy. UK: Elsevier; 2015.

94. Farina D, Leclerc F, Arendt-Nielsen L, et al. The change in spatial distribution of upper trapezius muscle activity is correlated to contraction duration. J Electromyogr Kinesiol 2008;18:16–25.

95. Falla D, Farina D. Periodic increases in force during sustained contraction reduce fatigue and facilitate spatial redistribution of trapezius muscle activity. Exp Brain Res 2007;182:99–107.

96. Tucker K, Falla D, Graven-Nielsen T, et al. Electromyographic mapping of the erector spinae muscle with varying load and during sustained contraction. J Electromyogr Kinesiol 2009;19:373–9.

97. Falla D, Gizzi L, Tschapek M, et al. Reduced task-induced variations in the distribution of activity across back muscle regions in individuals with low back pain. Pain 2014;155:944–53.

98. Falla D, Farina D. Non-uniform adaptation of motor unit discharge rates during sustained static contraction of the upper trapezius muscle. Exp Brain Res 2008;191:363–70.

99. Falla D, Farina D. Motor units in cranial and caudal regions of the upper trapezius muscle have different discharge rates during brief static contractions. Acta Physiol 2008;192:551–8.

100. Falla D, Andersen H, Danneskiold-Samsøe B, et al. Adaptations of upper trapezius muscle activity during sustained contractions in women with fibromyalgia. J Electromyogr Kinesiol 2010;20:457–64.

101. Madeleine P, Leclerc F, Arendt-Nielsen L, et al. Experimental muscle pain changes the spatial distribution of upper trapezius muscle activity during sustained contraction. Clin Neurophysiol 2006;117:2436–45.

102. Falla D, Farina D, Graven Nielsen T. Spatial dependency of trapezius muscle activity during repetitive shoulder flexion. J Electromyogr Kinesiol 2007;17:299–306.

103. Falla D, Arendt-Nielsen L, Farina D. The pain-induced change in relative activation of upper trapezius muscle regions is independent of the site of noxious stimulation. Clin Neurophysiol 2009;120:150–7.

104. Bouisset S, Zattara M. Biomechanical study of the programming of anticipatory postural adjustments associated with voluntary movement. J Biomech 1987;20:735–42.

105. Falla D, Rainoldi A, Merletti R, et al. Spatio-temporal evaluation of neck muscle activation during postural perturbations in healthy subjects. J Electromyogr Kinesiol 2004;14:463–74.

106. Falla D, Jull G, Hodges PW. Feedforward activity of the cervical flexor muscles during voluntary arm movements is delayed in chronic neck pain. Exp Brain Res 2004;157:43–8.

107. Boudreau S, Farina D, Kongstad L, et al. The relative timing of trunk muscle activation is retained in response to unanticipated postural-perturbations during acute low back pain. Exp Brain Res 2011;210:259–67.

108. Barton PM, Hayes KC. Neck flexor muscle strength, efficiency, and relaxation times in normal subjects and subjects with unilateral neck pain and headache. Arch Phys Med Rehabil 1996;77:680–7.

109. Fredin Y, Elert J, Britschgi N, et al. A decreased ability to relax between repetitive muscle contractions in patients with chronic symptoms after whiplash trauma of the neck. J Musculoskelet Pain 1997;5:55–70.

110. Elert J, Kendall SA, Larsson B, et al. Chronic pain and difficulty in relaxing postural muscles in patients with fibromyalgia and chronic whiplash associated disorders. J Rheumatol 2001;28: 1361–8.

111. Thorn S, Søgaard K, Kallenberg L, et al. Trapezius muscle rest time during standardized computer work–a comparison of female computer users with and without self-reported neck/shoulder complaints. J Electromyogr Kinesiol 2007;17:420–7.

112. Januario LB, Oliveira AB, Cid MM, et al. The coordination of shoulder girdle muscles during repetitive arm movements at either slow or fast pace among women with or without neck-shoulder pain. Hum Mov Sci 2017;55:287–95.

113. Laursen B, Jensen BR, Garde AH, et al. Effect of mental and physical demands on muscular activity during the use of a computer mouse and a keyboard. Scand J Work Environ Health 2002;28:215–21.

114. Pinheiro CF, dos Santos MF, Chaves TC. Flexion-relaxation ratio in computer workers with and without chronic neck pain. J Electromyogr Kinesiol 2016;26:8–17.

115. Maroufi N, Ahmadi A, Mousavi Khatir SR. A comparative investigation of flexion relaxation phenomenon in healthy and chronic neck pain subjects. Eur Spine J 2013;22:162–8.

116. Zabihhosseinian M, Holmes MW, Ferguson B, et al. Neck muscle fatigue alters the cervical flexion relaxation ratio in sub-clinical neck pain patients. Clin Biomech (Bristol, Avon) 2015;30:397–404.

117. O'Leary S, Falla D, Jull G. The relationship between superficial muscle activity during the cranio-cervical flexion test and clinical features in patients with chronic neck pain. Man Ther 2011;16:452–5.

118. Falla D, O'Leary S, Farina D, et al. Association between intensity of pain and impairment in onset and activation of the deep cervical flexors in patients with persistent neck pain. Clin J Pain 2011;27:309–14.

119. Muceli S, Falla D, Farina D. Reorganization of muscle synergies during multidirectional reaching in the horizontal plane with experimental muscle pain. J Neurophysiol 2014;111: 615–30.

120. Hodges PW, Coppieters MW, Macdonald D, et al. New insight into motor adaptation to pain revealed by a combination of modelling and empirical approaches. Eur J Pain 2013;17:1138–46.

121. Falla D, Hodges P. Individualized exercise interventions for spinal pain. Exerc Sport Sci Rev 2017;45:105–15.

122. Flodgren GM, Crenshaw AG, Alfredson H, et al. Glutamate and prostaglandin E2 in the trapezius muscle of female subjects with chronic muscle pain and controls determined by micro-dialysis. Eur J Pain 2005;9:511–15.

123. Gerdle B, Lemming D, Kristiansen J, et al. Biochemical alterations in the trapezius muscle of patients with chronic whiplash associated disorders (WAD) - A microdialysis study. Eur J Pain 2008;12:82–93.

124. Kadi F, Waling K, Ahlgren C, et al. Pathological mechanisms implicated in localized female trapezius myalgia. Pain 1998;78:191–6.

125. Lindman R, Hagberg M, Angqvist K, et al. Changes in muscle morphology in chronic trapezius myalgia. Scand J Work Environ Health 1991;17:347–55.

126. Larsson B, Bjork J, Elert J, et al. Fibre type proportion and fibre size in trapezius muscle biopsies from cleaners with and without myalgia and its correlation with ragged red fibres, cytochrome-c-oxidase-negative fibres, biomechanical output, perception of fatigue, and surface electromyography during repetitive forward flexions. Eur J Appl Physiol 2001;84:492–502.

127. Larsson B, Bjork J, Kadi F, et al. Blood supply and oxidative metabolism in muscle biopsies of female cleaners with and without myalgia. Clin J Pain 2004;20:440–6.

128. Larsson SE, Bengtsson A, Bodegard L, et al. Muscle changes in work-related chronic myalgia. Acta Orthop Scand 1998;59:552–6.

129. Larsson SE, Bodegard L, Henridsson KG, et al. Chronic trapezius myalgia: morphology and blood flow studied in 17 patients. Acta Physiol Scand 1990;61:394–8.

130. Uhlig Y, Weber BR, Grob D, et al. Fiber composition and fiber transformations in neck muscles of patients with dysfunction of the cervical spine. J Orthop Res 1995;13:240–9.

131. Falla D, Farina D. Muscle fiber conduction velocity of the upper trapezius muscle during dynamic contraction of the upper limb in patients with chronic neck pain. Pain 2005;116:138–45.

132. Falla D, Jull G, Rainoldi A, et al. Neck flexor muscle fatigue is side specific in patients with unilateral neck pain. Eur J Pain 2004;8:71–7.

133. Falla D, Rainoldi A, Merletti R, et al. Myoelectric manifestations of sternocleidomastoid and anterior scalene muscle fatigue in chronic neck pain patients. Clin Neurophysiol 2003;114:488–95.

134. Elliott J, Jull G, Noteboom JT, et al. Fatty infiltration in the cervical extensor muscles in persistent whiplash-associated disorders: a magnetic resonance imaging analysis. Spine 2006;31:847–55.

135. Elliott J, Noteboom JT, Sterling M, et al. The clinical presentation of chronic whiplash and the relationship to findings of MRI fatty infiltrate in the cervical extensor musculature. Eur Spine J 2009;18:1371–8.

136. Elliott J, O'Leary S, Sterling M, et al. Magnetic resonance imaging findings of fatty infiltrate in the cervical flexors in chronic whiplash. Spine 2009;35:948–54.

137. Elliott J, Pedler A, Kenardy J, et al. The temporal development of fatty infiltrates in the neck muscles following whiplash injury: an association with pain and posttraumatic stress. PLoS ONE 2011;6:e21194.

138. Elliott J, Sterling M, Noteboom JT, et al. Fatty infiltrate in the cervical extensor muscles is not a feature of chronic, insidious-onset neck pain. Clin Radiol 2008;63:681–7.

139. Uthaikhup S, Assapun J, Kothanm S, et al. Structural changes of the cervical muscles in elder women with cervicogenic headache. Musculoskelet Sci Pract 2017;29:1–6.

140. Kristjansson E. Reliability of ultrasonography for the cervical multifidus muscle in asymptomatic and symptomatic subjects. Man Ther 2004;9:83–8.

141. Fernández-de-las-Peñas C, Albert-Sanchís JC, Buil M, et al. Cross-sectional area of cervical multifidus muscle in females with chronic bilateral neck pain compared to controls. J Orthop Sports Phys Ther 2008;38:175–80.

142. Rezasoltani A, Ahmadipoor A, Khademi-Kalantari K, et al. The sign of unilateral neck semispinalis capitis muscle atrophy in

patients with chronic non-specific neck pain. J Back Musculoskelet Rehabil 2012;25:67–72.

143. Elliott J, Jull G, Noteboom T, et al. MRI study of the cross sectional area for the cervical extensor musculature in patients with persistent whiplash associated disorders (WAD). Man Ther 2008;13:258–65.

144. De Loose V, van den Oord M, Keser I, et al. MRI study of the morphometry of the cervical musculature in F-16 pilots. Aviat Space Environ Med 2009;80:727–31.

145. Elliott JM, Pedler AR, Jull GA, et al. Differential changes in muscle composition exist in traumatic and non-traumatic neck pain. Spine 2014;39:39–47.

146. Weber BR, Uhlig Y, Grob D, et al. Duration of pain and muscular adaptations in patients with dysfunction of the cervical spine. J Orthop Res 1993;11:805–11.

147. Gross AR, Paquin JP, Dupont G, et al. Exercises for mechanical neck disorders: a Cochrane review update. Man Ther 2016;24:25–45.

148. Fredin K, Lorås H. Manual therapy, exercise therapy or combined treatment in the management of adult neck pain - A systematic review and meta-analysis. Musculoskelet Sci Pract 2017;31:62–71.

149. Kay TM, Gross A, Goldsmith CH, et al. Exercises for mechanical neck disorders. Cochrane Database Syst Rev 2012;(15):CD004250.

150. Yamato TP, Saragiotto BT, Maher C. Therapeutic exercise for chronic non-specific neck pain: PEDro systematic review update. Br J Sports Med 2015;49:1350.

151. Bertozzi L, Gardenghi I, Turoni F, et al. Effect of therapeutic exercise on pain and disability in the management of chronic nonspecific neck pain: systematic review and meta-analysis of randomized trials. Phys Ther 2013;93:1026–36.

152. Linton SJ, van Tulder MW. Preventive interventions for back and neck pain problems: what is the evidence? Spine 2001;358:778–87.

153. Falla D, Jull G, Hodges P, et al. An endurance-strength training regime is effective in reducing myoelectric manifestations of cervical flexor muscle fatigue in females with chronic neck pain. Clin Neurophysiol 2006;117:828–37.

154. Falla D, Lindstrøm R, Rechter L, et al. Effectiveness of an 8-week exercise programme on pain and specificity of neck muscle activity in patients with chronic neck pain: a randomized controlled study. Eur J Pain 2013;17:1517–28.

155. O'Leary S, Jull G, Kim M, et al. Training mode-dependent changes in motor performance in neck pain. Arch Phys Med Rehabil 2012;93:1225–33.

156. Jull G, Falla D, Vicenzino B, et al. The effect of therapeutic exercise on activation of the deep cervical flexor muscles in people with chronic neck pain. Man Ther 2009;14:696–701.

157. Halvorsen M, Falla D, Gizzi L, et al. Short- and long-term effects of exercise on neck muscle function in cervical radiculopathy: a randomized clinical trial. J Rehabil Med 2016;48:696–704.

158. Andersen LL, Andersen CH, Skotte JH, et al. High-intensity strength training improves function of chronically painful muscles: case-control and RCT studies. Biomed Res Int 2014;187324.

159. O'Leary S, Falla D, Hodges P, et al. Specific therapeutic exercise of the neck induces immediate local hypoalgesia. J Pain 2007;8:832–9.

160. Lluch E, Schomacher J, Gizzi L, et al. Immediate effects of active cranio-cervical flexion exercise versus passive mobilisation of the upper cervical spine on pain and performance on the cranio-cervical flexion test. Man Ther 2014;19:25–31.

161. Lluch E, Arguisuelas MD, Calvente Quesada O, et al. Immediate effects of active versus passive scapular correction on pain and pressure pain threshold in patients with chronic neck pain. J Manipulative Physiol Ther 2014;37:660–6.

162. Falla D, O'Leary S, Farina D, et al. The change in deep cervical flexor activity after training is associated with the degree of pain reduction in patients with chronic neck pain. Clin J Pain 2012;28:628–34.

163. Jull G, Sterling M, Kenardy J, et al. Does the presence of sensory hypersensitivity influence outcomes of physical rehabilitation for chronic whiplash? - A preliminary RCT. Pain 2007;129:28–34.

164. Chiarotto A, Fortunato S, Falla D. Predictors of outcome following a short multimodal rehabilitation program for patients with whiplash associated disorders. Eur J Phys Rehabil Med 2015;51:133–41.

165. Ludvigsson ML, Petersen G, Dedering A, et al. Factors associated with pain and disability reduction following exercise interventions in chronic whiplash. Eur J Pain 2016;20:307–15.

166. Carroll LJ, Holm LW, Hogg-Johnson S, et al. Course and prognostic factors for neck pain in whiplash-associated disorders (WAD): results of the Bone and Joint Decade 2000-2010 Task Force on Neck Pain and Its Associated Disorders. Spine 2008;33:S83–92.

167. Adkins D, Boychuk J, Remple M, et al. Motor training induces experience-specific patterns of plasticity across motor cortex and spinal cord. J Appl Physiol 2006;101:1776–82.

168. Coffey V, Hawley J. The molecular bases of training adaptation. Sports Med 2007;37:737–63.

169. Fluck M. Functional, structural and molecular plasticity of mammalian skeletal muscle in response to exercise stimuli. J Exp Biol 2006;209:2239–48.

170. Gabriel D, Kamen G, Frost G. Neural adaptations to resistive exercise: mechanisms and recommendations for training practices. Sports Med 2006;36:133–49.

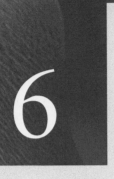

6

SENSORIMOTOR CONTROL DISTURBANCES IN NECK PAIN DISORDERS

Cervical afferent input is vital for the control of head and eye movement and postural stability. This chapter reviews the morphology, the central and reflex connections of cervical mechanoreceptors and the signs and symptoms caused when they are disturbed artificially. How disturbed cervical afferent input influences sensorimotor control is discussed, as well as the possible mechanisms and aetiology of disturbed cervical afferent input in people with neck pain disorders. Altered cervical afferent input may not only impair sensorimotor control but may also result in symptoms such as dizziness and visual disturbances. Understanding how and why sensorimotor control may be affected in people with neck pain, as well as being able to quantify sensorimotor impairments, provides direction for precise assessment and interventions for persons with neck pain disorders (see Chapters 9 and 16).

CERVICAL MECHANORECEPTORS

Morphology

Receptors in the cervical ligaments, joints and muscles convey afferent information that contributes to sensorimotor control. Muscle spindles are probably the most significant receptors. They are found in high densities, especially in the upper cervical region.[1,2] Joint and ligament receptors, via their influence on muscle spindles and the gamma motor neurons, initiate protective muscle activation to prevent joint degeneration and instability.[3,4]

The density of muscle spindles is highest in the suboccipital muscles. The average number of muscle spindles per gram of muscle is 242 in the obliquus capitis inferior, 190 in obliquus capitis superior, 98 in the rectus capitis posterior minor, 49 in the longus colli and 24 in the multifidus.[1,2] For comparison, the first lumbrical in the hand has 16 and the superficial region of the trapezius muscle contains 2 muscle spindles per gram of muscle.[1,2] Cervical muscle spindles, especially in the suboccipital muscles, are uniquely arranged and have high numbers of slow-twitch muscle fibres[5–7] to facilitate their role in movement precision, proprioception, control of head position and eye-head coordination.[5,8,9]

Central connections

Cervical afferents provide input to several areas of the spinal cord and central nervous system (CNS) to integrate and formulate appropriate efferent neuromuscular responses.[10] Areas include the central cervical nucleus, thalamus, cerebellum and somatosensory cortex. Cervical afferents also have unique connections to both the visual and vestibular systems via projections to the medial and lateral vestibular nuclei, as well as the superior colliculus, which is a reflex centre for coordination between eye and neck movement (Fig. 6.1).[11,12] The deep suboccipital muscles, in tandem with their important proprioceptive role, are vital for relaying and receiving this information to and from these CNS connections. Much of the descending information for head and eye movement control projects specifically to these muscles.[5,13]

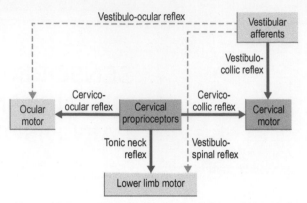

Fig. 6.2 ■ Sensorimotor control reflex activity relating to the cervical spine. *Bold lines* indicate reflex activity specific to the cervical spine. *Dashed lines* indicate reflex activity relating to the visual or vestibular system.

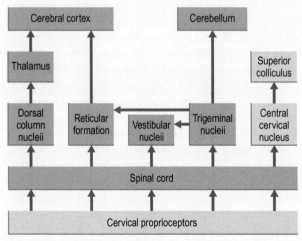

Fig. 6.1 ■ Central connections from the cervical afferents.

Reflex-mediated activity

Synaptic connections from the cervical receptors to other areas of the CNS also play an important role in neck reflex activity. Neck afferents are involved in reflexes, which influence head orientation, eye movement control and postural stability. These reflexes work in conjunction with other cervical, vestibular and visual reflexes acting on the neck or eye musculature, to coordinate postural stability and head and eye movement (Fig. 6.2).

The cervico-collic reflex (CCR) activates the neck muscles when they are stretched by head movement in relation to the body. The CCR is integrated with the vestibulo-collic reflex (VCR) to activate neck muscles to maintain head position and to limit unintentional head rotation displacements.[14,15] The CCR has high sensitivity to smaller, rather than larger neck rotations, which suggests that muscle spindles, rather than joint receptors, provide most input to the CCR.[16] The VCR is evoked by vestibular stimuli acting on the neck muscles, and is similar to the CCR, but responds to faster neck movements.[14,15]

The cervico-ocular reflex (COR) is evoked by stretch of the neck muscles. It acts together with the vestibulo-ocular (VOR) and optokinetic reflexes (OKR) to control the extraocular muscles. The COR serves to assist in maintaining eye position such that head movement results in equal but opposite movement of the eyes, creating clear vision with low-frequency movement.[17] Its importance in humans has been debated, but it can compensate when the VOR, which controls eye movement at higher head speeds, is impaired or diminished.[17–21] The OKR activates eye muscles in response to movement of the visual field over the retina.

Ocular influences on cervical muscles in humans are mediated by the frontal eye fields and the superior colliculus. They activate neck muscles in response to eye movements while the head is still. A close relationship has been observed between activity in the deep cervical extensor muscles and horizontal eye movement.[22,23]

Functional coupling between the eye-neck and scapular muscles is also thought to occur.[24,25]

The tonic neck reflex (TNR) is responsible for alteration in limb muscle activity when the body moves with respect to the head. The TNR integrates with the vestibulospinal reflex to achieve postural stability.[26]

Artificial disturbance to cervical somatosensory input

Experimental studies on healthy subjects have clearly demonstrated the nature of signs and symptoms that can be attributed to altered cervical afferent input. The association between disturbances of cervical afferent input and altered sensorimotor control has been demonstrated in several ways. For instance, injection of anaesthetic or sectioning of nerves in the upper cervical region has caused disequilibrium, ataxia and nystagmus.[27] Less invasive techniques, such as vibrating the neck muscles, which stimulates the muscle spindles, or restricting neck motion can induce eye position changes, illusory visual and head movements as well as altered velocity and direction of gait.[8,28–33] Furthermore, sustained isometric contraction causing neck muscle fatigue, affects postural sway, gait and head position awareness in healthy persons.[34–39] These findings demonstrate the significance of the cervical sensory system's contribution to head and eye movement control and postural stability.

MECHANISMS UNDERLYING DISTURBANCES IN SENSORIMOTOR CONTROL

The likely mechanism for disturbances in sensorimotor control in individuals with neck pain is conflict between converging inputs from the different sensory systems when cervical afferent activity is altered.[40] A changed or disturbed sensitivity of the muscle spindles may result in dizziness, altered head position or movement sense, eye-head coordination or postural stability. There is also some evidence that the neck may directly influence vestibular function[41,42] and may cause asymmetry of the VOR.[43,44] Any disturbance, either a decrease or increase of cervical somatosensory input, may result in altered sensorimotor control.[45,46]

Possible causes of altered cervical afferent input

Many mechanisms may disturb cervical afferent input in people with neck pain disorders, particularly after neck injury (Table 6.1). Afferent information from cervical receptors (mechanoreceptors and nociceptors) can be altered either by direct trauma or as a consequence of impaired or adapted muscle function,[47] for example, neck extensor and scapular muscle fatigue deleteriously affect standing balance.[34–37,39] Inflammatory mediators may activate chemosensitive nerve endings in joints and muscles leading to altered muscle spindle activity. For instance, several studies in cats show experimentally induced, long-lasting, increased muscle spindle activity following excitation of chemosensitive afferents in and around the cervical joint complex.[48–51]

Morphological changes may occur in neck muscles, particularly in the suboccipital muscles[8,52,53] which could affect their proprioceptive capability. Relationships between poor standing balance and fatty infiltrate in the rectus capitis posterior major muscle have been demonstrated in people with chronic neck pain.[53] Further, pain may affect sensorimotor control by modulating proprioceptive input at many levels; in the periphery (local information from mechanoreceptors), in the spinal cord and during supraspinal control and evaluation of cervical somatosensory information.[3,54]

TABLE 6.1			
Possible Mechanisms of Disturbed Cervical Afferent Input in Neck Pain Disorders			
Direct damage	**Functional impairment**	**Morphological change**	**Pain**
Mechanical disruption[179,180]	Altered protective muscle responses[55]	Changes from slow to fast twitch fibers[181]	Muscle inhibition
Excessive joint loading[182,183]	Inhibition of deep musculature[184]	Fatty infiltration into muscle[8,52]	Increased nociceptor input[185,186]
Muscle damage[187]	Altered feed-forward neuromuscular control[188]	Muscle atrophy (reduced cross-sectional area)	Somatosensory reorganization[59–61]
Local ischaemia[189]	Increase in superficial muscle activity[190,191]		Decreased non-nociceptive input[186,192]
Joint inflammation[193,194]	Altered neuromuscular efficiency[195]		Decreased primary motor cortex representation[54]
	Muscle fatigue[196]		Central inhibition
	Sympathetic nervous system activation[62,63]		Central sensitization[185]

FOCUS POINT

Altered head and eye movement control and postural stability are evident in neck disorders and should be considered in the examination of a patient with neck pain.

Experimentally induced neck pain can change cervical muscle activity[54–56] (including reflex activity[57,58]) and muscle spindle sensitivity. Pain may have a role in subcortical and cortical reorganization at many levels of the human somatosensory system.[59–61] There is also some evidence linking psychological stress and activation of the sympathetic nervous system, which may affect muscle spindle activity.[62] Experimental activation of the cervical sympathetic nerve has been shown to depress cervical muscle spindle afferents in animals.[63]

It is most probable that a combination of causes leads to an immediate, sustained alteration in cervical afferent input, which in turn influences sensorimotor control in individuals with neck pain disorders. The specific mechanisms for change are likely to be different between individuals.

SYMPTOMS OF ALTERED CERVICAL SENSORIMOTOR CONTROL

Dizziness or, more specifically, light headedness and unsteadiness are common symptoms associated with neck pain and disability, especially in people with chronic whiplash-associated disorders (WAD) where the incidence is up to 75%.[64–67] Visual complaints may also occur. We explored a number of possible visual symptoms and found that light sensitivity, needing to concentrate to read and visual fatigue were the most prevalent (> 50%) and troublesome in patients with both idiopathic and traumatic onset neck pain.[68] Tinnitus may likewise be a consequence of disturbed cervical afferent input in some patients.[69–71]

SIGNS OF ALTERED CERVICAL SENSORIMOTOR CONTROL

Altered sensorimotor control can encompass head and eye movement control, postural stability and coordination. Tests of head movement control primarily assess cervical proprioception either directly or indirectly, whereas tests of postural stability, eye movement control and coordination assess how a potential disturbance of cervical afferent information may have indirectly influenced each of these areas. Changes in sensorimotor control seem to occur to a greater extent in persons with neck pain of traumatic origin and in those complaining of dizziness. The presence of symptoms probably reflects a greater disturbance to cervical afferent input. Nevertheless, signs of altered sensorimotor control can be present in persons with neck pain of insidious onset and in some patients who do not specifically complain of dizziness and unsteadiness.

Cervical proprioception

Cervical proprioception is assessed traditionally by conscious tests, namely tests of cervical position, movement and force sense.[72] To date, most research on neck pain has evaluated position and movement sense. A systematic review of these measurements and their clinometric properties[73] found that test-retest reliability for joint position sense (JPS) was fair to excellent (Intraclass Correlation Co-efficients [ICC]: 0.35–0.87) and movement sense, using the fly test,[74] was moderate to excellent (ICC: 0.60–0.86). Both tests demonstrated discriminant validity.

Cervical joint position sense

The measure of JPS tests a patient's ability to relocate their head back to a natural head posture or to a predetermined target while vision is occluded.[19,73,75,76] There is now consistent evidence that JPS can be impaired in persons with neck pain regardless of the aetiology.[77,78] Evidence suggests that patients with greater pain, a traumatic onset of neck pain and symptoms of dizziness have poorer JPS.[67,79–82]

JPS testing is used as a measure of cervical proprioception, but deficits in JPS can be observed in association with vestibular pathology, although not always a consistent finding.[83,84] We recently investigated a test of trunk relocation with the head held still to stimulate cervical proprioceptors but limit vestibular involvement. Results suggested that this test was more specific to neck proprioception.[85] It has recently been used to identify cervical proprioceptive deficits associated with concussion risk.[86] These promising outcomes encourage more research to find tests which differentiate cervical from vestibular origins of symptoms.

Interestingly, JPS deficits may not be isolated to the neck. Proprioceptive deficits have also been measured at the shoulder, elbow and hand in persons with neck pain.[87–89] Such deficits are reasoned to reflect altered cervical afferent input affecting the coordination and movement of the upper limb.

Cervical movement sense or accuracy

Another measure of proprioception which tests fine control of neck movement is a test of movement sense, that is, the accuracy to follow either a stationary or moving target. Kristjansson and colleagues[74,90] found that persons with WAD had less accuracy in tracing a computer-generated moving pattern (the fly) when compared with both control and idiopathic neck pain groups. Woodhouse et al.[91] used a stationary movement pattern and again found that individuals with WAD demonstrated decreased accuracy to follow the pattern compared with idiopathic neck pain and control subjects. Sarig Bahat and colleagues[92] used a virtual environment to test accuracy to follow a moving target. The test depicted persons with neck pain but did not discriminate between traumatic onset and idiopathic neck pain.

Cervical force sense

Little research has been conducted to evaluate whether cervical force sense, a third dimension of proprioception, is affected in people with neck pain. Reduced force steadiness has been demonstrated during cervical muscle contractions especially at low load.[93,94] In addition, an inability to hold different pressure (force) levels steady in the craniocervical flexion test is evident in persons with neck pain.[95]

Kinematic disturbances

Other measures that could be related to altered cervical proprioception include disturbances in movement quality,[96–98] for example, changes in movement velocity profile.[96,99,100] Velocity profile includes the mean and peak velocity of movement as well as its smoothness and symmetry. Persons with neck pain consistently display deficits in most elements of the velocity profile. Symmetry of motion, measured as the time to peak velocity or the acceleration/deceleration ratio, may[99] or may not[101,102] be disturbed.

Vertical perception

The ability to correctly identify the true vertical, using the rod and frame test, is deemed to be another test of cervical proprioception.[103] Greater deficits have been found in association with WAD[103] whereas our study found altered vertical perception in participants with idiopathic neck pain but not WAD.[104] The measure has complexities, and in its current form, it may not be a suitable measure of cervical proprioception.[104]

Sensorimotor incongruence

Sensorimotor incongruence may occur as a result of impaired cervical proprioception and is more of an indirect measure exploring the cortical spatial representation of the body and motor planning.[105] Tests of sensorimotor incongruence are considered to assess the central tuning or regulation of proprioceptive information. It is tested by either perception of distorted visual feedback or judgement in laterality tasks. Participants with acute or chronic neck pain have demonstrated sensorimotor incongruence by either experiencing increased symptoms during a distorted arm coordination task or by having an impaired ability to identify incongruence between true head motion and a false visual reference.[106–108] In concert with vertical perception tasks, laterality judgement tasks were found to be impaired in idiopathic neck pain[105] but not WAD.[109] Indeed Richter et al.,[110] found that those with WAD had better laterality judgement reaction times and similar accuracy to controls, which they believe were strategies to compensate for altered proprioception.

Postural stability

Disturbed postural stability includes tests of various static standing tasks under several different conditions such as type of stance, visual and stability conditions. Dynamic measures such as influences on gait and functional balance tasks can also reveal impaired function.

Static measures

Disturbed postural control, commonly measured as increased sway in quiet stance, is not uncommon in patients with neck pain, and is common in the elderly with neck pain,[111–122] in patients with WAD and patients who have dizziness with their neck pain.[112,122] Deficits are demonstrated consistently in most standing tasks, namely comfortable, narrow and tandem stances, especially when vision is occluded. Sway is usually increased in the anterior posterior direction, which is indicative of somatosensory impairment.[123] Nevertheless in more difficult tests, some patients display less sway (a stiffening strategy).[124] These static balance disturbances in all likelihood reflect cervical afferent dysfunction rather than a disturbance of vestibular function because sway patterns are usually different in unilateral vestibular pathology (increased sway in the medial lateral direction).[125] Persons with neck pain also fail to maintain stability for 30 seconds in the more challenging tandem stance position more frequently than healthy individuals.[112,115,121,122] Changes in cervical muscle activity and

in muscle composition may make important contributions to altered postural stability. Relationships have been demonstrated between poorer postural stability and increased superficial muscle activity,[126] cervical muscle fatigue[127] and fatty infiltration of the suboccipital muscles.[53]

Although age is a factor that affects balance, we have determined that elderly subjects with neck pain have greater balance disturbances compared with elders without neck pain.[117,128] These deficits do not appear to be associated with age-related changes in vision or vestibular function. Rather they appear to be caused by the neck pain disorder.[129] Older patients have more profound deficits in balance than younger patients with neck pain. The impacts on balance of normal age-related changes in vision and in the vestibular system in addition to the impact of neck pain should be considered in assessment and management.

Recent studies have investigated the potential for adding a cervical spine bias to a balance test to help identify balance disturbances caused by altered cervical proprioception rather than for example, a vestibular cause. The bias was adding neck torsion to the balance test, that is, rotating the trunk on a stationary head to rotate the neck. Neck torsion has also been added to tests of cervical JPS[85] and smooth pursuit eye movement.[130] Adding neck torsion to the balance test revealed a greater balance deficit than when the neck was in neutral but only in persons with WAD, not in healthy controls[131] and not in persons with vestibular pathology.[132] This suggests that adding torsion to a balance test may make the test more specific to cervical-related balance deficits.

There is also interest in transforming postural sway signal into various frequency bands in an attempt to isolate proprioceptive disturbances. Different frequency bands are thought to represent different types of sensorimotor regulation with higher frequencies representing proprioceptive control.[118,119] Results of research to date suggest that persons with WAD and older adults with neck pain tend to use altered strategies to maintain balance or use low frequencies bands.[118,119] Research is in its infancy at this time, but these trends suggest that transforming postural sway signals into various frequency bands may be useful to identify the contribution of cervical afferent dysfunction to balance impairment in the future.

Dynamic and functional tasks

Postural control has also been investigated using functional tasks. Persons with WAD have demonstrated significant differences in the timed 10-m walk with head turns, the step test and tandem walk as well as delayed responses to perturbations while sitting and stepping on the spot.[133–135] Most research in the area has involved working age populations with WAD, yet similar findings for gait speed are observed in elders with neck pain.[128,136,137] This has important implications for falls assessment and prevention in the older population, especially because neck pain has been identified as a risk factor of concern for falling in elders.[138,139]

Eye movement control

Disturbances in eye movement control have been demonstrated across several types of eye movements particularly in persons with traumatic neck pain and in those reporting dizziness and/or visual disturbances. Control of vision can be divided into voluntary or involuntary eye movements to stabilize, fix or shift the gaze to track or maintain focus on visual stimuli. Gaze shift occurs when using either smooth pursuit (i.e., eye follow) to track a slow-moving target, or by using saccadic (rapid) eye movements to rapidly change a point of fixation. Vestibular ocular reflex, COR and OKR involuntarily move the eyes in the opposite direction to head movement so that images remain stable during head movements. Vergence eye movements differ. Here, each eye moves in the opposite direction, to maintain the image on each retina when targets are at different distances. Vergence eye movements (e.g., convergence and divergence) are used when focusing on objects at a distance or when objects are moving towards or away from the visual field. Vergence movements work with accommodation reflexes to change lens shape and pupil size to allow focusing between near and far targets. Deficits in eye movement control can lead to obvious symptoms as blurred vision, but such deficits can cause other symptoms including visual fatigue, sensitivity to light or headache as a result of increased load on the visual system as the individual struggles to maintain focus. It is possible that this may lead to a vicious circle where altered visual conditions lead to secondary cervical muscle overload and subsequent neck pain exacerbation.[140,141]

To date, deficits in oculomotor control such as decreased smooth pursuit velocity gain, altered velocity and latency of saccadic eye movements, altered convergence and an increased gain in the COR have been demonstrated in people with both insidious onset neck pain and WAD. Nevertheless, the majority of research has been conducted on people with WAD.[130,142–151] Convergence and accommodation insufficiency and eye alignment malfunctions occur in some individuals with either WAD,[148,152] or with idiopathic neck pain.[153] In addition, abnormal cervical muscle activity during eye movements with the head still was observed in persons with WAD when compared with control subjects,[154] as was a reduction in range of head movement during gaze fixation.[155,156]

An increased gain in the COR has been shown in individuals with WAD over a wide range of neck movement velocities but especially during slower movements.[145,146] This increased gain has also been observed in persons with idiopathic neck pain,[157] which supports the theory that cervical afferent disturbance is the cause of the deficits. Interestingly, when increased gain of the COR is observed in the elderly and in people with vestibular pathology, it is regarded as a compensation for a decrease in the VOR gain.[158] However, this compensatory response has not been observed in WAD and may be an important cause of disturbances to the visual system.[158]

Eye movement dysfunction may have prognostic value in WAD.[144,159] Hildingsson and colleagues [159] found that persons with eye movement dysfunction on smooth pursuit and/or saccadic eye movement on initial assessment soon after the car crash continued to have persistent disabling neck pain and disability at least 8 months postinjury. In contrast, individuals with normal eye movement on initial assessment recovered fully or had only minor discomfort at follow-up. It is possible that cognitive disturbance, another common complaint after whiplash, may manifest from disturbances in sensorimotor control as a result of abnormal cervical somatosensory input. Gimse et al.[160] found a close correlation between technical reading ability, information uptake and performance in the smooth pursuit neck torsion test. Similarly driving skills were associated with altered eye movement control in the absence of many other possible causes such as premorbid state and brain injury.[161]

Smooth pursuit neck torsion

Because there are several potential causes of oculomotor disturbances, Tjell and colleagues[149] developed the smooth pursuit neck torsion test (SPNT) to specifically differentiate eye movement disturbances related to altered cervical afferent input. The use of torsion in this test was the basis for investigating the use of torsion in the JPS and balance tests. A semiautomated analysis is used to measure the difference in smooth pursuit eye movement control with the head and trunk in a neutral position compared with when the trunk and neck are rotated relative to the stationary head.[150] A decrease in smooth pursuit velocity gain when the head is torsioned compared with the neutral position is only seen in individuals with neck pain, not in those with vestibular or CNS disorders or healthy controls.[125,149,150] SPNT deficits have been found in insidious onset neck pain particularly of upper cervical origin,[162] cervical vertigo and spondylosis but deficits are most evident in persons with WAD and in those complaining of dizziness.[130,149,150]

There is some debate about the SPNT because researchers using a fully automated analysis[163–165] have not found deficits to the same extent. This may reflect the importance of trained observers to extract the appropriate elements of the signal for analysis, by differentiating appropriate signals from blinks, square waves and other artefacts, rather than rely on a fully automated analysis. Alternatives have been explored. L'Heureux-Lebeau and colleagues[83] compared results with the SPNT and a test called the cervical torsion test where they monitored nystagmus following sustained neck torsion positions to left, neutral and the right. They found that both SPNT and nystagmus of greater than 2 degrees in any neck position was present in persons with neck pain and cervicogenic dizziness but not in those with a peripheral vestibular disorder. The authors suggested that the cervical torsion test might be an alternative method to the SPNT to demonstrate cervical afferent influence on eye movement control. To date, only individuals with cervicogenic dizziness have been studied and more research is required, particularly to differentiate vertebral artery insufficiency from cervical afferent dysfunction in this test.

Most tests of eye movement require quantification using sophisticated equipment. Recently, physiotherapists' ratings of visually assessed head and eye movement

control tests (gaze stability and eye-head coordination) were evaluated. Impairments were detected in persons with neck pain and importantly they were reliably detected in the clinical examination.[166] We recently expanded on this study and demonstrated the suitability of assessing the SPNT by clinical observational assessment compared with sophisticated measurement of eye movement (electro-oculography). Good agreement was present between electro-oculography and visual observation of blinded video analysis of the corrective saccadic eye movements.[167] Adding symptom reproduction is likely to enhance this clinical test, in a similar way to augmenting visual observation of eye movement in concussion.[168,169]

Coordination

Eye-head coordination

Altered eye-head coordination has been demonstrated in a variety of tasks in patients with neck pain. Patients with idiopathic neck pain have displayed an altered velocity profile in an eye-head coordination task involving moving their head to look at targets as fast and accurately as possible.[170] Patients with WAD displayed decreased head velocity during tasks of eye-head coordination and had compensatory head movements when requested to only rotate their eyes to the left or right.[156] Patients with both idiopathic neck pain and WAD displayed reduced precision in an eye-head-hand coordination task involving fast pointing movements to a visual target.[171]

Trunk-head coordination

Patients with neck pain can have impaired trunk-head coordination, that is, moving the head and trunk independently.[172] Specifically, they find it difficult to keep the head still while moving the trunk, which potentially could be related to altered CCR reflex activity.

ONSET OF DISTURBANCES IN SENSORIMOTOR CONTROL

Most studies investigating changes in sensorimotor control have been conducted in people with chronic neck pain disorders. Nevertheless, reports of dizziness and disturbances in balance, oculomotor control and JPS are found in patients in the acute phase following

FOCUS POINT

The observed changes in balance and head and eye movement control in persons with neck pain may reflect altered somatosensory input from a variety of structures in the cervical spine. Alterations in cervical somatosensory information in neck pain may be arising from a number of causes including direct trauma, functional impairment or morphological changes in the cervical muscles and the direct effects that pain has at many levels of the nervous system. Psychosocial and or work-related stresses may also affect cervical somatosensory function via activation of the sympathetic nervous system.

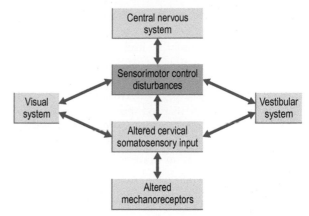

Fig. 6.3 ■ Impact of cervical somatosensory dysfunction on sensorimotor control. Several peripheral mechanisms can alter mechanoreceptor function and thus cervical somatosensory input to the sensorimotor control system. Such changes can alter the central nervous system and subsequent descending information, which further contributes to altered somatosensory input. Visual and vestibular input can be indirectly affected from altered cervical somatosensory input.

a whiplash injury [82,159,173–175] and often align with poorer outcomes and with higher levels of pain and disability. This evidence that disturbances in sensorimotor control begin early in the history of the disorder indicates that they are not a consequence of chronic pain. Cervical movement sense disorders in contrast, seem to develop over time, they often persist but again do not relate specifically to other signs and symptoms such as pain and disability of WAD.[176]

RELATIONSHIPS BETWEEN SENSORIMOTOR MEASURES

Disturbed cervical somatosensory input associated with neck pain may affect postural stability as well as head and eye movement control. A relationship between these measures might be expected because of similar mechanisms, however correlations between measures are not high,[177,178] even within tests with similar constructs, such as tests of cervical JPS and movement sense.[178] As a consequence, a patient with neck pain may present with disturbances to eye movement control but may not have any disturbance in cervical JPS or postural stability. This may reflect different control strategies and physical demands in the different tests. Thus assessment of each area is recommended. Further, the degree of dizziness reported by the patient does not necessarily determine the outcome of the physical measures. Although subjects with WAD complaining of dizziness appear to have greater deficits, 50% of subjects with WAD who did not complain of dizziness were shown to have deficits in two or more sensorimotor control tests.[177] At this time it is not known whether dizziness reflects an overall greater degree of cervical somatosensory dysfunction or relates to more specific areas of dysfunction (Fig. 6.3).

There is some evidence that patients with upper cervical impairment might be more prone to sensorimotor disturbances.[162] Assessment of cervical proprioception should always be undertaken in patients presenting with symptoms of dizziness, unsteadiness or visual disturbances. However, patients with sensorimotor deficits may not have overt symptoms.[112] Thus assessment of cervical proprioception should also be undertaken when patients are not responding as expected to traditional management.

CONCLUSION

Deficits in cervical JPS, balance and eye movement control have been demonstrated in patients with both insidious onset and traumatic neck pain and are, in all likelihood, reflecting disturbances in cervical somatosensory information. Cervical joint position and movement sense, eye movement control, coordination and postural stability need to be considered in the clinical reasoning process in patients with neck pain disorders. The lack of direct relationships between these measures and the lack of a direct relationship to patients' reported pain and disability indicates that each aspect of sensorimotor function should be assessed. The clinician should also be aware of other possible causes of dizziness (see Chapter 10). We advocate that assessment and management be tailored specifically to deficits in sensorimotor control. Concurrently, the potential causes of abnormal cervical somatosensory input need to be addressed. Rehabilitation strategies to enhance cervical proprioception, balance and eye movement control related to altered cervical afferent input are offered in Chapter 16.

REFERENCES

1. Kulkarni V, Chandy M, Babu K. Quantitative study of muscle spindles in suboccipital muscles of human foetuses. Neurol India 2001;49:355–9.
2. Boyd Clark L, Briggs C, Galea M. Muscle spindle distribution, morphology and density in the longus colli and multifidus muscles of the cervical spine. Spine 2002;27:694–701.
3. Ageborg E. Consequences of a ligament injury on neuromuscular function and relevance to rehabilitation- using the anterior cruciate ligament-injured knee as a model. J Electromyogr Kinesiol 2002;12:205–12.
4. Krogsgaard M, Dyre-Poulsen P, Fischer-Rasmussen T. Cruciate ligament reflexes. J Electromyogr Kinesiol 2002;12:177–82.
5. Liu J, Thornell L, Pedrosa-Domellof F. Muscle spindles in the deep muscles of the human neck: a morphological and immunocytochemical study. J Histochem Cytochem 2003;51:175–86.
6. Bolton PS, Holland CT. An in vivo method for studying afferent fibre activity from cervical paravertebral tissue during vertebral motion in anaesthetised cats. J Neurosci Methods 1998;85:211–18.
7. Richmond FJ, Bakker DA. Anatomical organization and sensory receptor content of soft tissues surrounding upper cervical vertebrae in the cat. J Neurophysiol 1982;48:49–61.
8. Andary M, Hallgren RC, Greenman PE, et al. Neurogenic atrophy of suboccipital muscles after a cervical injury: a case study. Am J Phys Med Rehabil 1998;77:545–9.
9. Selbie WS, Thomson DB, Richmond FJ. Suboccipital muscles in the cat neck: morphometry and histochemistry of the rectus capitis muscle complex. J Morphol 1993;216:47–63.
10. Swanik C, Lephart F, Giannantonio F, et al. Re-establishing proprioception and muscle control in the ACL injured athlete. J Sport Rehabil 1997;6:182–206.
11. Werner J. Neuroscience - a clinical perspective. Canada: W.B. Saunders; 1980.
12. Corneil BD, Olivier E, Munoz DP. Neck muscle responses to stimulation of monkey superior colliculus. I. Topography and manipulation of stimulation parameters. J Neurophysiol 2002;88:1980–99.
13. Hirai N, Hongo T, Sasaki S, et al. Neck muscle afferent input to spinocerebellar tract cells of the central cervical nucleus in the cat. Exp Brain Res 1984;55:286–300.
14. Peterson B, Goldberg J, Bilotto G, et al. Cervicocollic reflex: its dynamic properties and interaction with vestibular reflexes. J Neurophysiol 1985;54:90–108.
15. Peterson BW. Current approaches and future directions to understanding control of head movement. Prog Brain Res 2004;143:369–81.
16. Chan YS, Kasper J, Wilson VJ. Dynamics and directional sensitivity of neck muscle-spindle responses to head rotation. J Neurophysiol 1987;57:1716–29.
17. Bronstein AM, Morland AB, Ruddock KH, et al. Recovery from bilateral vestibular failure: Implications for visual and cervico-ocular function. Acta Otolaryngol Suppl 1995;520:405–7.
18. Doerr M, Hong SH, Thoden U. Eye movements during active head turning with different vestibular and cervical input. Acta Otolaryngol 1984;98:14–20.
19. Mergner T, Schweigart G, Botti F, et al. Eye movements evoked by proprioceptive stimulation along the body axis in humans. Exp Brain Res 1998;120:450–60.
20. Jurgens R, Mergner T. Interaction between cervico-ocular and vestibulo-ocular reflexes in normal adults. Exp Brain Res 1989;77:381–90.
21. Bouyer LJ, Watt DG. "Torso Rotation" experiments. 4: the role of vision and the cervico-ocular reflex in compensation for a deficient VOR. J Vestib Res 1999;9:89–101.
22. Vidal PP, Roucoux A, Berthoz A. Horizontal eye position-related activity in neck muscles of the alert cat. Exp Brain Res 1982;46:448–53.
23. Goonetilleke SC, Gribble PL, Mirsattari SM, et al. Neck muscle responses evoked by transcranial magnetic stimulation of the human frontal eye fields. Eur J Neurosci 2011;33:2155–67.
24. Richter HO, Banziger T, Abdi S, et al. Stabilization of gaze: a relationship between ciliary muscle contraction and trapezius muscle activity. Vision Res 2010;50:2559–69.
25. Richter HO, Zetterlund C, Lundqvist LO. Eye-neck interactions triggered by visually deficient computer work. Work 2011;39:67–78.
26. Yamagata Y, Yates BJ, Wilson VJ. Participation of Ia reciprocal inhibitory neurons in the spinal circuitry of the tonic neck reflex. Exp Brain Res 1991;84:461–4.
27. Ishikawa K, Matsuzaki Z, Yokomizo M, et al. Effect of unilateral section of cervical afferent nerve upon optokinetic response and vestibular nystagmus induced by sinusoidal rotation in guinea pigs. Acta Otolaryngol Suppl 1998;537:6–10.
28. Bove M, Courtine G, Schieppati M. Neck muscle vibration and spatial orientation during stepping in place in humans. J Neurophysiol 2002;88:2232–41.
29. Courtine G, Papaxanthis C, Laroche D, et al. Gait-dependent integration of neck muscle afferent input. Neuroreport 2003;14:2365–8.
30. Karnath HO, Reich E, Rorden C, et al. The perception of body orientation after neck-proprioceptive stimulation - effects of time and of visual cueing. Exp Brain Res 2002;143:350–8.

31. Karlberg M, Magnusson M, Johansson R. Effects of restrained cervical mobility on voluntary eye movements and postural control. Acta Otolaryngol 1991;111:664–70.

32. Lennerstrand G, Han Y, Velay JL. Properties of eye movements induced by activation of neck muscle proprioceptors. Graefes Arch Clin Exp Ophthalmol 1996;234:703–9.

33. Taylor JL, McCloskey DI. Illusions of head and visual target displacement induced by vibration of neck muscles. Brain 1991;114:755–9.

34. Duclos C, Roll R, Kavounoudias A, et al. Long-lasting body leanings following neck muscle isometric contractions. Exp Brain Res 2004;158:58–66.

35. Schmid M, Schieppati M. Neck muscle fatigue and spatial orientation during stepping in place in humans. J Appl Physiol 2005;99:141–53.

36. Schieppati M, Nardone A, Schmid M. Neck muscle fatigue affects postural control in man. Neuroscience 2003;121:277–85.

37. Gosselin G, Rassoulian H, Brown I. Effects of neck extensor muscles fatigue on balance. Clin Biomech (Bristol, Avon) 2004;19:473–9.

38. Owens EF Jr, Henderson CN, Gudavalli MR, et al. Head repositioning errors in normal student volunteers: a possible tool to assess the neck's neuromuscular system. Chiropr Osteopat 2006;5.

39. Vuillerme N, Pinsault N, Vaillant J. Postural control during quiet standing following cervical muscular fatigue: effects of changes in sensory inputs. Neurosci Lett 2005;378:135–9.

40. Baloh R, Halmagyi G. Disorders of the vestibular system. New York: Oxford University Press; 1996.

41. Hikosaka O, Maeda M. Cervical effects on abducens motoneurons and their interaction with vestibulo-ocular reflex. Exp Brain Res 1973;18:512–30.

42. Fischer A, Verhagen WIM, Huygen PLM. Whiplash injury. A clinical review with emphasis on neuro-otological aspects. Clin Otolaryngol 1997;22:192–201.

43. Hinoki M. Vertigo due to whiplash injury: a neuro-otological approach. Acta Otolaryngol 1975;419:9–29.

44. Padoan S, Karlberg M, Fransson PA, et al. Passive sustained turning of the head induces asymmetric gain of the vestibulo-ocular reflex in healthy subjects. Acta Otolaryngol 1998;118:778–82.

45. DeJong PI, DeJong JM. Ataxia and nystagmus induced by injection of local anaesthetics in the neck. Ann Neurol 1977;1977:240–6.

46. Hinoki M, Niki H. Neuro-otological studies on the role of the sympathetic nervous system in the formation of traumatic vertigo of cervical origin. Acta Otolaryngol Suppl 1975;330:185–96.

47. Heikkila H, Astrom PG. Cervicocephalic kinesthetic sensibility in patients with whiplash injury. Scand J Rehabil Med 1996;28:133–8.

48. Wenngren B, Pedersen J, Sjolander P, et al. Bradykinin and muscle stretch alter contralateral cat neck muscle spindle output. Neurosci Res 1998;32:119–29.

49. Pedersen J, Sjolander P, Wenngren B, et al. Increased intramuscular concentration of bradykinin increases the static fusimotor drive to muscle spindles in neck muscles of the cat. Pain 1997;70:83–91.

50. Thunberg J, Hellstrom F, Solander P, et al. Influences on the fusimotor-muscle spindle system from chemosensitive nerve endings in the cervical facet joints in the cat; possible implications for whiplash induced disorders. Pain 2001;91:15–22.

51. Hellstrom F, Thunberg J, Bergenheim M, et al. Elevated intramuscular concentration of bradykinin in law muscle increases the fusimotor drive to neck muscles in the cat. J Dent Res 2000;79:1815–22.

52. Elliott J, Jull G, Noteboom JT, et al. Fatty infiltration in the cervical extensor muscles in persistent whiplash-associated disorders-a magnetic resonance imaging analysis. Spine 2006;31:E847–55.

53. McPartland JM, Brodeur RR, Hallgren RC. Chronic neck pain, standing balance, and suboccipital muscle atrophy-a pilot study. J Manipulative Physiol Ther 1997;20:24–9.

54. Le Pera D, Graven-Nielsen T, Valeriani M, et al. Inhibition of motor system excitability at cortical and spinal level by tonic muscle pain. Clin Neurophysiol 2001;112:1633–41.

55. Holm S, Aage I, Solomonow M. Sensorimotor control of the spine. J Electromyogr Kinesiol 2002;12:219–34.

56. Zedka M, Prochazka A, Knight B, et al. Voluntary and reflex control of human back muscles during induced pain. J Physiol 1999;520:591–604.

57. Matre D, Arendt-Nielsen L, Knardahl S. Effects of localization and intensity of experimental muscle pain on ankle joint proprioception. Eur J Pain 2002;6:245–60.

58. Wang K, Svensson P, Arendt-Nielsen L. Effect of tonic muscle pain on short latency jaw-stretch reflexes in humans. Pain 2000;88:189–97.

59. Tinazzi M, Fiaschi A, Rosso T, et al. Neuroplastic changes related to pain occur at multiple levels of the human somatosensory system: a somatosensory-evoked potentials study in patients with cervical radicular pain. J Neurosci 2000;20:9277–83.

60. Gandevia SC, Phegan CM. Perceptual distortions of the human body image produced by local anaesthesia, pain and cutaneous stimulation. J Physiol 1999;514:609–16.

61. Flor H. Cortical reorganisation and chronic pain: Implications for rehabilitation. J Rehabil Med 2003;35:66–72.

62. Passatore M, Roatta S. Influence of sympathetic nervous system on sensorimotor function: whiplash associated disorders (WAD) as a model. Eur J Appl Physiol 2006;98:423–49.

63. Hellstrom F, Roatta S, Thunberg J, et al. Responses of muscle spindles in feline dorsal neck muscles to electrical stimulation of the cervical sympathetic nerve. Exp Brain Res 2005;165:328–42.

64. Heikkila H, Johansson M, Wenngren BI. Effects of acupuncture, cervical manipulation and NSAID therapy on dizziness and impaired head repositioning of suspected cervical origin: a pilot study. Man Ther 2000;5:151–7.

65. Humphreys BK, Bolton J, Peterson C, et al. A cross-sectional study of the association between pain and disability in neck pain patients with dizziness of suspected cervical origin. J Whiplash Assoc Disord 2003;1:63–73.

66. Jull G, Stanton W. Predictors of responsiveness to physiotherapy treatment of cervicogenic headache. Cephalalgia 2005;25:101–8.

67. Treleaven J, Jull G, Sterling M. Dizziness and unsteadiness following whiplash injury: characteristic features and relationship with cervical joint position error. J Rehabil Med 2003;35:36–43.

68. Treleaven J, Takasaki H. Characteristics of visual disturbances reported by subjects with neck pain. Man Ther 2014;19:203–7.

69. Jaramillo CA, Eapen BC, McGeary CA, et al. A cohort study examining headaches among veterans of Iraq and Afghanistan wars: associations with traumatic brain injury, PTSD, and depression. Headache 2016;56:528–39.

70. Michiels S, Van de Heyning P, Truijen S, et al. Does multi-modal cervical physical therapy improve tinnitus in patients with cervicogenic somatic tinnitus? Man Ther 2016;26:125–31.

71. Peng BG, Pang XD, Yang H. Chronic neck pain and episodic vertigo and tinnitus. Pain Med 2015;16:200–2.

72. Roijezon U, Clark NC, Treleaven J. Proprioception in musculoskeletal rehabilitation. Part 1: Basic science and principles of assessment and clinical interventions. Man Ther 2015;20: 368–77.

73. Michiels S, De Hertogh W, Truijen S, et al. The assessment of cervical sensory motor control: A systematic review focusing on measuring methods and their clinometric characteristics. Gait Posture 2013;38:1–7.

74. Kristjansson E, Hardardottir L, Asmundardottir M, et al. A new clinical test for cervicocephalic kinesthetic sensibility: "the fly." Arch Phys Med Rehabil 2004;85:490–5.

75. Blouin J, Okada T, Wolsley C, et al. Encoding target-trunk relative position: cervical versus vestibular contribution. Exp Brain Res 1998;122:101–7.

76. Revel M, Andre-Deshays C, Minguet M. Cervicocephalic kinesthetic sensibility in patients with cervical pain. Arch Phys Med Rehabil 1991;72:288–91.

77. de Vries J, Ischebeck BK, Voogt LP, et al. Joint position sense error in people with neck pain: a systematic review. Man Ther 2015;20:736–44.

78. Stanton TR, Leake HB, Chalmers KJ, et al. Evidence of impaired proprioception in chronic, idiopathic neck pain: systematic review and meta-analysis. Phys Ther 2016;96:876–87.

79. Feipel V, Salvia P, Klein H, et al. Head repositioning accuracy in patients with whiplash-associated disorders. Spine 2006;31: E51–8.

80. Humphreys B, Irgens P. The effect of a rehabilitation exercise program on head repositioning accuracy and reported levels of pain in chronic neck pain subjects. J Whiplash Relat Disord 2002;1:99–112.

81. Kristjansson E, Dall'Alba P, Jull G. A study of five cervicocephalic relocation tests in three different subject groups. Clin Rehabil 2003;17:768–74.

82. Sterling M, Jull G, Vicenzino B, et al. Development of motor system dysfunction following whiplash injury. Pain 2003;103: 65–73.

83. L'Heureux-Lebeau B, Godbout A, Berbiche D, et al. Evaluation of paraclinical tests in the diagnosis of cervicogenic dizziness. Otol Neurotol 2014;35:1858–65.

84. Treleaven J. Sensorimotor disturbances in neck disorders affecting postural stability, head and eye movement control. Man Ther 2008;13:2–11.

85. Chen X, Treleaven J. The effect of neck torsion on joint position error in subjects with chronic neck pain. Man Ther 2013;18:562–7.

86. Hides JA, Franettovich Smith MM, Mendis MD, et al. A prospective investigation of changes in the sensorimotor system following sports concussion. An exploratory study. Musculoskelet Sci Pract 2017;29:7–19.

87. Huysmans MA, Hoozemans MJM, van der Beek AJ, et al. Position sense acuity of the upper extremity and tracking performance in subjects with non-specific neck and upper extremity pain and healthy controls. J Rehabil Med 2010;42:876–83.

88. Knox JJ, Beilstein DJ, Charles SD, et al. Changes in head and neck position have a greater effect on elbow joint position sense in people with whiplash-associated disorders. Clin J Pain 2006;22:512–18.

89. Sandlund J, Djupsjobacka M, Ryhed B, et al. Predictive and discriminative value of shoulder proprioception tests for patients with whiplash-associated disorders. J Rehabil Med 2006;38:44–9.

90. Kristjansson E, Oddsdottir GL. "The fly": a new clinical assessment and treatment method for deficits of movement control in the cervical spine reliability and validity. Spine 2010;35: E1298–305.

91. Woodhouse A, Stavdahl O, Vasseljen O. Irregular head movement patterns in whiplash patients during a trajectory task. Exp Brain Res 2010;201:261–70.

92. Bahat HS, Chen XQ, Reznik D, et al. Interactive cervical motion kinematics: sensitivity, specificity and clinically significant values for identifying kinematic impairments in patients with chronic neck pain. Man Ther 2015;20:295–302.

93. Woodhouse A, Liljeback P, Vasseljen O. Reduced head steadiness in whiplash compared with non-traumatic neck pain. J Rehabil Med 2010;42:35–41.

94. Muceli S, Farina D, Kirkesola G, et al. Reduced force steadiness in women with neck pain and the effect of short term vibration. J Electromyogr Kinesiol 2011;21:283–90.

95. Jull G, Kristjansson E, Dall'Alba P. Impairment in the cervical flexors: a comparison of whiplash and insidious onset. Man Ther 2004;9:89–94.

96. Sarig-Bahat H, Weiss PL, Laufer Y. The effect of neck pain on cervical kinematics, as assessed in a virtual environment. Arch Phys Med Rehabil 2010;91:1884–90.

97. Grip H, Sundelin G, Gerdle B, et al. Cervical helical axis characteristics and its center of rotation during active head and upper arm movements-comparisons of whiplash-associated disorders, non-specific neck pain and asymptomatic individuals. J Biomech 2008;41:2799–805.

98. Sjölander P, Michaelson P, Jaric S, et al. Sensorimotor disturbances in chronic neck pain–range of motion, peak velocity, smoothness of movement, and repositioning acuity. Man Ther 2008;13: 122.

99. Roijezon U, Djupsjobacka M, Bjorklund M, et al. Kinematics of fast cervical rotations in persons with chronic neck pain: a cross-sectional and reliability study. BMC Musculoskelet Disord 2010;11.

100. Woodhouse A, Vasseljen O. Altered motor control patterns in whiplash and chronic neck pain. BMC Musculoskelet Disord 2008;9.

101. Sarig Bahat H, Chen X, Reznik D, et al. Interactive cervical motion kinematics: sensitivity, specificity and clinically significant values for identifying kinematic impairments in patients with chronic neck pain. Man Ther 2015;20:295–302.

102. Sarig Bahat H, Weiss PL, Laufer Y. The effect of neck pain on cervical kinematics, as assessed in a virtual environment. Arch Phys Med Rehabil 2010;91:1884–90.

103. Bagust J. Assessment of verticality perception by a rod-and-frame test: preliminary observations on the use of a computer monitor and video eye glasses. Arch Phys Med Rehabil 2005;86:1062–4.

104. Treleaven J, Takasaki H. High variability of the subjective visual vertical test of vertical perception, in some people with neck pain - should this be a standard measure of cervical proprioception? Man Ther 2015;20:183–8.

105. Elsig S, Luomajoki H, Sattelmayer M, et al. Sensorimotor tests, such as movement control and laterality judgment accuracy, in persons with recurrent neck pain and controls. A case-control study. Man Ther 2014;19:555–61.

106. Daenen L, Nijs J, Roussel N, et al. Altered perception of distorted visual feedback occurs soon after whiplash injury: an experimental study of central nervous system processing. Pain Physician 2012;15:405–13.

107. Daenen L, Nijs J, Roussel N, et al. Sensorimotor incongruence exacerbates symptoms in patients with chronic whiplash associated disorders: an experimental study. Rheumatology 2012; 51:1492–9.

108. Harvie DS, Hillier S, Madden VJ, et al. Neck pain and proprioception revisited using the proprioception incongruence detection test. Phys Ther 2016;96:671–8.

109. Pedler A, Motlagh H, Sterling M. Laterality judgments are not impaired in patients with chronic whiplash associated disorders. Man Ther 2013;18:72–6.

110. Richter HO, Roijezon U, Bjorklund M, et al. Long-term adaptation to neck/shoulder pain and perceptual performance in a hand laterality motor imagery test. Perception 2010;39:119–30.

111. Ålund M, Ledin T, Ödkvist L, et al. Dynamic posturography among patients with common neck disorders. A study of 15 cases with suspected cervical vertigo. J Vestib Res 1993;3: 383–9.

112. Field S, Treleaven J, Jull G. Standing balance: a comparison between idiopathic and whiplash-induced neck pain. Man Ther 2008;13:183–91.

113. Karlberg M, Magnusson M, Malmstrom EM, et al. Postural and symptomatic improvement after physiotherapy in patients with dizziness of suspected cervical origin. Arch Phys Med Rehabil 1996;77:874–82.

114. Karlberg M, Persson L, Magnusson M. Impaired postural control in patients with cervico-brachial pain. Acta Otolaryngol Suppl 1995;520(Pt 2):440–2.

115. Michaelson P, Michaelson M, Jaric S, et al. Vertical posture and head stability in patients with chronic neck. J Rehabil Med 2003;35:229–35.

116. Madeleine P, Prietzel H, Svarrer H, et al. Quantitative posturography in altered sensory conditions: A way to assess balance instability in patients with chronic whiplash injury. Arch Phys Med Rehabil 2004;85:432–8.

117. Poole E, Treleaven J, Jull G. The influence of neck pain on balance and gait parameters in community dwelling elders. Man Ther 2008;13:317–24.

118. Quek J, Brauer SG, Clark R, et al. New insights into neck-pain-related postural control using measures of signal frequency and complexity in older adults. Gait Posture 2014;39:1069–73.

119. Roijezon U, Bjorklund M, Djupsjobacka M. The slow and fast components of postural sway in chronic neck pain. Man Ther 2011;16:273–8.

120. Sjöström HJ, Allum J, Carpenter MG, et al. Trunk sway measures of postural stability during clinical balance tests in patients with chronic whiplash injury symptoms. Spine 2003;28:1725–34.

121. Treleaven J, Jull G, Murison R, et al. Is the method of signal analysis and test selection important for measuring standing balance in chronic whiplash? Gait Posture 2005;21:395–402.

122. Treleaven J, Jull G, Low Choy N. Standing balance in persistent WAD-comparison between subjects with and without dizziness. J Rehabil Med 2005;37:224–9.

123. Shumway-Cook A, Horak FB. Assessing the influence of sensory interaction on balance - suggestion from the field. Phys Ther 1986;66:1548–50.

124. Field S, Treleaven J, Jull G. Standing balance: A comparison between idiopathic and whiplash-induced neck pain. Man Ther 2008;13:183–91.

125. Treleaven J, LowChoy N, Darnell R, et al. Comparison of sensorimotor disturbance between subjects with persistent whiplash-associated disorder and subjects with vestibular pathology associated with acoustic neuroma. Arch Phys Med Rehabil 2008;89:522–30.

126. Juul-Kristensen B, Clausen B, Ris I, et al. Increased neck muscle activity and impaired balance among females with whiplash-related chronic neck pain: a cross-sectional study. J Rehabil Med 2013;45:376–84.

127. Stapley PJ, Beretta MV, Dalla Toffola E, et al. Neck muscle fatigue and postural control in patients with whiplash injury. Clin Neurophysiol 2006;47:610–22.

128. Uthaikhup S, Jull G, Sungkarat S, et al. The influence of neck pain on sensorimotor function in the elderly. Arch Gerontol Geriatr 2012;55:667–72.

129. Quek J, Treleaven J, Clark R, et al. An exploratory study examining factors underpinning postural instability in older adults with neck pain. Gait Posture 2018;60:93–8.

130. Treleaven J, Jull G, Low Choy N. Smooth pursuit neck torsion test in whiplash associated disorders-relationship to self reports of neck pain and disability, dizziness and anxiety. J Rehabil Med 2005;37:219–23.

131. Yu LJ, Stokell R, Treleaven J. The effect of neck torsion on postural stability in subjects with persistent whiplash. Man Ther 2011;16:339–43.

132. Williams K, Tarmizi A, Treleaven J. Use of neck torsion as a specific test of neck related postural instability. Musculoskelet Sci Pract 2017;29:115–19.

133. Cote JN, Patenaude I, St-Onge N, et al. Whiplash-associated disorders affect postural reactions to antero-posterior support surface translations during sitting. Gait Posture 2009;29: 603–11.

134. Stokell R, Yu AN, Williams K, et al. Dynamic and functional balance tasks in subjects with persistent whiplash: a pilot trial. Man Ther 2011;16:394–8.

135. Ciavarro GL, Nozza M, Zaccheddu M, et al. Assessment of whiplash injuries through 3D digital craniocorpography. J Biomech 2006;39:S149.

136. Poole E, Treleaven J, Jull G. The influence of neck pain on balance and gait parameters in community-dwelling elders. Man Ther 2008;13:317–24.

137. Uthaikhup S, Sunkarat S, Khamsaen K, et al. The effects of head movement and walking speed on gait parameters in patients with chronic neck pain. Man Ther 2014;19:137–41.

138. Kendall JC, Hartvigsen J, French SD, et al. Is there a role for neck manipulation in elderly falls prevention? An overview. J Can Chiropr Assoc 2015;59:53–63.

139. Kendall JC, Boyle E, Hartvigsen J, et al. Neck pain, concerns of falling and physical performance in community-dwelling Danish citizens over 75 years of age: a cross-sectional study. Scand J Public Health 2016;44:695–701.

140. Mork R, Bruenech JR, Thorud HMS. Effect of direct glare on orbicularis oculi and trapezius during computer reading. Optom Vis Sci 2016;93:738–49.

141. Richter HO, Banziger T, Forsman M. Eye-lens accommodation load and static trapezius muscle activity. Eur J Appl Physiol 2011;111:29–36.

142. Gimse R, Tjell C, Bjorgen IA, et al. Disturbed eye movements after whiplash due to injuries to the posture control system. J Clin Exp Neuropsychol 1996;18:178–86.

143. Heikkila HV, Wenngren BI. Cervicocephalic kinesthetic sensibility, active range of cervical motion, and oculomotor function in patients with whiplash injury. Arch Phys Med Rehabil 1998;79: 1089–94.

144. Hildingsson C, Wenngren B, Bring G, et al. Oculomotor problems after cervical spine injury. Acta Orthop Scand 1989;60: 513–16.

145. Kelders WPA, Kleinrensink GJ, Van der Geest JN, et al. The cervico-ocular reflex is increased in whiplash injury patients. J Neurotrauma 2005;22:133–7.

146. Montfoort I, Kelders WPA, van der Geest JN, et al. Interaction between ocular stabilization reflexes in patients with whiplash injury. Invest Ophthalmol Vis Sci 2006;47:2881–4.

147. Prushansky T, Dvir Z, Pevzner E, et al. Electro-oculographic measures in patients with chronic whiplash and healthy subjects: a comparative study. J Neurol Neurosurg Psychiatry 2004; 75:1642–4.

148. Storaci R, Manelli A, Schiavone N, et al. Whiplash injury and oculomotor dysfunctions: clinical-posturographic correlations. Eur Spine J 2006;15:1811–16.

149. Tjell C, Rosenhall U. Smooth pursuit neck torsion test: A specific test for cervical dizziness. Am J Otol 1998;19:76–81.

150. Tjell C, Tenenbaum A, Sandström S. Smooth pursuit neck torsion test- a specific test for whiplash associated disorders? J Whiplash Relat Disord 2003;1:9–24.

151. Wenngren B, Pettersson K, Lowenhielm G, et al. Eye motility and auditory brainstem response dysfunction after whiplash injury. Acta Orthop Scand 2002;122:276–83.

152. Brown S. Effect of whiplash injury on accommodation. Clin Exp Ophthalmol 2003;31:424–9.

153. Giffard P, Daly L, Treleaven J. Influence of neck torsion on near point convergence in subjects with idiopathic neck pain. Musculoskelet Sci Pract 2017;32:51–6.

154. Bexander CSM, Hodges PW. Cervico-ocular coordination during neck rotation is distorted in people with whiplash-associated disorders. Exp Brain Res 2012;217:67–77.

155. Grip H, Jull G, Treleaven J. Head eye co-ordination and gaze stability using simultaneous measurement of eye in head and head in space movements -potential for use in subjects with a whiplash injury. J Clin Monit Comput 2009;23:31–40.

156. Treleaven J, Jull G, Grip H. Head eye co-ordination and gaze stability in subjects with persistent whiplash associated disorders. Man Ther 2011;16:252–7.

157. de Vries J, Ischebeck BK, Voogt LP, et al. Cervico-ocular reflex is increased in people with nonspecific neck pain. Phys Ther 2016;96:1190–5.

158. Montfoort I, Van der Geest JN, Slijper HP, et al. Adaptation of the cervico- and vestibulo-ocular reflex in whiplash injury patients. J Neurotrauma 2008;25:687–93.

159. Hildingsson C, Toolanen G. Outcome after soft-tissue injury of the cervical spine: a prospective study of 93 car-accident victims. Acta Orthop Scand 1990;61:357–9.

160. Gimse R, Bjorgen IA, Tjell C, et al. Reduced cognitive functions in a group of whiplash patients with demonstrated disturbances in the posture control system. J Clin Exp Neuropsychol 1997;19:838–49.

161. Gimse R, Bjorgen I, Straume A. Driving skills after whiplash. Scand J Psychol 1997;38:165–70.

162. Treleaven J, Clamaron-Cheers C, Jull G. Does the region of pain influence the presence of sensorimotor disturbances in neck pain disorders? Man Ther 2011;16:636–40.

163. Dispenza F, Gargano R, Mathur N, et al. Analysis of visually guided eye movements in subjects after whiplash injury. Auris Nasus Larynx 2011;38:185–9.

164. Kongsted A, Jorgensen LV, Bendix T, et al. Are smooth pursuit eye movements altered in chronic whiplash-associated disorders? A cross-sectional study. Clin Rehabil 2007;21:1038–49.

165. Janssen M, Ischebeck BK, de Vries J, et al. Smooth pursuit eye movement deficits in patients with whiplash and neck pain are modulated by target predictability. Spine 2015;40:E1052–7.

166. Della Casa E, Helbling JA, Meichtry A, et al. Head-eye movement control tests in patients with chronic neck pain; inter-observer reliability and discriminative validity. BMC Musculoskelet Disord 2014;15.

167. Daley L, Giffard P, Thomas LC, et al. Validity of clinical measures of smooth pursuit eye movement control in patients with idiopathic neck pain. Musculoskelet Sci Pract 2017;33: 18–23.

168. McDevitt J, Appiah-Kubi KO, Tierney R, Wright WG. Vestibular and oculomotor assessments may increase accuracy of subacute concussion assessment. Int J Sports Med 2016;37:738–47.

169. Mucha A, Collins MW, Elbin RJ, et al. A brief vestibular/ocular motor screening (VOMS) assessment to evaluate concussions preliminary findings. Am J Sports Med 2014;42:2479–86.

170. Descarreaux M, Passmore S, Cantin V. Head movement kinematics during rapid aiming task performance in healthy and neck-pain participants: the importance of optimal task difficulty. Man Ther 2010;15:445–50.

171. Sandlund J, Roijezon U, Bjorklund M, et al. Acuity of goal-directed arm movements to visible targets in chronic neck pain. J Rehabil Med 2008;40:366–74.

172. Treleaven J, Takasaki H, Grip H. Trunk head co-ordination in neck pain. Quebec Canada: IFOMPT; 2012.

173. Cobo EP, Garcia-Alsina J, Almazan CG, et al. Postural control disorders in initial phases of whiplash. Med Clin 2009;132:616–20.

174. Dehner C, Heym B, Maier D, et al. Postural control deficit in acute QTF grade II whiplash injuries. Gait Posture 2008;28:113–19.

175. Jull G, Kenardy J, Hendrikz J, et al. Management of acute whiplash: a randomized controlled trial of multidisciplinary stratified treatments. Pain 2013;154:1798–806.

176. Oddsdottir GL, Kristjansson E. Two different courses of impaired cervical kinaesthesia following a whiplash injury. A one-year prospective study. Man Ther 2012;17:60–5.

177. Treleaven J, Jull G, LowChoy N. The relationship of cervical joint position error to balance and eye movement disturbances in persistent whiplash. Man Ther 2006;11:99–106.

178. Swait G, Rushton AB, Miall C, et al. Evaluation of cervical proprioceptive function. Spine 2007;32:E692–701.

179. Garret W, Nikolaou P, Ribbeck B, et al. The effect of muscle architecture on the biomechanical failure properties of skeletal muscle under passive extension. Am J Sports Med 1988;16:7–12.

180. Quick D. Acute lesion of the intrafusal muscle of muscle spindles. Ultrastructural and electrophysiological consequences. J Neurosci 1986;6:2097–105.

181. Uhlig Y, Weber BR, Grob D, et al. Fiber composition and fiber transformation in neck muscles of patients with dysfunction of the cervical spine. J Orthop Res 1995;13:240–9.

182. Loescher AR, Holland GR, Robinson PP. The distribution and morphological characteristics of axons innervating the periodontal ligament of reimplanted teeth in cats. Arch Oral Biol 1993;38:813–22.

183. Solomonow M, Zhou BH, Baratta RV, et al. Biomechanics of increased exposure to lumbar injury caused by cyclic loading: Part 1. Loss of reflexive muscular stabilization. Spine 1999; 24:2426–34.

184. Falla D, Jull G, Dall'Alba P, et al. An electromyographic analysis of the deep cervical flexor muscles in performance of craniocervical flexion. Phys Ther 2003;83:899–906.

185. Curatolo M, Petersen-Felix S, Arendt-Nielsen L, et al. Central hypersensitivity in chronic pain after whiplash injury. Clin J Pain 2001;17:306–15.

186. Seaman D. Dysafferentation: a novel term to describe the neuropathological effects of joint complex dysfunction - a look at likely mechanisms of symptom generation - in reply. J Manipulative Physiol Ther 1999;22:493–4.

187. Bani D, Bergamini M. Ultrastructural abnormalities of muscle spindles in the rat masseter muscle with malocclusion-induced damage. Histol Histopathol 2002;17:45–54.

188. Falla D, Jull G, Hodges PW. Feedforward activity of the cervical flexor muscles during voluntary arm movements is delayed in chronic neck pain. Exp Brain Res 2004;157:43–8.

189. Diwan F, Milburn A. The effects of temporary ischaemia on rat muscle spindles. J Embryol Exp Morphol 1986;92: 223–54.

190. Jull G. Deep cervical flexor muscle dysfunction in whiplash. J Musculoskelet Pain 2000;8:143–54.

191. Falla D. Unravelling the complexity of muscle impairment in chronic neck pain. Man Ther 2004;9:125–33.

192. Rossi S, Della Volpe R, Ginanneschi F, et al. Early somatosensory processing during tonic muscle pain in humans: Relation to loss of proprioception and motor "defensive" strategies. Clin Neurophysiol 2003;114:1351–8.

193. Gentle M, Thorp B. Sensory properties of ankle joint capsule mechanoreceptors in acute monoarthritic chickens. Pain 1994;57:361–74.

194. Gedalia U, Solomonow M, Zhou BH, et al. Biomechanics of increased exposure to lumbar injury caused by cyclic loading - part 2. Recovery of reflexive muscular stability with rest. Spine 1999;24:2461–7.

195. Falla D, Jull G, Edwards S, et al. Neuromuscular efficiency of the sternocleidomastoid and anterior scalene muscles in patients with chronic neck pain. Disabil Rehabil 2004;26: 712–17.

196. Falla D, Jull G, Rainoldi A, et al. Neck flexor muscle fatigue is side specific in patients with unilateral neck pain. Eur J Pain 2004;8:71–7.

7

PSYCHOLOGICAL AND SOCIAL CONSIDERATIONS IN NECK PAIN DISORDERS

The interest in psychosocial aspects of pain disorders has grown considerably over recent decades among researchers and clinicians alike. This reflects the move across all health professionals to consider behavioural, psychological and social dimensions in addition to biological features in understanding an individual's presenting pain disorder.[1,2] Unhelpful emotional, behavioural and cognitive features may influence management and prognosis. This chapter overviews a selection of psychological and social features that have been investigated in association with neck pain disorders, noting that it is artificial to separate them from biological features, as embraced in the biopsychosocial model. Nociception cannot be separated from emotions and behaviours. Likewise, emotions cannot be separated from a range of physiological responses, for example, anxiety and increased heart rate, stress and cortisol production. Indeed, much current research is focussing on psychophysical interactions towards better understanding and management of neck pain and other musculoskeletal disorders.[3–7]

PSYCHOLOGICAL FEATURES

Many emotions, behaviours and cognitions have been investigated in association with neck pain disorders. Commonly, these have included psychological distress (anxiety, depression and stress, including posttraumatic stress) as well as cognitive factors as catastrophizing, hypervigilance, fear avoidance beliefs (kinesiophobia, fear of pain), self-efficacy (general or pain self-efficacy) and expectations of recovery. The diverse nature of the studies makes it difficult to make general overall statements about the role of each of these features in the presentation or prognosis of neck pain disorders.[8] Neck pain populations have differed as have the psychological features investigated. Measurement tools differ and for some questionnaires there are no predetermined cut-off points, thus outcomes and interpretations of findings from these instruments differ. Psychological features often coexist and interact to moderate or mediate particular symptoms, behaviours or thoughts. They may be risk factors for chronicity.[9,10] Although recognizing these complexities, for clarity, selected, single psychological features will be considered, acknowledging that they frequently interact.

What is clearly evident is that there is variability in the frequency and magnitude of adverse psychological features within and between neck pain disorders and the individuals who present with them. For instance, two studies considering depression illustrate this variability. In a study of patients with chronic cervical radiculopathy attending a neurosurgery clinic, depression was not a major feature contributing to the disability or health status. Depression together with anxiety and catastrophizing, explained only 7.6% of the variance, and anxiety was the strongest-loading variable of the three.[11] In contrast, in a group of patients with chronic neck pain attending an interventional pain management clinic, a greater level of depression was the strongest predictor of clinical insomnia, and 28% of the group exceeded threshold scores for symptoms of depression.[12] Of note, both groups were described as suffering a chronic neck condition on the basis of pain for longer than 3 months. The findings not only illustrate the heterogeneity in psychological features among patients with neck pain disorders but illustrate the inadequacy of a time-based definition of chronicity to characterize a disorder (see Chapter 1).

Depression

Depression is commonly considered in studies of neck pain. Studies of general neck pain populations reveal that mean scores from questionnaires for depressive symptoms or low mood are well below threshold for depressive symptoms.[6,11,13,14] Thus the majority of individuals with neck pain (albeit not all) do not have significant depressive symptoms. Nevertheless, the frequency and level of depressive symptoms can be higher in particular patient groups, such as those with high pain levels relating to trauma induced neck pain (e.g., persisting whiplash-associated disorders or other recalcitrant neck pain disorders.[10,12,15–17]) It is therefore important to assess each patient on an individual basis.

Stress and anxiety

Stress and anxiety are common emotions associated with any pain, particularly in the acute phase. A systematic review and meta-analysis confirmed these relationships across various neck pain disorders.[18] Stress was found to be more frequently associated with neck pain than elevated anxiety, but there was insufficient evidence to support stress as a risk factor for chronic neck pain because of the low quality of the results in the studies reviewed at this time. Nevertheless, symptoms of posttrauma stress have been increasingly associated with recovery and nonrecovery in persons who have sustained a whiplash injury. Recovery trajectories have shown up to 20% of persons seeking treatment for whiplash-associated disorders (WAD) will have persisting and significant symptoms of posttrauma stress 12 months following the injury.[19] In particular, the hyperarousal subscale of the Posttraumatic Stress Diagnostic Scale has been shown to be one of the predictive factors for recovery or nonrecovery following a whiplash injury.[20] Symptoms such as stress and anxiety may be the result of pain. Conversely, premorbid anxiety may increase the risk of developing chronic pain as shown in the large longitudinal Norwegian Nord-Trøndelag Health Study (HUNT) where preaccident

baseline measures of anxiety were available.[21] Of the populations who did and did not develop a chronic WAD, 23.8% and 13.8% respectively exceeded the cut-off score for anxiety, suggesting that those individuals with preexisting anxiety are more likely to experience prolonged suffering. Nevertheless, anxiety levels are not necessarily high, even in individuals with chronic WAD.[22]

Catastrophization

Catastrophization is an emotion in which a negative perspective is placed on situations, for instance, believing that the neck pain or injury is far worse than it actually is and a feeling of hopelessness about the future. Similar to other psychological features, levels of pain catastrophization vary considerably.[22,23] In several studies, pain catastrophization has been reported to be low level with no major impact on pain or disability or treatment outcome.[11,14] Yet in another,[24] catastrophizing together with higher pain severity were found to modify treatment success, but the mean catastrophization score in this study was well below that regarded as clinically relevant catastrophization. Although less of a feature in idiopathic neck pain groups, higher pain catastrophization is one of the prognostic factors for poor outcome following a whiplash injury.[25] It appears to be a more frequent feature when pain originates from trauma as in a road traffic crash.[26] Higher levels of pain catastrophization in these patients may influence the likelihood of return to work,[9] although expectations for return to work partially mediate this relationship. High pain catastrophization can be associated with depression.[26,27] On a positive note, catastrophization levels can decrease as pain decreases and function returns, even in cases of recalcitrant WAD.[14,28]

Fear avoidance

Fear avoidance represents pain-related fear and anxiety causing an individual to avoid activities, to expect increased pain and to report more disability.[29,30] Fear of movement is a very normal reaction to acute neck pain and pain-related fear-avoidance beliefs and kinesiophobia are commonly found to be associated with neck pain disorders.[11,14,31–33] Fear of movement is one of several features that can mediate the relationship between pain intensity and disability.[34,35] As with other features, levels of avoidance and kinesiophobia are highly variable between individuals and range from negligible to well above threshold.[36–38] Notably, fear-avoidance beliefs and kinesiophobia seem to be the most consistent psychological feature(s) associated with neck pain disorders,[14,33,39] and unhelpful beliefs can influence outcomes.[39]

Patient expectations

Expectations should always be elicited from the patient in the initial interview because they can impact on the way the clinician communicates with the patient.[40] Positive and negative patient expectations about treatment outcomes can influence (albeit varaibly) recovery and nonrecovery respectively.[41–44] There may be a direct link between an expectation and the outcome of a treatment technique,[41] but often several factors shape an expectancy. For example, Ozegovic et al.[45] found that 10 different factors had an influence on expectations of recovery from a whiplash injury, the strongest being initial neck pain intensity and symptoms of depression. Similarly positive and negative expectations for return to work are shaped by several features.[46] In turn, patient expectations may mediate other associations, for example, the way in which pain catastrophizing and fear of movement affect return-to-work outcomes after a whiplash injury.[9]

Self-efficacy

Self-efficacy refers to a person's own beliefs about their ability to manage tasks and activities, even when difficulties are present.[47] Pain self-efficacy is related to the individual's beliefs about performing activities and tasks despite pain.[48] Low self-efficacy can directly affect neck pain and pain-related disability[13,49] and work ability.[50] Levels of self-efficacy again vary quite markedly between individuals and circumstances as reflected in dichotomous findings of relative minor to significant roles of self-efficacy in different neck pain groups.[11,49,51] Lower self-efficacy need not be a barrier to recovery as revealed by a negative association between pain self-efficacy at baseline and improvements in pain intensity and disability following a structured exercise intervention.[14] The authors reasoned that the professionally supported, structured exercise program might have offered effective support and relieved the participant's uncertainties in performing tasks in spite of pain.

Implications for assessment and management of psychological features

There are robust calls for consideration of various psychological features in the assessment and management of patients with neck pain[10,39,43,45] and this concurs with the biopsychosocial model. Patients are not inanimate objects, and the experience of neck pain will evoke various emotions, behaviours and thoughts. It is important to gain perspective on the balance between physical and mental/psychological health across the whole spectrum of individuals with neck pain.

A recent longitudinal study of 1100 community-based individuals with neck pain determined that neck pain was negativity associated with physical but not mental health related quality of life.[52] When the spectrum of individuals with neck pain is considered, the evidence suggests that it is the minority who have psychological features that are well outside population norms or cut-off values. The scores on various questionnaires of the studies reviewed for this chapter are frequently either well below thresholds for a certain psychological feature or are in the mild category, implying that many patients do not have substantive adverse emotions or behaviours. This is consistent with findings of a prospective study of 917 patients presenting to 97 chiropractic primary care practices for management of neck or low-back pain.[53] Only a minority of patients had high scores on psychological variables (for patients with neck pain, between <1% to 7.5% depending on the feature measured). Furthermore psychological features had little added value (about 1%) for predicting the outcome of treatment. The authors, in consequence, counselled against the use of extensive psychological screening tools at initial assessment.

The low incidence of persons with substantive psychological features presenting to community-based practices does not necessarily reflect the incidence in patients with neck pain disorders who are attending pain clinics or specialized intervention clinics[12,54] In addition, patients with persistent neck pain induced by trauma (e.g., whiplash) tend on average, to have greater sensory, physical and psychological responses than groups with insidious onset neck pain[55] and some may have other specific issues such as perceived injustice associated with loss and suffering.[10,26] A clinical trial of management for acute whiplash determined that general distress was one of the factors moderating neck pain and disability at baseline through to 12 months.[37] Yet, other trials of management of patients with chronic WAD found that psychological features were not associated with outcome.[56,57] This reinforces the fact that there can be no automatic assumptions about individual patients or conditions.

The opposite question to consider is whether treating psychological features improves outcomes for patients with neck pain disorders. Cognitive behaviour therapy can positively change emotions and behaviours associated with chronic musculoskeletal pain.[36,58,59] Yet, recent systematic reviews reveal that there is no strong or consistent evidence that psychological interventions for acute or chronic neck pain or WAD make any clinically relevant changes to neck pain and disability.[60–63] Topically, recent trials determined that the addition of cognitive behavioural therapy to an exercise program for patients with chronic neck pain compared with exercise alone produced no superior outcomes in neck pain and disability[22,64] or disability.[65] Nevertheless, in the latter trial, more participants made clinically meaningful reductions in pain with the combined program, and there were superior benefits in functional self-efficacy and pain-related fear. A further trial showed no differences postintervention, but there were significant advantages of the combined cognitive behavioural and exercise treatment at the 12 month follow-up across pain and disability and psychological features.[58] These results encourage further work on the nature of the combined intervention as well as who delivers the intervention. Other features such as "acceptance" are being studied for its potential role in rehabilitation outcomes of persons with chronic neck pain.[66]

Currently, information about psychosocial features is rather piecemeal and tends to be context specific for particular neck pain disorders at particular time points. Data at present is rather disparate. The ideal would be to develop an international mega database to build a full-bodied picture of psychological features across all domains of neck pain considering multiple variables including: neck disorders with pain and disability of mild, moderate to severe levels; whether neck pain is episodic or continuous; the stage of the condition; whether neck pain is of insidious onset or traumatic onset; whether the condition is compensable or non-compensable; whether the neck pain population is community based or attending specialized or tertiary clinics. Most importantly, a clear picture is needed of the incidence of "above threshold" scores within neck pain populations or preferably, the incidence of responses indicating normal, low, moderate or severe levels for the psychological features, which is currently unclear when population means only are presented.

The current lack of robust epidemiological data on the incidence of psychological features that are above normal thresholds does not detract from the need to help the patient with neck pain resolve unhelpful emotions, behaviours and beliefs when present, possibly even in sub-threshold levels. Variously, studies advocate the importance of addressing fear of movement,[33,39,67] catastrophization,[24,68] self-efficacy,[49,51] and expectations of recovery.[44] Neck pain disorders are heterogeneous in nature. There is variability in the nature and extent of emotional, behavioural and cognitive responses because there is variability in features as pain intensity, range of movement and muscle performance. Box 7.1 offers some factors that could be borne in mind when assessing and interpreting psychological features in a patient with a neck pain disorder.

SOCIAL FEATURES–THE WORK ENVIRONMENT

Social contexts can influence both the neck pain experience and the cervical spine disorder. Social features include aspects such as relationships with family and friends, cultural traditions, access to health care, education, socioeconomic status, work environment and lifestyle factors such as hobbies or recreational interests. Research has been undertaken into most of these features, but the area of greatest activity has been in relation to work environment. Social and psychological factors are inherently interwoven in the work environment and this will be the focus of this section. Both will be discussed, and biological associates will be included where relevant. Not surprisingly, each factor contributes to greater or lesser degrees and there is great variability in circumstances and individual features.

The changing face of work

The technological and digital revolutions are very rapidly changing the nature of work worldwide across the spectrum of occupations. Robots can make cars and

---

BOX 7.1

SOME FACTORS TO CONSIDER WHEN REASONING THE ROLE OF PSYCHOLOGICAL FEATURES IN NECK PAIN PATIENTS

- Many emotional reactions are normal responses rather than abnormal behaviours
  - It is understandable that a person may be anxious when they develop significant neck pain and they do not understand its cause. Normal anxiety is usually time limited. A patient's anxiety should lessen when the clinician explains the nature of their neck disorder and the pain, assures them of its benign nature and empowers the patient to be an active participant in their recovery.
  - Fear of movement or activity is understandable in an acute or severe state when, for example, a movement causes a sharp nauseating pain. There would be grave concerns about a patient who had no respect for their neck condition, and deliberately moved to cause themselves acute pain. When fear of movement is a normal response to pain, movement and activity usually return as pain resolves.[37,114,115]
  - The clinician must recognize when patients have unhelpful fear-avoidance beliefs and help them to modify these beliefs because they can be unhelpful to recovery.
  - The clinician can assist the patient quell emotional reactions through insightful explanations, education, assurance and due empathy and importantly, effective pain-relieving management.

- Differentiate between emotional and behavioural responses and psychopathologies
  - The diagnosis and management of the true psychopathologies is well beyond the scope of practice of the musculoskeletal clinician.
  - Temporary or mild low mood associated with neck pain should reasonably resolve with assurance and as pain, activity and participation in regular activities improve.
  - The diagnosis and management of a person with significant low mood, suggesting clinical depression requires the expertise of a clinical psychologist or psychiatrist.
- Questionnaires provide information on symptoms, not a diagnosis of a psychological disorder
  - Diagnoses of depression and a posttraumatic stress disorder, as examples, can only be made from a clinical examination by a trained practitioner. The scores on questionnaire only indicate the presence of symptoms.
- People and neck pain disorders are characterized by their heterogeneity
  - Pain is a personal experience.
  - Psychological responses and social determinants are not uniform. How a person perceives and reacts to a neck pain disorder is quite individual.

---

perform complex surgical procedures. The human role has in many circumstances, evolved to a sedentary occupation interfacing with a computer. The downside is that computer use has been linked with an increasing prevalence of neck pain.[69,70] No more than 6 hours computer use per day is linked to risk for developing neck pain.[71] In line with this, Shahidi and colleagues[6] found that 21% of workers commencing full-time office work, using a computer 75% of the time, developed chronic neck pain within the first 12 months of work. All work is not of a sedentary, sitting nature but there is an increased frequency of sedentary work compounded by the rapid rise in sedentary leisure pursuits across all ages with social media and other electronic devices. This work and lifestyle increases loads on the neck and contributes to other health problems. It is likely that the current sedentary nature of work and leisure, together with the aging population and possibly the

need to work longer, has contributed to neck pain joining back pain as the world's leading cause of years lived with a disability.[72]

Neck pain does not belong to any occupational category. Occupations involving sustained neck postures or awkward neck postures, high mechanical workload, lifting in awkward postures, working with the arms raised to, or above shoulder level, working with the arms in sustained positions have all been associated with neck pain.[73–78] Many occupations across the spectrum of work are linked with significant neck pain including the professions (e.g., dentists and dental assistants, laparoscopic surgeons; nurses, ophthalmologists and optometrists, ultra-sonographers), the trades (e.g., hairdressing, electricians, plumbers, dress makers), desk and office workers as well as craft workers.[74–77,79–83] Nevertheless, office workers appear to be particularly prone to neck pain.[69,70,84]

Although various features combine to be associated with neck pain, the physical nature of the work is one of the major risk factors.[73,76,78,81,85] A clinician must thoroughly understand the work undertaken by their patient and the physical requirements and demands of that work. Often, modifications can be made to the work, or to how the individual performs the work, to limit adverse strains on the neck and shoulders. Likewise, simple preventative strategies can be helpful to break up any prolonged work activity. This was illustrated with surgeons' reports of lessening of pain and fatigue in the neck and shoulder region with the inclusion of simple, targeted, stretching micro breaks within an operative procedure.[82] How easily neck pain can develop was illustrated in a longitudinal study by Hanvold and colleagues.[76] They tracked young adults over 6.5 years as they proceeded through technical training college, apprenticeship and into the work environment. They found that the transition from technical school to working life was accompanied by increased neck and shoulder pain in several occupations. Time alone increased the tendency to develop moderate to severe pain levels. It is logical to try to prevent this predictable work-related pain onset. Prevention is the ideal and it might be possible with the provision not only of information about ways to protect the body from undue strains, but with the routine inclusion of supervised practice in good work technique in technical and professional training programs of occupations where there is a known risk of developing neck pain.

Workplace psychosocial factors and the development of neck pain

Several social issues have been investigated around work for their association with neck pain. Studies vary in the breadth and nature of the features measured, the occupations investigated and the population considered. Findings, not surprisingly, differ and illustrate the variety of psychosocial features that can potentially influence the neck pain experience. As examples, Yang et al.[86] derived data for nearly 14,000 Americans from the 2010 National Health Interview and Occupational Health Supplementary Surveys. Their analysis indicated that workplace risk factors for neck pain included work-family imbalance, exposure to a hostile work environment, job insecurity, non-standard work arrangements, multiple jobs and long work hours. The large prospective

Norwegian HUNT study of 29,496 workers[87] found that work stress was an independent predictor of chronic neck pain, although more so in men than women, but poor job control was not a risk factor. Christian et al.[73] in another large population study (> 4000 workers) found that initially the greatest social risk factor for neck pain was role conflict. Over a period of 4 years, the risk factors for the pain persisting or a new episode of neck pain developing, were role conflict, social climate and decision control.[85] Factors that also seem to be fairly consistently associated with neck pain are high job demands and low levels of supportive leadership (i.e., job strain).[78,81] Socioeconomic circumstances seem not to be a major factor,[88] which is understandable given the variety of occupations linked with neck pain.

Factors that may protect a worker from neck pain are of particular interest in establishing optimal work environments. These, as could be expected, are the opposite to provocative factors. For instance, Christensen and colleagues[73] found that empowering leadership and decision control protected against neck pain. A Swedish study,[89] albeit in relation to musculoskeletal pain in general, found that less sickness leave was associated with less stress, more support from superiors, having an influence on working hours and, as opposed to common logic, working long and irregular hours. Certainly, prospective studies have shown a preventative effect of higher social support in reducing the development of neck pain.[90,91] The clinician must be aware of the variables in social features that might come into play with neck pain disorders, assess the individual patient's circumstances and, when in a position to do so, discuss issues with management.

Biological associates of work-related social and psychological factors

Within the spirit of the biopsychosocial model, investigators have been considering possible biological associates of neck pain associated with psychological and social features. Several studies have identified perceived muscular tension as either an early sign of musculoskeletal symptoms or a predictive factor for future neck pain.[76,92,93] The feeling of muscle tension might be a physical manifestation related to work stress, or could reflect altered neuromuscular control via increased co-contraction of neck muscles, identified in individuals with neck pain including office workers.[94,95] There is functional coupling between vision and the neck, thus the muscle tension perceived could reflect the effect on neck musculature, of unfavourable visual conditions such as glare exposure.[96–98] Lesser neck extensor endurance at baseline, has also been found to be a risk factor for developing new onset, chronic neck pain within 12 months of commencing work.[6]

Greater pain intensity and disability at baseline are usually strong predictors of persisting pain or poorer outcomes.[8,99] Pain mechanisms are starting to be measured in association with other psychological or social variables to determine any influence of changes in central nervous system processing in a worker's pain state. Although there is variability between studies, minor signs of widespread mechanical and cold hyperalgesia have been found in office workers with neck pain.[100] Reduced diffuse noxious inhibitory controls or impaired endogenous pain inhibition were also found to be a predisposing factor for neck pain in office workers.[6] In addition, the level of pain experienced in response to a physical task, termed *sensitivity to movement-evoked pain*, was shown to be related to work disability level following a whiplash injury.[101] The findings of these studies are beginning to reveal the potential role of psychophysical features and highlight the need to consider variables and their interactions within a biopsychosocial context.

An area of rapidly increasing interest in neck and low-back pain is sleeping patterns and pain-associated sleep interference. Sleep disturbances can impact on neck pain and neck pain can impact on sleep quality.[102] Psychological features, such as low mood, may contribute to poor sleep as may social factors, such as low support at work and imbalances in effort and reward.[12,103] Sleep disturbance is also associated with increased sick leave[104] and, not surprisingly, poorer response to physical therapy treatments.[105,106] Thus it is important that patients are questioned about their sleep quality and that any sleep disturbances or insomnia are addressed as part of pain management.

Return to work

Individuals with neck pain often continue to work (presenteeism) rather than take time off work (absenteeism), which is opposite to many cases of low-back pain. Presenteeism, regardless of the reason, is associated with costs in terms of lost productivity,[107] as well as social costs, for instance, straining worker relationships if extra work has to be taken on by colleagues for a prolonged period. It appears that the costs of presenteeism may exceed those of absenteeism when all factors are considered.[108]

Studies examining features associated with return to work often included cohorts of people with either neck pain or low-back pain,[99,109] and thus have obvious limitations from physical perspectives. Yet there does appear to be commonalties in relation to individual and social perspectives. Factors associated with a greater likelihood of return to work include positive expectations, greater self-efficacy, active coping skills, higher education and socioeconomic status and lower severity of pain/injury/functional disability.[9,99,101,109,110] Lesser likelihood of return to work is associated with the opposite attributes. In addition, older age, female gender, depression and higher physical work demands can mitigate against return to work or return to full-time work.[46,99,111]

It is vital for the clinician to understand the work status of the patient. Some features are nonmodifiable, such as age and gender but others are modifiable. The clinician can assist with strategies to either improve workplace performance or facilitate return to work, with good management methods to alleviate pain, to restore physical function and to encourage active coping through effective self-management strategies for work and home. It seems that such an approach is more effective, or at least as effective, as work-focused interventions.[112,113]

CONCLUSION

Neck pain and disability can be moderated or mediated by psychological and social factors. It is clear that the relative contributions of biological, psychological and social features vary remarkably between and within patients depending on changing circumstances, within and between various disorders, and in acute and persistent pain states. Each patient must be understood as an individual and there should be no preconceived judgements. More research is required that considers, simultaneously, the relative contributions of a range of biological, psychological and social features, rather consider them in relative isolation. Such research is proceeding.

REFERENCES

1. Engel G. The need for a new medical model: a challenge for biomedicine. Science 1977;196:129–36.
2. Waddell G. 1987 Volvo award in clinical sciences. A new clinical model for the treatment of low-back pain. Spine 1987;12:632–44.
3. Dunne-Proctor R, Kenardy J, Sterling M. The impact of post-traumatic stress disorder on physiological arousal, disability, and sensory pain thresholds in patients with chronic whiplash. Clin J Pain 2016;32:645–53.
4. Feinberg R, Hu J, Weaver M, et al. Stress-related psychological symptoms contribute to axial pain persistence after motor vehicle collision: path analysis results from a prospective longitudinal study. Pain 2017;158:682–90.
5. Pedler A, Sterling M. Patients with chronic whiplash can be subgrouped on the basis of symptoms of sensory hypersensitivity and posttraumatic stress. Pain 2013;154:1640–8.
6. Shahidi B, Curran-Everett D, Maluf K. Psychosocial, physical, and neurophysiological risk factors for chronic neck pain: a prospective inception cohort study. J Pain 2015;16:1288–99.
7. Walton D, Kwok T, Mehta S, et al. Cluster analysis of an international pressure pain threshold database identifies 4 meaningful subgroups of adults with mechanical neck pain. Clin J Pain 2017;33:422–8.
8. Walton D, Carroll L, Kasch H, et al. An overview of systematic reviews on prognostic factors in neck pain: results from the International Collaboration on Neck Pain (ICON) Project. Open Orthop J 2013;7(Suppl. 4: M9):494–505.
9. Carriere J, Thibault P, Milioto M, et al. Expectancies mediate the relations among pain catastrophizing, fear of movement, and return to work outcomes after whiplash injury. J Pain 2015;16:1280–7.
10. Scott W, Trost Z, Milioto M, et al. Barriers to change in depressive symptoms after multidisciplinary rehabilitation for whiplash: the role of perceived injustice. Clin J Pain 2015;31:145–51.
11. Halvorsen M, Kierkegaard M, Harms-Ringdahl K, et al. Dimensions underlying measures of disability, personal factors, and health status in cervical radiculopathy: a cross-sectional study. Medicine 2015;94:e999.
12. Kim S, Lee D, Yoon K, et al. Factors associated with increased risk for clinical insomnia in patients with chronic neck pain. Pain Physician 2015;18:593–8.
13. Falla D, Peolsson A, Peterson G, et al. Perceived pain extent is associated with disability, depression and self-efficacy in individuals with whiplash-associated disorders. Eur J Pain 2016;20:1490–501.
14. Karlsson L, Gerdle B, Takala E, et al. Associations between psychological factors and the effect of home-based physical exercise in women with chronic neck and shoulder pain. SAGE Open Med 2016;4:1–12.
15. Börsbo B, Peolsson M, Gerdle B. Catastrophizing, depression, and pain: correlation with and influence on quality of life and health - a study of chronic whiplash-associated disorders. J Rehabil Med 2008;40:562–9.
16. Degen R, MacDermid J, Grewal R, et al. Prevalence of symptoms of depression, anxiety, and posttraumatic stress disorder in workers with upper extremity complaints. J Orthop Sports Phys Ther 2016;46:590–5.
17. Young S, Aprill C, Braswell J, et al. Psychological factors and domains of neck pain disability. Pain Med 2009;10:310–18.
18. Ortego G, Villafañe J, Doménech-García V, et al. Is there a relationship between psychological stress or anxiety and chronic nonspecific neck-arm pain in adults? A systematic review and meta-analysis. J Psychosom Res 2016;90:70–81.
19. Sterling M, Hendrikz J, Kenardy J. Similar factors predict disability and posttraumatic stress disorder trajectories after whiplash injury. Pain 2011;152:1272–8.
20. Ritchie C, Hendrikz J, Jull G, et al. External validation of a clinical prediction rule to predict full recovery and continued moderate/severe disability following acute whiplash injury. J Orthop Sports Phys Ther 2015;45:242–50.
21. Myrtveit S, Wilhelmsen I, Petrie K, et al. What characterizes individuals developing chronic whiplash?: The Nord-Trøndelag Health Study (HUNT). J Psychosom Res 2013;74:393–400.
22. Overmeer T, Peterson G, Ludvigsson ML, et al. The effect of neck-specific exercise with or without a behavioral approach on psychological factors in chronic whiplash-associated disorders: a randomized controlled trial with a 2-year follow-up. Medicine 2016;95:e4430.
23. Sullivan M, Adams H, Rhodenizer T, et al. A psychosocial risk factor-targeted intervention for the prevention of chronic pain and disability following whiplash injury. Phys Ther 2006;86:8–18.
24. Verhagen A, Karels C, Schellingerhout J, et al. Pain severity and catastrophising modify treatment success in neck pain patients in primary care. Man Ther 2010;15:267–72.
25. Walton D, Macdermid J, Giorgianni A, et al. Risk factors for persistent problems following acute whiplash injury: update of a systematic review and meta-analysis. J Orthop Sports Phys Ther 2013;43:31–43.
26. Margiotta F, Hannigan A, Imran A, et al. Pain, Perceived injustice, and pain catastrophizing in chronic pain patients in Ireland. Pain Pract 2017;17:663–8.
27. Park S, Lee R, Yoon D, et al. Factors associated with increased risk for pain catastrophizing in patients with chronic neck pain: a retrospective cross-sectional study. Medicine 2016;95:e4698.
28. Smith A, Jull G, Schneider G, et al. Cervical radiofrequency neurotomy reduces psychological features in individuals with chronic whiplash symptoms. Pain Physician 2014;17:265–74.
29. Vlaeyen J, Linton S. Fear-avoidance model of chronic musculoskeletal pain: 12 years on. Pain 2012;153:1144–7.
30. Zale E, Lange K, Fields S, et al. The relation between pain-related fear and disability: a meta-analysis. J Pain 2013;14:1019–30.
31. Bahat HS, Weiss P, Sprecher E, et al. Do neck kinematics correlate with pain intensity, neck disability or with fear of motion? Man Ther 2014;19:252–8.
32. Lindstroem R, Graven-Nielsen T, Falla D. Current pain and fear of pain contribute to reduced maximum voluntary contraction

of neck muscles in patients with chronic neck pain. Arch Phys Med Rehabil 2012;93:2042–8.

33. Pool J, Ostelo R, Knol D, et al. Are psychological factors prognostic indicators of outcome in patients with sub-acute neck pain? Man Ther 2010;15:111–16.

34. Kamper S, Maher C, Lda C, et al. Does fear of movement mediate the relationship between pain intensity and disability in patients following whiplash injury? A prospective longitudinal study. Pain 2012;153:113–19.

35. Pedler A, Kamper S, Sterling M. Addition of posttraumatic stress and sensory hypersensitivity more accurately estimates disability and pain than fear avoidance measures alone after whiplash injury. Pain 2016;157:1645–54.

36. Jay K, Brandt M, Jakobsen M, et al. Ten weeks of physical-cognitive-mindfulness training reduces fear-avoidance beliefs about work-related activity: randomized controlled trial. Medicine 2016;95:e3945.

37. Jull G, Kenardy J, Hendrikz J, et al. Management of acute whiplash: a randomized controlled trial of multidisciplinary stratified treatments. Pain 2013;154:1798–806.

38. Sterling M, Kenardy J, Jull G, et al. The development of psychological changes following whiplash injury. Pain 2003;106: 481–9.

39. Robinson J, Theodore B, Dansie E, et al. The role of fear of movement in subacute whiplash-associated disorders grades I and II. Pain 2013;154:393–401.

40. Stenneberg M, Rood M, de Bie R, et al. To what degree does active cervical range of motion differ between patients with neck pain, patients with whiplash, and those without neck pain? A systematic review and meta-analysis. Arch Phys Med Rehabil 2017;98:1407–34.

41. Bishop M, Mintken P, Bialosky J, et al. Patient expectations of benefit from interventions for neck pain and resulting influence on outcomes. J Orthop Sports Phys Ther 2013;43:457–65.

42. Groeneweg R, Haanstra T, Bolman C, et al. Treatment success in neck pain: the added predictive value of psychosocial variables in addition to clinical variables. Scand J Pain 2017;14: 44–52.

43. Oka H, Matsudaira K, Fujii T, et al. Risk factors for prolonged treatment of whiplash-associated disorders. PLoS ONE 2015;10:e0132191.

44. Palmlöf L, Holm L, Alfredsson L, et al. Expectations of recovery: a prognostic factor in patients with neck pain undergoing manual therapy treatment. Eur J Pain 2016;20:1384–91.

45. Ozegovic D, Carroll L, Cassidy J. Factors associated with recovery expectations following vehicle collision: a population-based study. J Rehabil Med 2010;42:66–73.

46. Ozegovic D, Carroll L, Cassidy J. What influences positive return to work expectation? Examining associated factors in a population-based cohort of whiplash-associated disorders. Spine 2010;35:E708–13.

47. Altmaier E, Russell D, Kao C, et al. Role of self-efficacy in rehabilitation outcome among chronic low back pain patients. J Couns Psychol 1993;40:335–9.

48. Nicholas M. The pain self-efficacy questionnaire: taking pain into account. Eur J Pain 2007;11:153–63.

49. Söderlund A, Sandborgh M, Johansson A. Is self-efficacy and catastrophizing in pain-related disability mediated by control over pain and ability to decrease pain in whiplash-associated disorders? Physiother Theory Pract 2017;33:376–85.

50. Agnew L, Johnston V, Ludvigsson ML, et al. Factors associated with work ability in patients with chronic whiplash-associated disorder grade II-III: a cross-sectional analysis. J Rehabil Med 2015;47:546–51.

51. Gustavsson C, Bergström J, Denison E, et al. Predictive factors for disability outcome at twenty weeks and two years following a pain self-management group intervention in patients with persistent neck pain in primary health care. J Rehabil Med 2013;45:170–6.

52. Nolet P, Côté P, Kristman V, et al. Is neck pain associated with worse health-related quality of life 6 months later? A population-based cohort study. Spine J 2015;15:675–84.

53. Ailliet L, Rubinstein S, Hoekstra T, et al. Adding psychosocial factors does not improve predictive models for people with spinal pain enough to warrant extensive screening for them at baseline. Phys Ther 2016;96:1179–89.

54. Elbinoune I, Amine B, Shyen S, et al. Chronic neck pain and anxiety-depression: prevalence and associated risk factors. Pan Afr Med J 2016;24:89.

55. Ris I, Juul-Kristensen B, Boyle E, et al. Chronic neck pain patients with traumatic or non-traumatic onset: differences in characteristics. A cross-sectional study. Scand J Pain 2017;14: 1–8.

56. Ludvigsson M, Peterson G, Dedering A, et al. Factors associated with pain and disability reduction following exercise interventions in chronic whiplash. Eur J Pain 2016;20:307–15.

57. Michaleff Z, Maher C, Lin C, et al. Comprehensive physiotherapy exercise programme or advice for chronic whiplash (PROMISE): a pragmatic randomised controlled trial. Lancet 2014;384: 133–41.

58. Monticone M, Ambrosini E, Rocca B, et al. Group-based multimodal exercises integrated with cognitive-behavioural therapy improve disability, pain and quality of life of subjects with chronic neck pain: a randomized controlled trial with one-year follow-up. Clin Rehabil 2017;37:742–52.

59. O'Moore K, Newby J, Andrews G, et al. Internet cognitive behaviour therapy for depression in older adults with knee osteoarthritis: a randomized controlled trial. Arthritis Care Res 2018;70:61–70.

60. Gross A, Kaplan F, Huang S, et al. Psychological care, patient education, orthotics, ergonomics and prevention strategies for neck pain: a systematic overview update as part of the ICON Project. Open Orthop J 2013;7:530–61.

61. Markozannes G, Aretouli E, Rintou E, et al. An umbrella review of the literature on the effectiveness of psychological interventions for pain reduction. BMC Psychol 2017;5:31.

62. Monticone M, Ambrosini E, Cedraschi C, et al. Cognitive-behavioral treatment for subacute and chronic neck pain: a Cochrane Review. Spine 2015;40:1495–504.

63. Shearer H, Carroll L, Wong J, et al. Are psychological interventions effective for the management of neck pain and whiplash-associated disorders? A systematic review by the Ontario Protocol

for Traffic Injury Management (OPTIMa) Collaboration. Spine J 2016;16:1566–81.

64. Monticone M, Baiardi P, Vanti C, et al. Chronic neck pain and treatment of cognitive and behavioural factors: results of a randomised controlled clinical trial. Eur Spine J 2012;21:1558–66.

65. Thompson D, Oldham J, Woby S. Does adding cognitive-behavioural physiotherapy to exercise improve outcome in patients with chronic neck pain? A randomised controlled trial. Physiotherapy 2016;102:170–7.

66. Thompson D, Woby S. Acceptance in chronic neck pain: associations with disability and fear avoidance beliefs. Int J Rehabil Res 2017;40:220–6.

67. Vangronsveld K, Peters M, Goossens M, et al. The influence of fear of movement and pain catastrophizing on daily pain and disability in individuals with acute whiplash injury: a daily diary study. Pain 2008;139:449–57.

68. Thompson D, Woby S. The processes underpinning reductions in disability among people with chronic neck pain. A preliminary comparison between two distinct types of physiotherapy intervention. Disabil Rehabil 2018;40:779–83.

69. Côté P, van der Velde G, Cassidy J, et al. The burden and determinants of neck pain in workers: results of the Bone and Joint Decade 2000-2010 Task Force on Neck Pain and its Associated Disorders. Spine 2008;33:S60–74.

70. Tornqvist E, Hagberg M, Hagman M, et al. The influence of working conditions and individual factors on the incidence of neck and upper limb symptoms among professional computer users. Int Arch Occup Environ Health 2009;82:689–702.

71. Blatter B, Bongers P. Duration of computer use and mouse use in relation to musculoskeletal disorders of neck or upper limb. Int J Ind Ergon 2002;30:295–306.

72. Vos T, Barber R, Bell B, et al. Global, regional, and national incidence, prevalence, and years lived with disability for 301 acute and chronic diseases and injuries in 188 countries, 1990-2013: a systematic analysis for the Global Burden of Disease Study 2013. Lancet 2015;386:743–800.

73. Christensen J, Knardahl S. Work and neck pain: a prospective study of psychological, social, and mechanical risk factors. Pain 2010;151:162–73.

74. Dianat I, Karimi M. Musculoskeletal symptoms among handicraft workers engaged in hand sewing tasks. J Occup Health 2016;58:644–52.

75. Feng Q, Liu S, Yang L, et al. The prevalence of and risk factors associated with musculoskeletal disorders among sonographers in central China: a cross-sectional study. PLoS ONE 2016;11:e0163903.

76. Hanvold T, Wærsted M, Mengshoel A, et al. A longitudinal study on risk factors for neck and shoulder pain among young adults in the transition from technical school to working life. Scand J Work Environ Health 2014;40:597–609.

77. Simonsen J, Axmon A, Nordander C, et al. Neck and upper extremity pain in sonographers. Associations with occupational factors. Appl Ergon 2017;58:245–53.

78. Sterud T, Johannessen H, Tynes T. Work-related psychosocial and mechanical risk factors for neck/shoulder pain: a 3-year

follow-up study of the general working population in Norway. Int Arch Occup Environ Health 2014;87:471–81.

79. Al-Juhani MA-M, Khandekar R, Al-Harby M, et al. Neck and upper back pain among eye care professionals. Occup Med 2015;65:753–7.

80. Carroll LJ, Hogg-Johnson S, Cote P, et al. Course and prognostic factors for neck pain in workers - Results of the bone and joint decade 2000-2010 task force on neck pain and its associated disorders. Spine 2008;33:S93–100.

81. Jun D, Michaleff Z, Johnston V, et al. Physical risk factors for developing non-specific neck pain in office workers: a systematic review and meta-analysis. Int Arch Occup Environ Health 2017;90:373–410.

82. Park A, Zahiri H, Hallbeck M, et al. Intraoperative "Micro Breaks" with targeted stretching enhance surgeon physical function and mental focus: a multicenter cohort study. Ann Surg 2017;265:340–6.

83. Radanović B, Vučinić P, Janković T, et al. Musculoskeletal symptoms of the neck and shoulder among dental practitioners. J Back Musculoskelet Rehabil 2017;30:675–9.

84. Hush J, Michaleff Z, Maher C, et al. Individual, physical and psychological risk factors for neck pain in Australian office workers: a 1-year longitudinal study. Eur Spine J 2009;18:1532–40.

85. Christensen J, Knardahl S. Time-course of occupational psychological and social factors as predictors of new-onset and persistent neck pain: a three-wave prospective study over 4 years. Pain 2014;155:1262–71.

86. Yang H, Hitchcock E, Haldeman S, et al. Workplace psychosocial and organizational factors for neck pain in workers in the United States. Am J Ind Med 2016;59:549–60.

87. Fanavoll R, Nilsen T, Holtermann A, et al. Psychosocial work stress, leisure time physical exercise and the risk of chronic pain in the neck/shoulders: longitudinal data from the Norwegian HUNT Study. Int J Occup Med Environ Health 2016;29:585–95.

88. Leclerc A, Chastang J, Taiba R, et al. Musculoskeletal pain at various anatomical sites and socioeconomic position: results of a national survey. Rev Epidemiol Sante Publique 2016;64:331–9.

89. Schell E, Theorell T, Nilsson B, et al. Work health determinants in employees without sickness absence. Occup Med 2013;63:17–22.

90. van den Heuvel S, van der Beek A, Blatter B, et al. Psychosocial work characteristics in relation to neck and upper limb symptoms. Pain 2005;114:47–53.

91. Ostergren P, Hanson B, Balogh I, et al. Incidence of shoulder and neck pain in a working population: effect modification between mechanical and psychosocial exposures at work? Results from a one year follow up of the Malmo shoulder and neck study cohort. J Epidemiol Community Health 2005;59:721–8.

92. Huysmans M, Blatter B, van der Beek A. Perceived muscular tension predicts future neck-shoulder and arm-wrist-hand symptoms. Occup Environ Med 2012;69:261–7.

93. Paksaichol A, Lawsirirat C, Janwantanakul P. Contribution of biopsychosocial risk factors to nonspecific neck pain in office workers: a path analysis model. J Occup Health 2015;57:100–9.

94. Johnston V, Jull G, Darnell R, et al. Alterations in cervical muscle activity in functional and stressful tasks in female office workers with neck pain. Eur J Appl Physiol 2008;103:253–64.

95. Lindstrøm R, Schomacher J, Farina D, et al. Association between neck muscle coactivation, pain, and strength in women with neck pain. Man Ther 2011;16:80–6.

96. Mork R, Bruenech J, Thorud H. Effect of direct glare on orbicularis oculi and trapezius during computer reading. Optom Vis Sci 2016;93:738–49.

97. Richter H, Zetterlund C, Lundqvist L. Eye-neck interactions triggered by visually deficient computer work. Work 2011;39:67–78.

98. Zetterberg C, Forsman M, Richter H. Effects of visually demanding near work on trapezius muscle activity. J Electromyogr Kinesiol 2013;23:1190–8.

99. Cancelliere C, Donovan J, Stochkendahl M, et al. Factors affecting return to work after injury or illness: best evidence synthesis of systematic reviews. Chiropr Man Therap 2016;24:32.

100. Johnston V, Jimmieson NL, Jull G, et al. Quantitative sensory measures distinguish office workers with varying levels of neck pain and disability. Pain 2008;137:257–65.

101. Mankovsky-Arnold T, Wideman T, Thibault P, et al. Sensitivity to movement-evoked pain and multi-site pain are associated with work-disability following whiplash injury: a cross-sectional study. J Occup Rehabil 2017;27:413–21.

102. Christensen J, Johansen S, Knardahl S. Psychological predictors of change in the number of musculoskeletal pain sites among Norwegian employees: a prospective study. BMC Musculoskelet Disord 2017;18:140.

103. Johannessen H, Sterud T. Psychosocial factors at work and sleep problems: a longitudinal study of the general working population in Norway. Int Arch Occup Environ Health 2017;90:587–608.

104. Aili K, Nyman T, Hillert L, et al. Sleep disturbances predict future sickness absence among individuals with lower back or neck-shoulder pain: a 5-year prospective study. Scand J Public Health 2015;43:315–23.

105. Kovacs F, Seco J, Royuela A, et al. Patients with neck pain are less likely to improve if they experience poor sleep quality: a prospective study in routine practice. Clin J Pain 2015;31:713–21.

106. Paanalahti K, Wertli M, Held U, et al. Spinal pain–good sleep matters: a secondary analysis of a randomized controlled trial. Eur Spine J 2016;25:760–5.

107. Vänni K, Neupane S, Nygård C. An effort to assess the relation between productivity loss costs and presenteeism at work. Int J Occup Saf Ergon 2017;23:33–43.

108. Pereira M, Johnston V, Straker L, et al. An investigation of self-reported health-related productivity loss in office workers and associations with individual and work-related factors using an employer's perspective. J Occup Environ Med 2017;59:e138–44.

109. Rinaldo U, Selander J. Return to work after vocational rehabilitation for sick-listed workers with long-term back, neck and shoulder problems: a follow-up study of factors involved. Work 2016;55:115–31.

110. Ng E, Johnston V, Wibault J, et al. Factors associated with work ability in patients undergoing surgery for cervical radiculopathy. Spine 2015;40:1270–6.

111. Ahlstrom L, Dellve L, Hagberg M, et al. Women with neck pain on long-term sick leave-approaches used in the return to work process: a qualitative study. J Occup Rehabil 2017;27:92–105.

112. Marchand G, Myhre K, Leivseth G, et al. Change in pain, disability and influence of fear-avoidance in a work-focused intervention on neck and back pain: a randomized controlled trial. BMC Musculoskelet Disord 2015;16:94.

113. Myhre K, Marchand G, Leivseth G, et al. The effect of work-focused rehabilitation among patients with neck and back pain: a randomized controlled trial. Spine 2014;39:1999–2006.

114. Pedler A, Sterling M. Assessing fear-avoidance beliefs in patients with whiplash-associated disorders. A comparison of 2 measures. Clin J Pain 2011;27:502–7.

115. Smith A, Jull G, Schneider G, et al. Cervical radiofrequency neurotomy reduces central hyperexcitability and improves neck movement in individuals with chronic whiplash. Pain Med 2014;15:128–41.

Section 3

CLINICAL ASSESSMENT

This section on clinical assessment considers the interview and physical examination of patients with neck pain disorders and emphasizes the importance of skills in clinical reasoning. High level skills in clinical reasoning ensures an accurate interpretation of the patient's presenting disorder and is the basis for developing a relevant and comprehensive patient-centred management program.

Chapters within this section have also been devoted to the differential diagnosis of dizziness and sensorimotor control disturbances as well as the differential diagnosis of headache. These symptoms have multiple potential causes, one of which is a cervical musculoskeletal cause. Accurate examination is required to rule a cervical cause in or out so that patients receive relevant care for their disorders.

8

CLINICAL ASSESSMENT: THE PATIENT INTERVIEW

■ ■

Skill in clinical reasoning is one of the pillars for good clinical practice. It is a constant and ongoing process through all facets of the examination and patient management program. Clinical reasoning in the patient interview is an intricate process that requires integration of multiple features from many different perspectives. There are many layers of enquiry to gain an understanding of the patient, their needs and preferences, their neck pain disorder and how it is impacting on them personally and in their activities of daily living and work. Information is used to propose provisional diagnoses, to direct the physical examination, to establish patient-centred goals of treatment, to identify relevant outcome measures and to plan management.

The clinical reasoning process is now well imbedded in physiotherapy education and practice.[1] Research is continuing in various aspects of clinical reasoning from clinician[2,3] and patient management perspectives[4,5] and in different practice environments.[6] In this chapter, the elements of the clinical interview of a patient with a neck pain disorder will be outlined and desired outcomes of the interview will be discussed.

ELEMENTS OF THE PATIENT INTERVIEW

Patient-centred care is advocated as a best-practice model,[7] in which patients are involved in decisions about their care, and care is provided that respects and responds to their individual preferences, needs, beliefs and treatment goals. The elements of the patient interview begin to establish the patient-clinician relationship and provide a comprehensive understanding of the patient, their neck pain disorder, its impact on their work and quality of life, as well as diagnostic, physical examination and treatment directives. The reader is referred to established texts to review the structuring of questions.[1,8] Common models of clinical reasoning are hypothetico-deductive reasoning, pattern recognition and narrative reasoning.[1] These models are not mutually exclusive and a clinician could use parts of all three methods in their assessment. Whatever reasoning model(s) are used, there is some assurance "when the pattern fits" or, in other words, when the mechanism of onset fits with the nature of symptoms, when symptoms fit with the nature of physical or participation limitations, and ultimately when the pattern of symptoms and functional limitations fit with the findings of the physical examination. When the pattern fits, there is greater confidence in interpretation and in constructing a management program. When the pattern does not fit, the clinician should use hypothetico-deductive reasoning, reset and test new hypotheses and rethink the whole case to ensure an accurate understanding of the patient and their neck pain disorder.

OUTCOMES OF THE PATIENT INTERVIEW

There are several outcomes desired from the patient interview, and information gained about one feature often informs several outcomes (Box 8.1). For each outcome, examples will be given on how decisions are derived. Importantly, the patient interview directs the physical examination. The discussion is by no means exhaustive, rather the aim is to give some insight into the process.

The patient-clinician rapport and collaborative relationship

The clinical examination lays the basis for the therapeutic relationship between patient and clinician and the importance of this initial communication cannot be overestimated. Excellent communication is vital to the success of management. Although specific information is required about the patient's neck pain, the clinician should not dominate the interview.[9] Rather in the spirit of patient-centred care, clinicians should let the patient tell their story, listen attentively, clarify points and request more detail or specific information as required. Patients wish to be listened to, be understood and be assured that their neck pain is acknowledged or validated.[10] For instance, patients might rightfully perceive injustice if their neck symptoms are doubted following a whiplash injury.[11] They may feel that their pain and disability

has not been understood or acknowledged if the discord between their disabling neck pain and "normal" findings x-rays is not explained well. Likewise, statements such as: "Your pain is in your brain" can easily be misinterpreted leaving the patient quite distressed, thinking that the clinician feels their pain is "in their head".

Engaging with the patient, demonstrating empathy, interest and friendliness are important clinician attributes.[12] As the patient tells their story, the clinician must listen and interpret the meaning of the information towards making clinical decisions. When focusing on gaining specific information, the clinician must be mindful not to ignore or fail to respond to any concerns or fears that the patient may express.[13] Sensitivity to patients' concerns and needs works towards developing a successful collaborative relationship.

Musculoskeletal disorder recognition

Neck pain is a symptom of various origins. Even though musculoskeletal causes or "mechanical neck pain" is by far the most common, neck pain can also be a symptom of non-musculoskeletal sources. A primary outcome of the initial examination is to be assured that the patient is presenting with a musculoskeletal disorder. Even though presentations and pain syndromes may be complex in some patients, initial basic assurance can be gained if pain is felt in the posterior neck region (with or without spread to neighbouring areas) and symptoms have familiar patterns of being aggravated or eased with neck movements and postures. Likewise, a clear understanding of history of onset and its relation to adverse mechanical loading whether insidious onset (postures or activities) or trauma (minor or major) adds to the picture of a musculoskeletal disorder. Neck pain disorders are often recurrent, and it is important to understand the pattern or temporal behaviour of this recurrence and provocative features. There is usually a familiar pattern of exacerbations and remissions. The clinician needs to beware when histories of onset do not fit a familiar pattern. Thus in the patient interview, the clinician must listen for a history, presenting features and behaviours of symptoms that are consistent with a "mechanical" cervical musculoskeletal disorder.

Red flag recognition

Recognition of unusual histories, symptoms or symptom behaviours is essential to identify any potential "red flags" that may indicate either serious underlying musculoskeletal pathology (e.g., a fracture) or non-musculoskeletal pathologies. Fractures must be considered in cases of neck trauma especially in older persons or when there is a dangerous injuring mechanism and when neurological signs are present.[14] Red flag pathologies do occur in the cervical spine but are relatively rare. Nevertheless the cervical spine can be the site of primary tumours and metastases,[15,16] but these are not common in patients presenting primarily with posterior neck pain without other neurological or systemic symptoms.[17] Clinicians are very aware of the potentially devastating consequences of a vertebral or carotid arterial dissection. Recent onset, moderate to severe unusual headache or neck pain that is progressing, a history of transient neurological symptoms and recent exposure to infection or even minor head/neck trauma should alert the clinician to possible arterial dissection.[18,19] The neck can also be a site of referred visceral pain. Cardiac pain may be felt in the anterior neck region.[20] Immediate referral for medical investigation is mandatory when there is any indication or suspicion of serious underlying pathology and the pattern does not fit a musculoskeletal disorder.

Vertebral and ligament anomalies of the upper cervical spine are well documented in congenital conditions such as Down syndrome.[21] Children presenting with acute torticollis (wry neck) may require referral for radiology because imaging is necessary to confirm or rule out atlanto-axial rotary fixation.[22] Atlanto-axial rotary fixation is not common but can occur spontaneously after trivial trauma. It also might occur secondary to ligamentous laxity and inflammation following infection (e.g., tonsillitis) or head or neck surgery (e.g., adeno-tonsillectomy) (Grisel syndrome). Atlanto-axial rotary fixation is usually treated conservatively, but on occasions surgical fixation is required.[23]

Conditions requiring caution

Some neurological and rheumatological conditions do not negate physiotherapy management but require due care. As examples, cervical dystonia has many causes and is characterized by abnormal head posture, involuntary muscle contractions of the neck muscles (which causes abnormal movements) and awkward posture of the head and neck. Neck pain may be a feature. First-line treatment is usually botulinum toxin type A injections

but other methods (electromyography biofeedback training, muscular elongation, postural exercises and electrotherapy) can be helpful adjunct treatments.[24] Neck pain can present in inflammatory arthropathies, such as rheumatoid arthritis or ankylosing spondylitis.[25,26] Upper cervical involvement is not uncommon in rheumatoid arthritis and may result in atlanto-axial subluxation. Such conditions require that any treatment proceed with due safety.

Questions are also asked about the patient's general health, medications and any relevant surgical or medical history to seek any comorbidities or other considerations that require proper regard and care when management plans for the neck disorder are developed.

Provisional decision on pain mechanism(s)

The patient is asked to describe many aspects of their pain to provide information on its distribution, intensity and quality, how it reacts to movements and postures, its general pattern over 24 hours and history of onset. This information has several functions including an initial estimate of the pain severity and the possible regional source of pain (upper, mid, lower cervical region). An important interpretation relates to pain mechanisms (nociceptive, inflammatory, neuropathic, peripheral and central nervous system sensitization). Pain mechanisms (Chapter 2) inform assessment. For instance, the presence of severe pain and pain with associated central sensitization indicates caution in the physical examination because pain may be easily exacerbated. Central sensitization may occur in any condition. It is not uniquely associated with chronic pain and can be present in acute pain states.[27] It is more prevalent following trauma and is present in a small proportion of patients with whiplash-associated disorders (WAD) and in patients with cervical radiculopathy.[28] It is rarely found in patients with idiopathic neck pain.[29]

The clinician listens for pain descriptors and behaviours, which help to characterize each pain mechanism. Nociceptive pain is suspected with reports of local pain in the neck shoulder region (there may be referral into the arm and/or thorax), the pain in any 24 hours is intermittent or a continuous dull ache often interspersed with sharp pains. There is a typical mechanical pattern with movements and postures aggravating and easing symptoms.[30] Inflammatory pain is considered in association with nociceptive pain especially when there is pronounced or prolonged aching with or following activity.

Peripheral neuropathic pain is present in cervical radiculopathy. The pain is referred usually, but not always, into the arm in a dermatomal distribution. The quality is a sharp shooting pain or a burning pain, it is often relentless and difficult to obtain relief. There may be other sensations such as pins and needles or numbness.[31]

Peripheral and central nervous system sensitization is suspected when there is a wider spread of pain and allodynia and hyperalgesia (mechanical, thermal) are present. There is often marked pain sensitivity to movement and once pain is aggravated, it may take hours to subside.

Multiple mechanisms may be present simultaneously in a patient's neck pain disorder, for example, local neck pain on movement (nociceptive) in the presence of a cervical radiculopathy (neuropathic). Local nociceptive pain, neuropathic pain and central sensitization may present in patients with moderate to severe pain in both acute and chronic WAD.[27,32] In cervicogenic headache, there is nociception from local joint dysfunction (C0–1, C1–2 or C2–3) although it is thought that the headache reflects a rostral neuraxial spread of central sensitization to the trigeminocervical nucleus.[33]

Provisional decision on other symptoms

Sensorimotor disturbances

There is a variety of symptoms other than pain that may accompany neck pain disorders. These include symptoms of light headedness or dizziness, unsteadiness, visual disturbances and cognitive deficits such as decreased concentration. They are frequently associated with impaired cervical sensorimotor control when closely related to neck pain. Nevertheless, dizziness is a common symptom and can be associated with a mild brain injury in traumatic origin neck pain (motor vehicle crash, concussion in a sporting injury), a central or peripheral vestibular disorder or vascular disorders (such as vertebral artery insufficiency or cervical arterial dissection). The origins and differential diagnoses of these symptoms are explored in detail in Chapters 6 and 10. The clinician must carefully elicit the nature and behaviour of presenting symptoms to provisionally decide on their possible source as well as direct further physical examination.

Sleep

Fatigue is another symptom state and patients' sleep patterns should be explored routinely in questions concerning general wellbeing. The role of poor sleep is receiving extensive interest in relation to musculoskeletal pain states. There is evidence to indicate that persons with neck pain who report poor sleep quality are less likely to respond to treatment than those with good sleep quality.[34,35] Poor sleep quality may not only affect neck health but general health.[36] In patients with chronic neck pain receiving interventional pain management, greater levels of depression were linked with clinical insomnia.[37] If patients report problems with sleep, the relationship between poor sleep quality and neck pain needs to be explored because neck pain may be contributing to interruption of sleep or conversely a sleep disorder may be adversely affecting the neck pain condition. Improving sleep should become an important aspect of overall patient management and referral to an appropriate specialist may be required especially if the patient has a primary sleep disorder.

Knowledge of physical provocative factors and functional limitations

Understanding which movements, postures or activities aggravate as well as ease symptoms informs on several factors. One, as mentioned, is pain mechanisms, another is which movement directions, forces or loads are not being tolerated by the structures of the cervical region. A third is to inform on meaningful outcomes by which the impact of interventions can be determined. Box 8.2 gives examples of provocative factors and possible interpretations, which in turn begin to direct the physical examination and what findings might be expected. If the expected findings are confirmed in the physical examination, then clinical reasoning is accurate and importantly, "the pattern fits". It is of equal value to understand what postures, movements and activities ease symptoms. This information can contribute to physical diagnosis and provides material to help patients problem solve on neck care.

The history should provide a clear understanding of movements, functional activities and work practices that might be possible sources of adverse strains contributing to the development of the neck pain disorder.[38] Health care is often reactive and the focus is on the acute episode rather than being concerned with the

BOX 8.2
POSSIBLE INTERPRETATIONS OF PROVOCATIVE FACTOR

1. Neck pain when looking down reading or using a device for a prolonged period
   - adverse strain on posterior elements, compression of anterior elements
   - neck extensor endurance inadequate for the task
2. Catching pain, suboccipital region on quick turning, (e.g., driving)
   - C1–2 dysfunction
   - poor movement sense
3. Neck pain and later headache develops with prolonged computer use
   - adverse loading and dysfunction upper cervical joints
   - poor control of posture
   - poor endurance of deep neck flexors
   - poor scapular muscle control
4. Looking up causes neck pain and light headedness, unsteadiness
   - upper cervical joint dysfunction
   - poor control and strength of neck flexors
   - poor sensorimotor function – proprioception, balance
   - rule out Vertebrobasilar insufficiency (VBI)
5. Carrying bags of groceries increases neck pain
   - excessive compressive loads on cervical joints
   - poor scapular muscle control
   - poor neck flexor and extensor control
   - adverse load on the brachial plexus
6. Neck and arm pain on reaching backwards
   - adverse strain on neural tissues
   - adverse loading on cervical joints
   - adverse strain on glenohumeral joint

bigger picture. The bigger picture is that neck pain is a recurrent disorder and perpetuation of any adverse strains from work or recreational postures and practices must be addressed if there is any possibility to lessen recurrences and slow progression of the neck disorder. An important management outcome will be to successfully reduce adverse strains and achieve more suitable work or recreational practices towards a concerted and comprehensive rehabilitation effort to manage the disorder in the long term.

The clinician must not only understand which features aggravate neck pain but have a full appreciation of the impact of the condition on a patient's participation in work, activities of daily living and recreation.

Has the patient withdrawn, reduced or modified their work or general activities as a result of their neck pain disorder? Likewise, what are their expectations regarding return to former participation levels? Both the clinician and the patient should discuss whether expectations are a realistic outcome goal.

Knowledge of psychological or social moderators

There are several emotions that may be associated with a neck pain disorder. Listening to the patient is important as what a clinician believes will be psychological features/concerns does not always match the patient's actual concerns.[39] Clinicians must be mindful that many emotions are normal and reasonable behaviours for a person who is experiencing a neck pain disorder, especially in the early stages. "Pathologizing" patient's emotions must be avoided.[40] Labelling normal behaviours as maladaptive can be harmful for the patient and counterproductive to good rehabilitation.[41]

There are abundant psychological questionnaires available to provide indications of various emotional states. They have been used extensively in research to better understand the moderating role of psychological features on treatment effectiveness and prognosis. Nevertheless, the extensive use of these questionnaires in clinical trials and prognostic studies should not be misunderstood as endorsing their routine use in everyday clinical practice. Rather, psychological questionnaires should be used judiciously, and not routinely especially in initial consultations. The clinician should carefully consider if and when their use is indicated as well as the timing of their use. Psychological questionnaires have limitations and are not diagnostic. Inappropriate use and interpretation of questionnaires can lead to a poor service for the patient.[40,41]

Some patients may have unhelpful emotions and beliefs that can hinder/moderate their recovery from the neck pain disorder but better therapeutic alliances are likely to result if the clinician focusses on listening to and understanding the patient, their condition and their beliefs in the first instance.[41] Hearing how the patient describes their condition, if they are guarding their necks, how neck pain is affecting their work, how they are coping at work and home as well as asking questions about any concerns, their expectancies of treatments and outcome goals provides the clinician with an initial sound insight into patient's anxieties, fears, mood and coping skills. Initial patient management can be designed and implemented on this knowledge. In addition, when patients consult a clinician for treatment of their neck pain, they have an expectation of receiving advice, hands-on physical examination and treatment and exercise, that is, physical therapies. If, with this expectation, patients are suddenly confronted with questionnaires probing them about their psychological state, they may well react with thoughts of: "I have come to have my neck treated, not my head". Therapeutic relationships can be irrevocably harmed, and patients may not be assured that their neck pain is acknowledged.[10]

If at a later stage in treatment, patients are not progressing as expected and the clinician is concerned that psychological features such as depression, an anxiety state, posttraumatic stress or a personal trait are adversely moderating symptoms and hindering recovery, the clinician can explain their concerns to the patient and, in context, ask them to complete a relevant questionnaire to allay or confirm the clinician's concerns. This lays a cooperative basis for managing emotional features that might influence recovery, with the help of the clinician or other appropriate practitioner.

Provisional diagnosis

Patients desire a diagnosis so they understand "what is wrong" with their neck, and clinicians require a diagnosis to implement an appropriate treatment program. Physiotherapists make a diagnosis based on presenting symptoms, functional limitations, movement dysfunctions and pathophysiological processes to direct their management (i.e., pain mechanisms, impaired kinematics, impaired neuromuscular and sensorimotor control).

Pathological or pathoanatomic diagnoses are discouraged in many quarters, but this "blanket ban" could be questioned. The terms *nonspecific neck pain* or *nonspecific low-back pain* have been adopted to express a limited understanding of the pathological source of pain in a patient presenting with spinal pain especially because radiological imaging often cannot identify a lesion of proven relevance, and clinical tests are not sensitive or specific enough to define a pathoanatomic lesion. The adoption of the biopsychosocial model may have suppressed research in investigations into pathology as an important component of the spinal pain experience;[42]

as possibly, have opinions that peripheral nociception automatically ceases after the usual time for tissue healing has passed. Indeed, there have been increasing calls to put the "bio" back into the biopsychosocial model in both neck pain and low-back pain.[42–44]

Pathological processes do occur in particular anatomic structures in the generation of neck pain as noted in painful extremity disorders. Lesions in discs, zygapophysial joints, ligaments and bone can result from injury.[45] Some research is proceeding to understand the relationships between structural change and neck pain.[46,47] Medical interventional management, whether surgery or radiofrequency neurotomies, relies on accurately identifying the anatomic source of symptoms. Surgery relies on a clinical presentation which is complemented by radiological identification of pathoanatomy such as lateral canal stenosis from a disc fragment or osteophyte. Neither plain x-rays nor clinical tests can identify lesser pathologies, but clinical examination methods can reliably detect a segmental source of symptoms when present. The flexion rotation test has proven validity to identify C1–2 segmental dysfunction.[48,49] Manual examination can identify a symptomatic zygapophysial joint and its accuracy has been proven against anaesthetic blocks.[50–52] Manual examination may also be able to determine painful central joint (discal) dysfunction when present, but this has not been tested because there is no gold standard on which it can be judged.

Clinical tests cannot provide a pathoanatomic diagnosis but an argument can be put for the value of a basic segmental diagnosis to complement the physical diagnosis of pathophysiological mechanisms. A clinical examination of the cervical region, which includes a skilled manual examination, can provide at the least a basic diagnosis of painful facet (zygapophysial) joint dysfunction or possibly central joint (discal) dysfunction as relevant. This is valuable from several perspectives. First, it can direct local active and passive management techniques and guide advice on management. Second, manual examination can assist to determine pain processes (e.g., the presence or not of a peripheral nociceptive source of pain). Third, it can inform on the extent to which the cervical spine is involved in complaints such as headache and dizziness by determining the presence or not of cervical segmental dysfunction and if present, matching the severity of the symptoms with the degree of dysfunction (i.e., does the pattern fit). Fourth, the manual skill to examine the neck and accurately identify the symptomatic segment is invaluable in cost-effective diagnostic screening for anaesthetic blocks or radiofrequency neurotomies for cervical zygapophysial pain.[53,54] Fifth, patients desire a diagnosis, and nonspecific neck pain is an unsatisfactory label and does not necessarily validate their neck pain with some form of tangible evidence.[10] Eliciting symptomatic joint dysfunction with manual examination effectively serves this purpose and provides a very basic diagnosis that the clinician can discuss with the patient.

Prognostic features

Prognosis is a key component of clinical decision making. Knowing which features indicate a good, fair or poor prognosis helps in understanding the possible course of a patient's complaint. It may also help in deciding who requires more in-depth investigations and targeted intervention in the early stages to potentially influence prognosis and prevent a transition to a recurrent or persistent pain state. Knowledge of features consistently indicating a good, fair or poor prognosis is far from absolute. Many features have been researched and at this stage many of the predictors identified have low or very low confidence or have inconclusive predictive value. More research is required to confirm or discard them as important features.[55] Perhaps not unexpectedly, different features are nominated depending on whether occupational neck pain, whiplash-induced neck pain or nontraumatic neck pain is being investigated.[55–60]

There is little evidence as yet of the benefits of making decisions about management of neck pain based on prognostic indicators. A challenge is that many prognostic features are not modifiable, for instance, being female or having a previous history of neck pain.[58,61] High initial neck pain intensity and high disability are two factors with high confidence to foreshadow a poor prognosis. Yet at present, there is a lack of evidence and consensus on effective pharmacological management of severe musculoskeletal pain. Likewise, every person with high initial pain intensity does not have a poor prognosis, some recover well as we have identified in our clinical trials.[62]

Prognostic studies are important, and more research is required to document features in which there can be strong confidence. Likewise, research is necessary to determine any benefit of targeted intervention based on prognostic features that might help meet the great challenge of preventing transition from an acute state to a recurrent or persistent pain state.

TREATMENT GOALS AND OUTCOME MEASURES

Goal setting is an important component of patient-centred care.[63,64] Active engagement of the patient in goal setting and management planning is considered to promote compliance and to facilitate ongoing self-management or maintenance programs, which is so important with the recurrent nature of neck pain disorders.[65] Goal setting takes place initially after the patient interview and physical examination. A helpful outcome measure that can be an initial basis for discussing goal setting is the Patient Specific Functional Scale (PSFS) where the patient nominates and rates the functions with which they are having difficulty.[66] The scale can be used to set and evaluate progress in achieving goal. Goals should focus on activity and participation and it is often helpful to set and attain progressive goals to reach a desired outcome.

In tandem, a clear set of outcomes should be established at the conclusion of the interview that will capture, as relevant to the individual patient and their goals, changes in symptoms, physical functioning, psychological functioning as well as work and social participation. There are several well-established measures that the clinician can use, including measures of pain intensity (numerical rating scale), the PSFS,[66] the Neck Disability Index[67] and a less used, but region-specific questionnaire, the Pictorial Fear of Activity Scale-Cervical.[68] Other outcomes and goals depend on patient circumstances and could be, for instance, related to dizziness severity and its impact on function (Dizziness Handicap Inventory),[69] fatigue, posttraumatic stress symptoms, return to customary participation levels or return to work. Carroll and colleagues[70] confirmed the value of a simple single outcome question: "How well are you recovering?" to obtain a brief overall assessment of recovery especially of patients with longer recovery periods as with some persons with WAD. Recovery was rated using six response options from "all better" to "getting much worse". Outcome measures must be as patient specific as possible and capable of measuring relevant clinical change.

CONCLUSION

An effective and quality patient interview fulfils several principal functions. It begins to establish the important patient-clinician relationship. It allows the patient to tell their story and express any concerns. It provides the clinician with a comprehensive understanding of the patient and the neck pain disorder on which they can plan the physical examination as well as begin to plan management strategies. The patient and clinician, as part of this initial communication, should be beginning to discuss expectancies and goals of management to have a clear pathway of rehabilitation.

REFERENCES

1. Jones M, Rivett D, editors. Clinical reasoning in musculoskeletal practice. 2nd ed. London: Elsevier; 2018.
2. Chowdhury A, Bjorbækmo W. Clinical reasoning-embodied meaning-making in physiotherapy. Physiother Theory Pract 2017;33:550–9.
3. Langridge N, Roberts L, Pope C. The role of clinician emotion in clinical reasoning: balancing the analytical process. Man Ther 2016;21:277–81.
4. Elvén M, Hochwälder J, Dean E, et al. A clinical reasoning model focused on clients' behaviour change with reference to physiotherapists: its multiphase development and validation. Physiother Theory Pract 2015;31:231–43.
5. Jones L, O'Shaughnessy D. The pain and movement reasoning model: introduction to a simple tool for integrated pain assessment. Man Ther 2014;19:270–6.
6. Langridge N, Roberts L, Pope C. The clinical reasoning processes of extended scope physiotherapists assessing patients with low back pain. Man Ther 2015;20:745–50.
7. Committee on Quality of Health Care in America. Institute of Medicine. Crossing the quality chasm: a new health system for the 21st century. Washington, DC: National Academy Press; 2001.
8. Hengeveld E, Banks K. Maitland's vertebral manipulation: management of neuromusculoskeletal disorders. 8th ed. UK: Churchill Livingstone, Elsevier; 2013.
9. Hiller A, Guillemin M, Delany C. Exploring healthcare communication models in private physiotherapy practice. Patient Educ Couns 2015;98:1222–8.
10. MacDermid J, Walton D, Miller J, et al. What is the experience of receiving health care for neck pain? Open Orthop J 2013;7(Suppl. 4: M5):428–39.
11. Sullivan M, Adams H, Martel M, et al. Catastrophizing and perceived injustice: risk factors for the transition to chronicity after whiplash injury. Spine 2011;36:S244–9.
12. O'Keeffe M, Cullinane P, Hurley J, et al. What influences patient-therapist interactions in musculoskeletal physical therapy? Qualitative systematic review and meta-synthesis. Phys Ther 2016;96:609–22.
13. Josephson I, Woodward-Kron R, Delany C, et al. Evaluative language in physiotherapy practice: how does it contribute to the therapeutic relationship? Soc Sci Med 2015;143:128–36.
14. Stiell I, Clement C, McKnight D, et al. The Canadian C-Spine Rule versus the NEXUS low-risk criteria in patients with trauma. N Engl J Med 2003;349:2510–18.
15. Katsuura Y, Cason G, Osborn J. Rare cause of neck pain: tumours of the posterior elements of the cervical spine. BMJ Case Rep 2016 in press.
16. Luksanapruksa P, Buchowski J, Wright N, et al. Outcomes and effectiveness of posterior occipitocervical fusion for suboccipital spinal metastases. J Neurosurg Spine 2017;26:554–9.
17. Bogduk N. Regional musculoskeletal pain. The neck. Baillière's best practice & research. Clin Rheumatol 1999;13:261–85.
18. Cassidy J, Boyle E, Côté P, et al. Risk of carotid stroke after chiropractic care: a population-based case-crossover study. J Stroke Cerebrovasc Dis 2017;26:842–50.
19. Thomas L. Cervical arterial dissection: an overview and implications for manipulative therapy practice. Man Ther 2016;21:2–9.
20. Bakhshi M, Rezaei R, Baharvand M, et al. Frequency of craniofacial pain in patients with ischemic heart disease. J Clin Exp Dent 2017;9:e91–5.
21. Dlouhy B, Policeni B, Menezes A. Reduction of atlantoaxial dislocation prevented by pathological position of the transverse ligament in fixed, irreducible os odontoideum: operative illustrations and radiographic correlates in 41 patients. J Neurosurg Spine 2017;27:20–8.
22. Roche C, O'Malley M, Dorgan J, et al. A pictorial review of atlanto-axial rotatory fixation: key points for the radiologist. Clin Radiol 2001;56:947–58.
23. Morales L, Alvarado F, Corredor J, et al. Bilateral C1 laminar hooks combined with C2 pedicle screw fixation in the treatment of atlantoaxial subluxation after Grisel syndrome. Spine J 2016;16:e755–60.
24. De Pauw J, Van der Velden K, Meirte J, et al. The effectiveness of physiotherapy for cervical dystonia: a systematic literature review. J Neurol 2014;261:1857–65.
25. Holden W, Taylor Stephens H, et al. Neck pain is a major clinical problem in ankylosing spondylitis, and impacts on driving and safety. Scand J Rheumatol 2005;34:159–60.
26. Kim D, Hilibrand A. Rheumatoid arthritis in the cervical spine. J Am Acad Orthop Surg 2005;13:463–74.
27. Sterling M, Jull G, Vicenzino B, et al. Sensory hypersensitivity occurs soon after whiplash injury and is associated with poor recovery. Pain 2003;104:509–17.
28. Chien A, Eliav E, Sterling M. Whiplash (grade II) and cervical radi5culopathy share a similar sensory presentation: an investigation using quantitative sensory testing. Clin J Pain 2008;24:595–603.
29. Malfliet A, Kregel J, Cagnie B, et al. Lack of evidence for central sensitization in idiopathic, non-traumatic neck pain: a systematic review. Pain Physician 2015;18:223–36.

30. Smart K, Blake C, Staines A, et al. Mechanisms-based classifications of musculoskeletal pain: part 3 of 3: symptoms and signs of nociceptive pain in patients with low back (± leg) pain. Man Ther 2012;17:352–7.

31. Smart K, Blake C, Staines A, et al. Mechanisms-based classifications of musculoskeletal pain: part 2 of 3: symptoms and signs of peripheral neuropathic pain in patients with low back (± leg) pain. Man Ther 2012;17:345–51.

32. Smith A, Jull G, Schneider G, et al. Cervical radiofrequency neurotomy reduces central hyperexcitability and improves neck movement in individuals with chronic whiplash. Pain Med 2014;15:128–41.

33. Chua N, van Suijlekom H, Vissers K, et al. Differences in sensory processing between chronic cervical zygapophysial joint pain patients with and without cervicogenic headache. Cephalalgia 2011;31:953–63.

34. Kovacs F, Seco J, Royuela A, et al. Patients with neck pain are less likely to improve if they experience poor sleep quality: a prospective study in routine practice. Clin J Pain 2015;31:713–21.

35. Paanalahti K, Wertli M, Held U, et al. Spinal pain-good sleep matters: a secondary analysis of a randomized controlled trial. Eur Spine J 2016;25:760–5.

36. Aili K, Nyman T, Hillert L, et al. Sleep disturbances predict future sickness absence among individuals with lower back or neck-shoulder pain: a 5-year prospective study. Scand J Public Health 2015;43:315–23.

37. Kim S, Lee D, Yoon K, et al. Factors associated with increased risk for clinical insomnia in patients with chronic neck pain. Pain Physician 2015;18:593–8.

38. Hanvold T, Wærsted M, Mengshoel A, et al. A longitudinal study on risk factors for neck and shoulder pain among young adults in the transition from technical school to working life. Scand J Work Environ Health 2014;40:597–609.

39. van Randeraad-van der Zee CH, Beurskens A, Swinkels R, et al. The burden of neck pain: its meaning for persons with neck pain and healthcare providers, explored by concept mapping. Qual Life Res 2016;25:1219–25.

40. Maujean A, Sterling M. 'De-pathologising' the psychological responses to injury and pain. Musculoskelet Sci Pract 2017;30:vii–viii.

41. Stewart J, Kempenaar L, Lauchlan D. Rethinking yellow flags. Man Ther 2011;16:196–8.

42. Hancock M, Maher C, Laslett M, et al. Discussion paper: what happened to the "bio" in the bio-psycho-social model of low back pain? Eur Spine J 2011;20:2105–10.

43. Petersen T, Laslett M, Juhl C. Clinical classification in low back pain: best-evidence diagnostic rules based on systematic reviews. BMC Musculoskelet Disord 2017;18:188.

44. Sterling M. Balancing the 'bio' with the psychosocial in whiplash associated disorders. Man Ther 2006;11:180–1.

45. Taylor J. The Cervical Spine. An atlas of normal anatomy and the morbid anatomy of ageing and injuries. Australia: Elsevier; 2017.

46. Farrell S, Osmotherly P, Cornwall J, et al. Morphology of cervical spine meniscoids in individuals with chronic whiplash-associated disorder: a case-control study. J Orthop Sports Phys Ther 2016;46:902–10.

47. Farrell S, Osmotherly P, Cornwall J, et al. Cervical spine meniscoids: an update on their morphological characteristics and potential clinical significance. Eur Spine J 2017;26:939–47.

48. Hall T, Briffa K, Hopper D, et al. Comparative analysis and diagnostic accuracy of the cervical flexion-rotation test. J Headache Pain 2010;11:391–7.

49. Takasaki H, Hall T, Oshiro S, et al. Normal kinematics of the upper cervical spine during the Flexion-Rotation Test - In vivo measurements using magnetic resonance imaging. Man Ther 2011;16:167–71.

50. Jull G, Bogduk N, Marsland A. The accuracy of manual diagnosis for cervical zygapophysial joint pain syndromes. Med J Aust 1988;148:233–6.

51. Phillips D, Twomey L. A comparison of manual diagnosis with a diagnosis established by a uni-level lumbar spinal block procedure. Man Ther 1996;1:82–7.

52. Schneider G, Jull G, Thomas K, et al. Intrarater and interrater reliability for select clinical tests in patients referred for diagnostic facet joint blocks in the cervical spine. Arch Phys Med Rehabil 2013;94:1628–34.

53. Rabey M, Hall T, Hebron C, et al. Reconceptualising manual therapy skills in contemporary practice. Musculoskelet Sci Pract 2017;29:28–32.

54. Schneider G, Jull G, Thomas K, et al. Derivation of a clinical decision guide in the diagnosis of cervical facet joint pain. Arch Phys Med Rehabil 2014;95:1695–701.

55. Walton D, Carroll L, Kasch H, et al. An overview of systematic reviews on prognostic factors in neck pain: results from the International Collaboration on Neck Pain (ICON) Project. Open Orthop J 2013;7(Suppl. 4: M9):494–505.

56. Bruls V, Bastiaenen C, Bie RD. Prognostic factors of complaints of arm, neck, and/or shoulder: a systematic review of prospective cohort studies. Pain 2015;156:765–88.

57. Jun D, Michaleff Z, Johnston V, et al. Physical risk factors for developing non-specific neck pain in office workers: a systematic review and meta-analysis. Int Arch Occup Environ Health 2017;90:373–410.

58. Paksaichol A, Janwantanakul P, Purepong N, et al. Office workers' risk factors for the development of non-specific neck pain: a systematic review of prospective cohort studies. Occup Environ Med 2012;69:610–18.

59. Sterud T, Johannessen H, Tynes T. Work-related psychosocial and mechanical risk factors for neck/shoulder pain: a 3-year follow-up study of the general working population in Norway. Int Arch Occup Environ Health 2014;87:471–81.

60. Walton D, Macdermid J, Giorgianni A, et al. Risk factors for persistent problems following acute whiplash injury: update of a systematic review and meta-analysis. J Orthop Sports Phys Ther 2013;43:31–43.

61. Nolet P, Côté P, Cassidy J, et al. The association between a lifetime history of a work-related neck injury and future neck pain: a population based cohort study. J Manipulative Physiol Ther 2011;34:348–55.

62. Jull G, Kenardy J, Hendrikz J, et al. Management of acute whiplash: a randomized controlled trial of multidisciplinary stratified treatments. Pain 2013;154:1798–806.

63. Stevens A, Köke A, van der Weijden T, et al. The development of a patient-specific method for physiotherapy goal setting: a user-centered design. Disabil Rehabil 2017;17:618.

64. Stevens A, Moser A, Köke A, et al. The use and perceived usefulness of a patient-specific measurement instrument in physiotherapy goal setting. A qualitative study. Musculoskelet Sci Pract 2017;27:23–31.

65. Lenzen S, Daniels R, Bokhoven MV, et al. Setting goals in chronic care: shared decision making as self-management support by the family physician. Eur J Gen Pract 2015;21:138–44.

66. Westaway MD, Stratford PW, Blinkley JM. The patient-specific functional scale: validation of its use in persons with neck dysfunction. J Orthop Sports Phys Ther 1998;27:331–8.

67. Vernon H. The Neck Disability Index: patient assessment and outcome monitoring in whiplash. J Musculskel Pain 1996;4:95–104.

68. Turk D, Robinson J, Sherman J, et al. Assessing fear in patients with cervical pain: development and validation of the Pictorial Fear of Activity Scale-Cervical (PFActS-C). Pain 2008;139:55–62.

69. Tesio L, Alpini D, Cesarani A, et al. Short form of the dizziness handicap inventory. Am J Phys Med Rehabil 1999;78:233–41.

70. Carroll L, Jones D, Ozegovic D, et al. How well are you recovering? The association between a simple question about recovery and patient reports of pain intensity and pain disability in whiplash-associated disorders. Disabil Rehabil 2012;34:45–52.

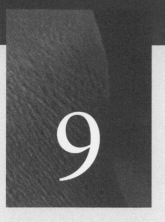

9 CLINICAL ASSESSMENT: PHYSICAL EXAMINATION

The physical examination of the patient with a neck pain disorder includes a local and regional examination. There is an interdependency in posture and motion between the different regions of the cervical spine, as well as between the cervical, thoracic, craniomandibular and shoulder girdle regions.

The clinical reasoning process continues in the physical examination. The hypotheses formed from the patient interview are tested and are either accepted or rejected and reformulated. The desired outcomes of the physical examination are: (1) a physical diagnosis that identifies the source of symptoms, confirms pain mechanisms and defines associated impairments in the sensory, articular, nervous, neuromuscular and sensorimotor systems; (2) a functional diagnosis which defines how postures, movement and activity immediately aggravate or relieve neck pain; (3) a practical understanding of how work practices, the work environment, sport or functional activity could be contributing to the disorder; (4) clear directions for the development of a management program, (5) a suite of appropriate outcome measures on which to evaluate and progress treatment.

Sound clinical reasoning throughout the physical examination is paramount for good decision making. Normal variations from an ideal posture are common and there is variability in cervical range of movement and muscle strength between healthy individuals. Thus the relevance of findings to the patient's neck pain condition must always be considered. An indicator of relevance that is commonly used is "reproduction of the patient's pain" on a particular test. At a deeper level, relevance is evident when a clear pattern emerges between the patient's presenting complaint, the aggravating features and findings from the physical examination. No decision can or should be made on single or isolated findings. Presentation of a single, isolated impairment is not the nature of musculoskeletal disorders. The questions: "Is a pattern present?" or "Does the pattern fit?" should be foremost in the clinician's thoughts.

The physical examination is a continual process of evaluation, intervention, reevaluation and reflection.[1] Patient-centred outcome measures such as estimates of symptom change on a numeric rating scale or changes in scores on the Patient Specific Functional Scale[2,3] are important and relevant. However, symptom resolution does not mean that the impairments contributing to those symptoms have resolved automatically.[4-6] It is essential to derive a suite of outcome measures from the physical examination relevant to patients' symptoms and functional complaints, when aims of management are not just symptom relief but to rehabilitate the person's neck pain disorder. Such a suite of outcome measures also directs treatment progression and dosage, as well as providing target goals for the patient, which can offer incentives for compliance with self-management programs.

On the theme of incentives for compliance with self-management, the physical examination is an excellent opportunity for patient education. Demonstrating the link between symptoms and functional complaints, such as a poor posture, altered movement or muscle function, is a powerful tool in helping the patient both understand their condition and the treatment rationale. Showing how a change in a static or functional posture can decrease their neck pain is a convincing lesson. It provides the basis for a change in behaviour (e.g., how they sit or work) as well as highlighting the need for their participation in a self-management program to address the features that may be contributing, or perpetuating, to their neck pain.

In this chapter, we present a comprehensive physical examination of the cervical region, which considers postural analysis and examination of articular, nervous, neuromuscular and sensorimotor systems as well as consideration of adjacent regions as necessary. An order for testing is suggested (Table 9.1). It avoids excess positional changes for the patient and importantly, it facilitates understanding of how findings of different elements may interact. The examination will be presented in this order, but the order can be changed depending on the patient's presentation and the clinician's line of reasoning. Although the examination proforma is comprehensive, in practice, the information gained from the patient interview should guide the direction of the physical examination. Not all tests are relevant or necessary for all patients. Clinicians should prioritize examination procedures as part of the clinical reasoning process, matching the physical examination to the patient's complaint and most importantly, then matching the examination findings to a meaningful management approach. Case examples are presented in Chapter 18 to demonstrate this process.

ANALYSIS OF PROVOCATIVE MOVEMENT OR POSTURE

One of the most patient-centred and relevant analyses in the physical examination is the analysis of the posture, movement or activity that the patient reports is provocative of their symptoms. Such an analysis often reveals the heart of the problem and leads the clinician to other tests. Fig. 9.1 presents examples of a possible analysis of a patient's provocative activity and illustrates initial clinical reasoning in the physical examination, including first thoughts on possible management options. This analysis often guides the direction of further examination, making it relevant to the patient's presentation. Placing first priority on the analysis of the patient's nominated provocative activity is not only a crucial examination strategy, but it also assures the patient that the clinician is listening and hearing their concerns and

TABLE 9.1

Scheme for a comprehensive examination of the cervical region

Position	Assessment
Standing, sitting	Patient reported provocative movement or posture Postural analysis

Sitting	Postural analysis
	Analysis of active range of motion
	  Assessment of cardinal planes of motion
	  Movement speed and velocity profile
	  Movement tests to further direct management
	  Movement diagnostic tests
	Positional tests for vertebral artery insufficiency

Supine	Sensory testing and pain mechanisms
	Examination of the nervous system
	  Clinical neurological examination
	  Tests of nerve tissue mechanosensitivity
	  Nerve palpation
	Manual examination
	  Passive physiological intervertebral movements
	Craniocervical ligament tests

Prone	Manual examination
	  Posteroanterior glides
	Muscle tests
	  Scapular muscle tests

Supine	Scapular muscle tests Craniocervical flexion test Neck flexor strength and endurance
Four-point kneeling	Neck extensor tests Neck extensor strength and endurance

Sensorimotor tests	Cervical position and movement sense
	  Cervical position sense
	  Cervical movement sense
	Standing balance
	Oculomotor assessment
	  Gaze stability
	  Eye follow: smooth pursuit neck torsion
	Eye-head coordination; trunk-head coordination

giving them significance in examination and management. The patient's nominated activity also becomes an outcome measure.

ANALYSIS OF POSTURE

The forward head posture (FHP) has traditionally received attention as the adverse postural position in

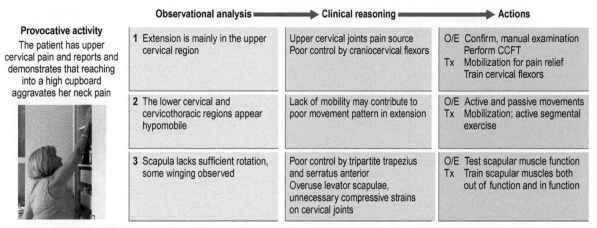

Provocative activity	Observational analysis ➡	Clinical reasoning ➡	Actions
The patient has upper cervical pain and reports and demonstrates that reaching into a high cupboard aggravates her neck pain	**1** Extension is mainly in the upper cervical region	Upper cervical joints pain source Poor control by craniocervical flexors	O/E Confirm, manual examination Perform CCFT Tx Mobilization for pain relief Train cervical flexors
	2 The lower cervical and cervicothoracic regions appear hypomobile	Lack of mobility may contribute to poor movement pattern in extension	O/E Active and passive movements Tx Mobilization; active segmental exercise
	3 Scapula lacks sufficient rotation, some winging observed	Poor control by tripartite trapezius and serratus anterior Overuse levator scapulae, unnecessary compressive strains on cervical joints	O/E Test scapular muscle function Tx Train scapular muscles both out of function and in function

Fig. 9.1 ■ Example of clinical reasoning of a patient's provocative activity. *CCFT*, Craniocervical flexion test; *O/E*, on examination; *Tx*, treatment.

neck pain disorders. The FHP places the upper cervical spine in extension and flexes the lower cervical region. In tandem, modelling has confirmed that a FHP is associated with shortness of the suboccipital extensors and lengthening of the longus capitis, multifidus and semispinalis cervicis.[7] The FHP is usually associated with a greater thoracic or cervicothoracic kyphosis[8,9] and reduced cervical range of motion.[9,10] However, not all patients with neck pain disorders have a FHP and the strength of its association is debatable.[8,11–13] Although initial observation of posture may be undertaken in standing, it is important that the head and neck posture is assessed in sitting, particularly when patients nominate activities in sitting as aggravating their disorder. People without a FHP in standing often display a FHP when sitting.[14] The adoption of a FHP in sitting seems to be the major problem as verified in several studies of neck pain patients undertaking computer work.[14–17] Pertinently, a slouched FHP is associated with higher neck extensor activity (and load on cervical structures).[18] As a positive point, rehabilitation of a patient's habitual FHP posture has a better chance of success than trying to change a fixed or structural posture.

Other postures may be problematic. The head flexed posture has likewise been associated with neck pain especially in this era of technology with prolific use of various mobile handheld devices.[19] In the flexed posture, the mechanical demand on extensor muscles increases 3 to 5 times.[20] A posture that does not seem to necessarily relate to neck pain is a radiological measure

of a straightened or even slightly kyphotic cervical curve. Lordotic, straight and kyphotic cervical curves have all been measured in healthy men, women and children.[21,22]

Spinal posture is analyzed in standing by judging the posture of the lumbopelvic region, the shape of the thoracic and cervical spinal curves, the position of the head and shoulder girdle. Aberrant postures (e.g., a poor scapular or thoracic posture) may be immediately modified to determine if correction lessens symptoms. Posture is then assessed in unsupported sitting. The patient may sit with the lumbopelvic region and spine in the preferred neutral position or they may sit in an undesirable extended or, conversely and commonly, a slumped or flexed posture. The patient is asked to sit in what they consider a perfect posture. The better strategy to observe is the pelvis rolling up into a neutral position restoring the normal lumbar lordosis (with evident use of the lumbar multifidus). The kyphosis forms in the thoracic region and there is a neutral head on neck posture. It is undesirable when an upright posture is gained with dominant use of the thoracolumbar extensors, and the lordosis forms in the thoracolumbar or the lower thoracic region while the lumbopelvic region remains in a flexed position.[23] This pattern of correction is considered to signify a poor pattern of control in the lumbar region.[24]

Scapular posture is observed. The "ideal" scapular posture is such that the superior angles are level with the T2 or T3 spinous process, the spines of the scapulae are level with the T3 or T4 spinous process and the inferior angles are level with the T7–9 spinous process.[25] The spine of the scapulae and clavicles have a slight superolateral orientation and the scapulae sit flush against the chest wall in both the sagittal and transverse planes. Variations in scapular orientation and asymmetries are common and are often seen in asymptomatic people. Common observations in people with neck pain, often in combinations, include a downward scapular rotation, scapular protraction, winging of the medial border (excessive internal scapular rotation) or a prominence of the inferior angle (excessive anterior tilt). Change in orientation may indicate dysfunction in scapular muscles and thus scapular position is observed in association with changes in muscle form. Overactivity or altered resting tone of muscles, such as the levator scapulae, rhomboids and pectoralis minor may be implicated in a downwardly rotated and protracted scapular position in association with impaired activity in the tripartite trapezius and serratus anterior muscles. An elevated scapular position might reflect shortness in the upper trapezius, but it may be a posture

protective of mechanosensitive nerve tissue. In the latter case, the scapula appears to be held in a raised position. It is associated with a "thickening" appearance of the anterior scalene muscle or an apparent subtle lateral shift of the mid to lower cervical region (towards the side of the mechanosensitivity). The initial interpretation of a protective posture is later confirmed with neurodynamic tests (see subsequent section). When changes in scapular posture are protective of nerve mechanosensitivity, attempts to correct it may aggravate symptoms. In this case, attention to scapular posture correction is delayed until the nerve mechanosensitivity has been addressed.

There is considerable individual variation in spinal posture and positions of the scapulae. Thus it is necessary to investigate the relevance of any spinal or scapular postural variation to the patient's presenting neck pain. The relevance is gauged by determining any difference in neck pain and range of cervical rotation when tested in the patient's natural posture compared with a corrected postural position (Fig. 9.2A–C). Cervical rotation

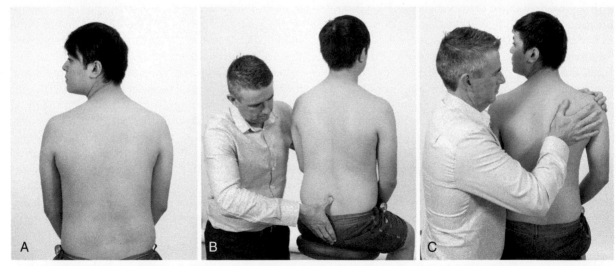

Fig. 9.2 ■ (A) Spinal and scapular posture is assessed in sitting. The patient is requested to rotate their head to each side. The clinician notes the range and any pain provoked. (B) Facilitation of spinal posture. An upright neutral spinal posture is facilitated by the clinician with manual guidance through L5 and the lumbopelvic region. Cervical rotation is then reassessed to both directions in the upright neutral spinal posture and any change in range and pain is noted. (C)Testing the effect of positioning the scapula in a neutral position. Scapular posture is observed. Each scapula is then positioned manually so that the scapula sits flush on the chest wall (neutral position). The clinician notes the movement corrections necessary to achieve this neutral scapular posture as these will inform the postural correction strategy in management. Cervical rotation is reassessed to both directions in the corrected scapular posture and any change in range and pain is noted. Scapular correction is performed on both sides.

is the movement direction chosen for testing because it is affected by both an FHP [9,10] and the length of axioscapular muscles.[26,27] A working interpretation is made from the outcome that may help to direct treatment. Alternatives are that correction of posture (spinal or scapular) results in the following.

- A marked reduction in pain and increase in range of cervical rotation.

  Interpretation: poor spinal and/or scapular posture is adversely loading cervical structures; it is a significant contributor to the neck pain disorder; segmental joint pain may be a consequence of this adverse loading.

  Implication for management: train a neutral posture (1) to decrease cervical segmental loading and pain; (2) as an exercise for the deep cervical flexors and/or axioscapular postural muscles (see Chapter 15).

- A slight reduction in pain and slight increase in range of cervical rotation

  Interpretation: poor spinal and/or scapular posture is a part contributor to the neck pain disorder. It is probable that other factors (e.g., painful segmental dysfunction) are also relevant to the disorder.

  Implication for management: train a neutral posture (1) to decrease cervical segmental loading and pain and (2) as an exercise for the deep cervical flexors and/or axioscapular postural muscles.

- No reduction in pain and no increase in range of cervical rotation

  Interpretation: poor spinal/scapular posture has little or no direct role in the neck pain disorder. Other factors are more relevant to the disorder (e.g., painful segment dysfunction, nerve mechanosensitivity).

  Implication for management: train a neutral posture as an exercise for the deep cervical flexors and/or axioscapular postural muscles.

Control of scapular posture

Control of scapular posture is further explored, particularly when scapular postures were linked with pain in the previous test. A lack of active scapular control may become more obvious when the scapulae are loaded.

Three functional tests are performed. First, the patient is asked to slowly flex, abduct and then externally rotate the arms. Arm movements should be less than 30 degrees to assess scapular control in a neutral functional position. In the first 30 to 40 degrees of arm elevation, minimal scapular motion is expected.[28] Thus the scapulae should remain relatively stable if the scapular muscles are providing adequate control. Second, the patient performs isometric contractions against mild resistance with the shoulder held in minimal elevation. Gently resisted isometric shoulder abduction may expose an inability to maintain upward rotation of the scapula, suggesting weakness of the upper trapezius. If resisted flexion reveals an inability to maintain posterior tilt of the scapular, it suggests weakness in lower trapezius, serratus anterior and if resisted external rotation shows an inability to control internal rotation of the scapula (winging), it suggest weakness in serratus anterior and the lower trapezius (Fig. 9.3). Second, scapular control is assessed under low load in a closed chain condition in a small wall push up. The shoulders are held in the same minimally elevated position to that of the isometric

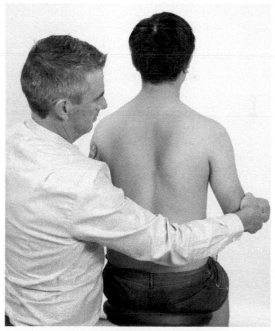

Fig. 9.3 ■ The clinician gently resists isometric shoulder abduction and observes for movement of the scapula. Tests are also performed for arm flexion and external rotation.

tests. Third, scapular control is assessed through the full range of upper limb elevation during which the scapula should progressively upwardly rotate, posteriorly tilt and externally rotate. The clinician observes for reduced or delayed scapular rotation in arm elevation and lowering which signals poor function of the trapezius-serratus anterior force couple.[29] Scapular rotation is manually facilitated in different planes of motion (i.e., scapular upward rotation, external rotation, posterior tilt) to identify the specific direction of any loss of scapular control during arm elevation and its relationship to symptoms.

Adjacent regions

There are neurophysiological, biomechanical and functional links between the cervical spine and both the craniomandibular complex and upper limb. The cervical spine has been implicated in craniomandibular disorders,[30–35] shoulder disorders,[36] lateral epicondylalgia[37] and carpal tunnel.[38] Thus a screening examination of the neck (active movement examination and a manual segmental examination) is an essential first step in the presence of any of these disorders. The examination can be extended to a more detailed assessment of the cervical region if these examinations reveal positive results. Likewise, adjacent regions should be examined in patients presenting with primarily a neck complaint (e.g., a screening examination of the craniomandibular complex in a patient presenting with a cervicogenic headache.[34])

The biomechanical relationships between spinal and arm movement are revealed when full arm elevation is impossible without motion occurring in the cervicothoracic, thoracic and even the lumbar spine.[39–42] However, there is inconsistency in reports for biomechanical, postural, kinesiological and functional links between disorders of the craniomandibular complex and the neck, which probably reflects the heterogeneity in nature and presentation of craniomandibular disorders,[32] a problem shared by neck pain disorders. There is popular opinion that neurophysiological interrelationships and the presence and influence of central nervous system sensitization commonly underpin links between neck pain and pain in the craniomandibular complex or indeed painful disorders of the shoulder or elbow.[32,35,37,43] A neurophysiological link would explain findings of neck tenderness or mechanical hyperalgesia

and a general restriction of motion but without signs of cervical musculoskeletal dysfunction (e.g., no deficit when performing the craniocervical flexion test, no positive cervical flexion rotation test) in a temporomandibular disorder.[32,35] Clinical reasoning can be complex in determining the origin of symptoms in such patients and where to direct primary treatment. Often a trial of treatment with careful assessment of effect over the first one to two treatments provides the answer.

ANALYSIS OF CERVICAL MOTION

The analysis of cervical motion is a fundamental component of the examination of a patient presenting with neck pain. Changes in motion are pathognomic of a cervical disorder.[44,45] The range, pain provoked, the nature and pattern of motion loss help to define the disorder and directly informs management as well as provide an outcome measure. The analysis of cervical motion provides information on the following.

- Range of available motion and its relationship to symptoms.
- Reasons for limitations of motion: biological (pain, articular restrictions, neural mechanosensitivity or extensibility, poor neuromuscular control, muscular restrictions [spasm, extensibility]), psychological (fear of movement).
- Patterns of movement restriction for diagnostic and management purposes.[46–48]
- Disturbances in control of movement (acceleration, velocity, movement smoothness).[49–51]

Motion analysis is designed to consider all components of the functional cervical spine, the craniocervical (C0–2) cervical (C2–7), and cervicothoracic regions (C7–T4). Even though there is some interdependence between the regions, each region is assessed separately, recognizing the independence of the regions (see Chapter 3). The focus on cervical regions does not dismiss any assessment of the thoracic or lumbar regions as relevant to the individual patient.

ASSESSMENT OF CARDINAL PLANES OF MOTION

The relationship between movement and pain or other symptoms such as light headedness is documented for all movement tests. Here, we describe possible observations and analyses of motion and neuromuscular control of movement.

Cervical and craniocervical motion

Cervical flexion. Request the patient to look down to flex the cervical region. A smooth flattening of the cervical lordosis should be observed down to the upper thoracic region with the head remaining in a neutral position. Points to note include the following.

- A tendency to extend the craniocervical region beyond that expected from passive restraints of the posterior structures as full flexion is approached could be protective of nerve tissue mechanosensitivity. To confirm, ask the patient to flex their chin and assess pain response; or add a nerve tissue sensitizing, straight leg raise position and assess any change in pain.
- The pattern of return is usually initiated from the lower cervical region with the head in a neutral position. Initiation of return with excessive craniocervical extension (chin up first) may signal

dominance by the superficial extensor muscles (e.g., splenius capitis, semispinalis capitis).

Cervical extension. Request the patient to look up towards the ceiling and follow the ceiling back with their eyes as far as possible. Points to note include the following.

- The mass of the head should be posterior to the line of the shoulders. If it remains in line with the shoulder, the patient is probably moving largely in their upper cervical region only (Fig. 9.4A and B). Possible reasons for this pattern include reluctance to move a painful segment into extension and/or weakness of the flexors and an inability to eccentrically control the weight of the head.
- The head moves backwards but at a point of extension, the neck appears to "translate backwards". Possible reasons are "segmental instability" or more commonly, poor control of the head movement by the deep and superficial cervical flexors. The moment arm of sternocleidomastoid (SCM) reduces with progressive extension and if

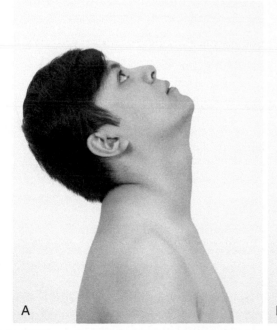 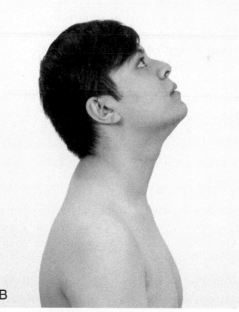

Fig. 9.4 ■ (A) The patient displays an appropriate pattern of cervical extension and the head's centre of gravity is posterior to the line of the shoulders. (B) Extension is principally occurring in the upper cervical region only. Note the head's centre of gravity is in the line of the shoulders, not posterior to them.

there is weakness of the deep cervical flexors, they cannot control the movement.[52] Occasionally the patient may passively assist their head back to the upright position.

- The return of the head from a fully extended position to a neutral upright position should be initiated with craniocervical flexion. If the return to the neutral position is initiated by an anterior translation type movement in the lower cervical region (SCM action) and craniocervical flexion is the last movement, this indicates weakness of the deep cervical flexors.

Craniocervical flexion and extension. The cervical spine remains in neutral and the patient is requested to first, nod their chin down and second to lift their chin up as far as possible. Points to note include the following.

- Upper cervical flexion: restriction of range and a pulling sensation. Possible reasons are articular restrictions, shortness of the suboccipital extensors, neural tissue mechanosensitivity. The latter is differentiated by presensitizing neural tissues with either the addition of a straight leg raise, flexion of the trunk (slump sitting) or presetting craniocervical flexion and adding cervical flexion.[53]
- Upper cervical extension: restriction of range. The most common reason is articular. Note any production of dizziness or light headedness.
- Upper cervical flexion or extension: symptoms of dizziness or light headedness. Possible reasons are cervicogenic dizziness, or possible signs of altered blood flow in the vertebral artery. Relate to the nature of the dizziness and other symptoms and historical factors in differential diagnosis (see Chapter 10).

Craniocervical and cervical lateral flexion. Request the patient to curl their head sideways towards their shoulder. The movement is tested bilaterally. Points to note include the following.

- Lateral flexion of the head on the neck (C0–2). Most lateral flexion in the craniocervical region is at C0–1. Note the contralateral pattern of lateral flexion and rotation in the two upper cervical joints. If there is a restriction in (L) craniocervical

lateral flexion, the pattern would fit with a reduction in (R) craniocervical rotation.

- Observe the shape of the lateral curve of the neck. A segmental restriction may be relatively discreet and can be identified by an interruption to the shape of the curve.
- Lateral flexion of the cervical region appears restricted en-bloc from C2 downwards, as a result of hypertonicity or shortness of the scalene muscles. Possible reasons include: (1) a protective response to mechanosensitive nerve tissue (the range of lateral flexion and pain response will be altered when neural tissue is presensitized by placing the arm in slight abduction and external rotation with the wrist and fingers in extension); (2) an upper costal breathing pattern; and (3) compensatory activity for weak deep cervical flexors.[54]

Craniocervical and cervical rotation. Request the patient to turn their head to look over the shoulder. Points to consider include the following.

- C1–2 provides almost one-half of the range of head rotation and the movement should be initiated with the head. When motion is limited, a lack of free spin of the head suggests an upper cervical restriction; the presence of free spin suggests a lower cervical restriction. In the latter case, the head may rotate with some ipsilateral lateral flexion, reflecting a loss of the normal C0–2 contralateral lateral flexion that accompanies C0–2 rotation.
- Rotation at C1–2 can be tested specifically with the flexion-rotation test.[55]
- The head cannot rotate fully unless there is up to a 10-degree contribution from the upper thoracic spine.[56]

Movement speed and velocity profile

Assessment of axial rotation provides the opportunity to test for other qualities of movement performance. To this point of the assessment, the patient has performed movements at self-selected speeds. Impairments in the mean and peak velocity of neck motion have been identified in people with neck pain disorders, that is, they have slower neck movements but not necessarily reduced range of motion. This deficit has significant implications for dynamic functional tasks such as involved with driving and reacting to visual and auditory stimuli.[51,57] It is important to identify.

For an initial qualitative assessment of neck movement velocity profile:

- Request the patient to move as quickly as they can to a specific point in range (i.e., 45-degree rotation), stop, hold the position and then return to the starting position as quickly as possible. Judge the speed of the movement.
- Assess overall speed and velocity profile. Observe how quickly and how smoothly the movement is performed. The clinician should observe a smooth acceleration followed by a smooth deceleration rather than stilted movements.

Cervicothoracic region

Adequate mobility in the cervicothoracic and thoracic spinal regions is necessary for normal motion in the cervical spine and shoulder complex.

Cervicothoracic flexion and extension. Movement at the cervicothoracic region is examined in conjunction with cervical flexion and extension. Points to consider include the following.

- Observe for a spreading (flexion) and closing (extension) of the interspinous spaces from C7 to approximately T3–4.
- In extension, note any hinging appearance through the lower cervical region which may occur when the cervicothoracic region is hypomobile.
- If observation is unsatisfactory, the clinician may palpate the interspinous motion at each segment during the movement.

Cervicothoracic rotation and lateral flexion. Movement at the cervicothoracic region is examined in conjunction with cervical rotation and arm elevation. Palpation of spinous process movement with these tests is an easier and more exacting assessment than observation.

- Palpate for the lateral displacement of the thoracic spinous processes (rotation) while the patient rotates the head (Fig. 9.5).
- Single arm elevation induces rotation and ipsilateral lateral flexion in the upper thoracic

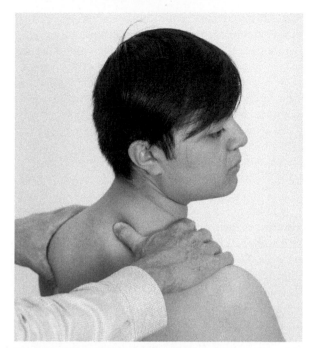

Fig. 9.5 ■ The patient performs repeated head rotation while the clinician palpates for the lateral displacement of the thoracic spinous processes (rotation) at each thoracic segment (C7–T1 to T3–4 or T4–5). Movement is examined in each direction. This examination technique can be used as a treatment technique. The clinician performs a transverse glide through the spinous process of the hypomobile thoracic segments as the patient rotates the head.

segments.[41,42] Palpate for the displacement of the thoracic spinous processes while the patient performs assisted unilateral arm elevation (see Fig. 3.4).

Movement tests to further direct management

Two movement examination schemes extend examination of movement in cardinal planes to further direct specific management approaches. One scheme is the combined movement examination which was originally described by Edwards.[46] It is built on a theory which considers the combined nature of functional movements, the coupled nature of spinal segmental movements and the relationship between movements that load the segments in similar ways. A comprehensive theory has developed to underpin the combined movement approach.[58] The active movement component of the approach aims to identify the primary movement and the primary combination of movements that most accurately reproduce the patients' pain, or in the case of severe pain, most accurately relieves pain. It provides the basis and rationale for the starting position and progression of manipulative therapy techniques. Inter-examiner reliability has been established for the main components of the active combined movements assessment.[59]

Another scheme of active movement examination is related to the mechanical diagnosis and therapy approach. The primary objective is to determine if neck pain or related arm symptoms can be abolished or reduced with the use of repeated movements or sustained postures. A principal of assessment is the use of direction-specific loading strategies to relieve pain or stimulate "centralization", that is, shift peripherally located pain to a more central location. Any movement direction might be used, based on a patient's presentation but a key movement is neck retraction. Assessment outcomes may help classify patients into one of three syndromes, derangement, dysfunction or postural syndrome, which assists in directing treatment. The reliability of the assessment method has been established for persons trained in the McKenzie method.[60]

Movement diagnostic tests

There is often contention about the ability of physical examination tests to assist diagnosis. There is now evidence that either a single test or a combination of physical tests can reliably detect cervical facet/zygapophysial joint dysfunction.

Cervical flexion rotation test. The flexion rotation test will identify C1–2 dysfunction. Its basis is that C1–2 axial rotation is separated from cervical axial rotation by fully flexing the neck before performing head rotation (see Fig. 3.1A and B).[61] The test was first described some 40 years ago,[62] but more recent research has proven its construct validity, reliability and discriminant ability.[47,55,63,64] It is a valuable test to identify cervicogenic headache associated with C1–2 dysfunction and to discriminate persons with cervicogenic headache from those with migraine or no headache complaint.[47,64]

Extension rotation test, manual segmental examination, palpation of segmental tenderness. This combination of tests is able to detect a symptomatic cervical

zygapophysial joint as tested against diagnostic facet joint anaesthetic blocks: sensitivity (79% confidence interval [CI], 72–86), specificity (84% CI, 77–90), positive likelihood ratio 4.94 (CI 2.80–8.20) and negative likelihood ratio .25 (CI .15–43).[48] The study was conducted with people with chronic neck pain attending an interventional pain management clinic. Interestingly, the presence of catastrophization and psychological distress did not modify or confound the outcome of the physical examination. The validity of this clinical examination contributes both to diagnosis of the neck pain disorder, and to identify patients potentially suitable for facet joint interventions.[65]

Spurling's test. This test is used to help identify if a patient's arm pain is related to a cervical radiculopathy. The neck is placed in either rotation or lateral flexion and extension is added, which narrows the intervertebral foramen. The clinician applies a compressive force through the head. A positive test response is reproduction of arm pain. It is a vigorous test and is only indicated when the presence of a cervical radiculopathy is not obvious from other aspects of the examination. Although Spurling's test has high specificity, it has low sensitivity.[66] Thus at best, the test is only able to contribute to a clinical diagnosis.

Positional tests for vertebral artery insufficiency

The presence of dizziness or unsteadiness in association with neck pain may have its origins in vestibular, cervical or vascular disorders (see Chapter 10). The vascular disorders of concern include the relatively rare presentation of cervical arterial dissection (CAD) or vertebrobasilar insufficiency (VBI). Points to note include the following.

■ When there are any concerns about the presence of CAD or VBI, then priority must be given to investigating these factors before conducting any other part of the physical examination.

■ In the rare event of a strong suspicion of CAD, clinicians are advised not to undertake a potentially provocative cervical movement examination. Rather, the patient should be referred immediately to a hospital emergency department with documentation about the concerns (younger patients aged under 55 years, acute, sudden onset of unfamiliar moderate to severe headache or neck pain often progressing, history of recent minor neck or head trauma, respiratory infection or onset of neurological features [e.g., 5Ds—dizziness and/or unsteadiness; diplopia; dysarthria/dysphasia; dysphagia; drop attacks or 3Ns—nystagmus; nausea; perioral numbness or paraesthesia], disturbances to balance or vision).[67]

■ Perform VBI tests as the first tests when there is suspicion of VBI; usually an older patient who reports symptoms of the 5Ds or 3Ns. Historically, there have been many tests proposed for VBI. None have high sensitivity and specificity or predictive value to identify risk of CAD or adverse events associated with manipulative therapy. Nevertheless, sustained end-range rotation is regarded as the most provocative and reliable test for those individuals with VBI.[68] The test is performed in sitting and end range rotation is sustained for at least 10 seconds. Positive responses include the production of dizziness, feelings of faintness, nystagmus which does not settle within a few seconds, or any of the 5Ds. A period of 10 seconds is advocated before rotation is tested to the other side in case there is any latency in responses.

The second indication for VBI testing is in patients for whom cervical manipulation or end range, firm mobilization techniques are considered in management. Premanipulative screening includes the sustained rotation test and also sustaining the position of the neck in which manipulation is to be performed to potentially identify any individuals with asymptomatic VBI. A comprehensive framework was developed by the International Federation of Orthopaedic Manipulative Physical Therapists for the examination of the cervical region in patients with suspected vascular dysfunction,[69] and readers are referred to this framework and its scheduled updates.

SENSORY TESTING AND PAIN MECHANISMS

Quantitative sensory testing (QST) can assist in understanding pain mechanisms (see Chapter 2). These tests are undertaken particularly in those patients whose history and pain descriptions suggest the possibility of central pain mechanisms. This occurs in some subjects with whiplash-associated disorders (WAD),[70] cervical radiculopathy,[71] headache including cervicogenic headache[72] or another neuropathic pain state. These sensory changes occur early so testing is relevant in patients both in acute and persistent stages of their disorder.[70] There are many sensory tests that can be performed but two that have been used extensively in research into neck pain disorders are tests to elicit signs of mechanical and thermal hyperalgesia. Tests are conducted over the local neck region to detect any potential peripheral sensitization and tests are also conducted at remote sites, commonly over the tibialis anterior, to detect evidence of widespread hyperalgesia which suggest the presence of central sensitization.

Measures of mechanical pain thresholds can be made with commercially available, low-cost pressure algometers. Thermal sensitivity (heat and cold pain thresholds) can be examined with thermorollers, which can be set at predetermined temperatures.[73] Cold hyperalgesia is proving to be important in identifying central sensitization and also as a potential predictor of recovery following a whiplash injury. Maxwell and Sterling[74] rated a simple, clinically friendly, ice application over the neck (two ice cubes in a plastic bag) against a laboratory thermotest system. They found that a pain intensity rating of greater than 5 out of 10 with the ice test gave a positive likelihood ratio of 8.44 suggesting the likely presence of cold hyperalgesia.

EXAMINATION OF THE NERVOUS SYSTEM

A battery of tests is undertaken to detect the presence of neuropathy and changes in nerve function. Multiple tests, as opposed to any single test, improves diagnostic accuracy for cervical radiculopathy[75] and upper limb neuropathy.[76,77] The test battery routinely includes a clinical neurological examination and tests of nerve tissue mechanosensitivity. Elements of QST may be included to investigate nerve conduction integrity (e.g., small fibre function).

Clinical neurological examination

A neurological examination is undertaken to evaluate nerve conduction integrity when symptoms (1) extend beyond the shoulder into the upper limb, or (2) include paranesthesia, anaesthesia, weakness, reduced dexterity within the upper quadrant or (3) if there are specific descriptions of pain indicating nerve irritation (e.g., burning, shooting, itching). These symptoms may have been reported in specific questionnaires for neuropathic pain (e.g., Self-Administered Leeds Assessment of Neuropathic Symptoms and Signs (S-LANSS); Neuropathic Pain Questionnaire (NPQ); painDETECT questionnaire).[78,79] Other factors such as muscle wasting or changes in balance and gait also indicate the need for a neurological examination.

A standard neurological examination includes evaluation of spinal reflexes (biceps C5, C6; brachioradialis C6; triceps C7), strength of muscles in related myotomes (upper trapezius C4; middle deltoid C5; biceps brachii C6; triceps brachii C7; extensor pollicis longus C8; palmer interossei T1), and tests of sensation in related dermatomes[80] (light touch, pin prick, vibration). The clinical neurological examination has acceptable test reliability.[81]

The neurological examination may expand in response to variations in clinical presentation. Examples include the following.

- Sensory testing to differentiate dermatomal[80,82] from peripheral nerve distribution when nerve entrapment is suspected (e.g., median nerve in carpal tunnel syndrome, ulnar nerve in cubital tunnel syndrome).
- QST may be indicated when an entrapment neuropathy is suspected but changes in nerve function are not detected by conventional neurological examination. Further testing may include vibration thresholds for Aβ fibres; as well as cold and warm detection for Aδ and C-fibres, respectively.[83]
- Upper motor neurone tests are added if spinal cord compromise is suspected (cervical myelopathy). These include Hoffman, Babinski and clonus tests, as well as an evaluation of balance and gait. Detection of myelopathy should not depend on any single test because cord signal changes may correlate poorly with upper limb reflexes and other pathological reflexes.[84] In a sample of patients with cervical myelopathy and cord signal change on magnetic resonance imaging (MRI), 67% had a Hoffman sign, 16% had clonus, 44% had Romberg sign and 60% had a gait abnormality.[84]

- Evaluation of cranial nerve function[85] may be indicated in clinical presentations where patients report or display neurological symptoms such as a change in balance or coordination, slurred or altered speech patterns, changes in the senses, blurred vision, changes in behavior and/or fatigue. Such symptoms could be suggestive of concussion when the patient has had a traumatic head and neck injury or CAD when the patient presents with an acute onset, moderate to severe, unusual headache.

Tests of nerve mechanosensitivity

Nerve tissue mechanosensitivity may be associated with antalgic postures, painful restriction of active and passive movements including neurodynamic tests, tenderness on nerve palpation, and relevant local signs (e.g., joint dysfunction).[86-88] Active movements and neurodynamic tests are positive for nerve tissue mechanosensitivity if they reproduce symptoms, and symptoms can be altered by structural differentiation. Structural differentiation delineates nerve tissue mechanosensitivity as a cause, by changing symptoms when selectively loading or unloading the nervous system with manoeuvres at a site remote to the symptoms.[89-91] Examples include the following: when manual correction of a depressed or downwardly rotated scapula reduces distal arm pain, it may indicate postural based tensile strain on the brachial plexus in a relaxed upright posture; shoulder and upper arm pain increases when shoulder abduction is repeated with the wrist in extension compared with a neutral position; there is an increase in pain with cervical flexion when it is performed in sitting with the knees straightened.

Neurodynamic tests

The four variants of the upper limb neurodynamic test[87,90] (Fig. 9.6) and the slump test[91] are relevant for the upper quadrant. As mentioned, a test is considered positive if it reproduces symptoms that can be altered by structural differentiation.[89-91] Neurodynamic tests of the upper limb are reliable when these criteria for a positive test are used.[75,81,87,92] The point of excursion of a test movement at which symptoms are reproduced (e.g., elbow extension during the median nerve bias test) is a reliable measure[93] and usually indicates a positive test of nerve tissue mechanosensitivity. Yet this

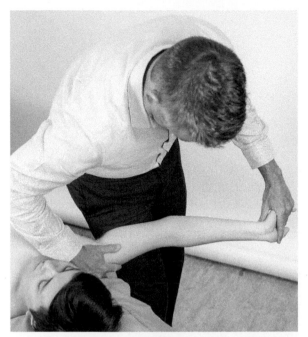

Fig. 9.6 ▪ Neurodynamic tests include the conventional test, which biases the brachial plexus and median nerve (*pictured here*) as well as tests that bias the median, radial and ulnar nerves. In the conventional test, the movement sequence is gentle shoulder girdle fixation in a neutral position, followed by shoulder abduction and lateral rotation, elbow extension, forearm supination and wrist extension. The sequence of test movements may be altered, and the test is often performed with wrist extension preceding elbow extension, so that one angle, elbow extension, can be measured in assessment. Sensitizing movements include contralateral cervical lateral flexion or craniocervical flexion.

might not always be the case. Range of motion is reflective of protective muscle responses that are elicited in both symptomatic[94] and asymptomatic states.[95] A study in patients with chronic WAD showed bilateral loss of elbow extension during neurodynamic testing irrespective of the presence or not of arm pain.[96] The reduction in mobility in these patients may have reflected a hypersensitive flexor withdrawal response.

Nerve tissue mechanosensitivity may be a feature of cervicogenic headache where its incidence is estimated as roughly 10% of cases.[5,97] Here the provocative movement is craniocervical flexion and the mechanosensitivity purportedly involves movement of the dura. Described as a myodural bridge, the dura mater is attached to the foramen magnum and to the body of the C2 vertebra.

There are also fibrous connections between the rectus capitis posterior minor and the ligamentum flavum in this region.[98-100] The test for neural tissue mechanosensitivity involves passive craniocervical flexion. A restriction in range could reflect deficient dural movement in a cephalad direction, tightness in the suboccipital extensors or hypomobility into flexion of the C0–1 and C1–2 joints. To structurally differentiate a neural tissue origin of the restriction, craniocervical flexion is repeated with the nerve tissue presensitized by placing the lower limb in a straight leg raise and then the upper limb in the neurodynamic test position (Fig. 9.7A and B).[101] Reproduction of neck or headache symptoms with the test is a positive neural tissue response. This test is mandatory before the craniocervical flexion test to avoid any exacerbation of symptoms of a neuropathic origin. There has been no formal evaluation of the inter-examiner reliability of this test, but reliability has been established for a similar test of neural tissue provocation using craniocervical flexion with added flexion.[53]

Nerve palpation

Nerve palpation is a further component of the assessment of nerve tissue mechanosensitivity. Palpation of the trunks of the brachial plexus and peripheral nerves has moderate to substantial measurement reliability.[81] Nerves palpated include the median, ulnar and radial nerves in cases of cervicobrachial pain, and the C2 nerve and greater and lesser occipital nerves in cases of cervicogenic headache. In the presence of sensitized peripheral nerve tissue, the nerves are tender to gentle palpation, that is, they exhibit mechanical allodynia. Such findings reinforce the necessity for the physical examination and physical treatments to be undertaken with care to avoid provoking the patient's symptoms.

MANUAL EXAMINATION

The cervical segments from C0–1 to at least T3–4 or T4–5 are examined. A variety of manual examination techniques can be used in a variety of positions and for a variety of reasons. The reader is referred to relevant texts for detailed rationales and technique descriptions.[46,102-104] Techniques may be performed in sitting, supine or prone lying. They may be performed purely as passive movements in single (Fig. 9.8) or combined (Fig. 9.9) planes or with the addition of active movement

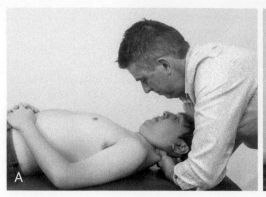
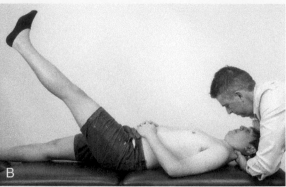

Fig. 9.7 ■ (A) The test for nerve tissue mechanosensitivity in the craniocervical region. The clinician passively flexes the craniocervical region and notes the range, end feel and pain response. Craniocervical flexion is repeated up to 4 times, (i.e., with each leg in a straight leg raise position and with each arm in an upper limb neurodynamic position). (B) The patient holds a straight leg raise position and the clinician again performs craniocervical flexion and judges the range, end feel and pain response. A slight change in available flexion range is not uncommon. Reproduction of neck or head pain is a positive sign and is usually associated with a firm end feel and a definite reduction in range of movement.

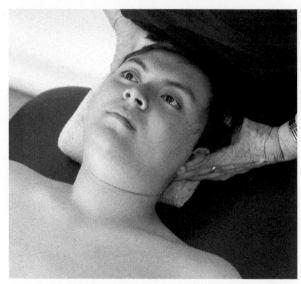
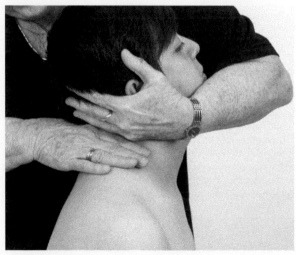

Fig. 9.8 ■ Test of left lateral flexion at the occipito-atlantal joint (C0–1) in supine lying. The tip of the index finger is placed on the transverse process of C1 and the pad palpates the mastoid process. Lateral flexion of the skull on C1 is performed and the clinician feels for the approximation of mastoid process to the transverse process.

Fig. 9.9 ■ Test of C3–4 right lateral flexion in extension as a component of a combined movement examination. C4 is stabilized by gripping the lamina between the index finger and thumb. The head to C3 is gripped by the opposite hand (hypothenar eminence on C3) and the lateral flexion movement is produced by the arm and shoulder girdle.

(Fig. 9.10).[105] Techniques may emphasize the examination of physiological planes of motion (Fig. 9.11) or maybe regarded as more "provocative" movement tests (Fig. 9.12). A number of techniques are usually used in clinical decision making. Despite the variety of techniques, the desired outcomes of the manual examination are similar, namely to determine the symptomatic segment(s) and to further inform the management approach. No one method(s) is necessarily superior. One commonality is that each method requires skilled

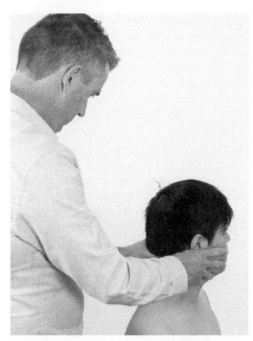

Fig. 9.10 ■ Test of C4–5 left rotation using a sustained natural apophysial glide. The medial border of the (R) thumb is placed on the lamina of C5 and the (L) thumb is placed on C4 perpendicular to the (R) thumb in the facet plane. A passive glide is applied as the patient actively rotates.

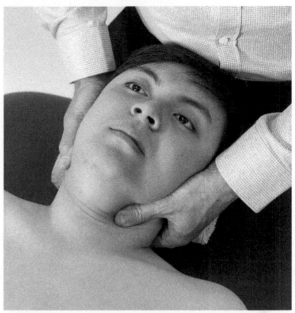

Fig. 9.11 ■ An anteroposterior glide is performed in the facet plane to assess the downward glide of the C2 on C3 (extension). Care must be taken to ensure that C2 is well supported with a gentle lumbrical grip with the thumb on the anterior aspect of the transverse process and the index and remaining fingers gripping the lamina. The movement is produced by gentle elbow extension and flexion as direct force by the thumb will be painful. The direction of the glide is in a cephalad direction and a medial bias can be introduced which emphasizes a lateral flexion component.

application to deliver optimal outcomes. Skill is gained through concentration and repetitive practice as required for acquisition of any physical skill be it hitting a golf ball in an intended direction, performing arthroscopic surgery or assessing cervical intersegmental motion. An important aspect of manual handling skill is that the clinician can perform all techniques with no or negligible clinician-induced local discomfort because this can lead to false positive interpretations.

Manual examination of segmental motion is a qualitative assessment and not an absolute measure. It has had an unsteady history from a scientific perspective. In the past, it was treated as a semiquantitative measure of segmental motion and tissue compliance. In these earlier times, there were enthusiastic beliefs about the accuracy of manual examination techniques with respect to tissue compliance. This is evident in the design of the inter-therapist reliability studies to test a clinician's ability to rate segmental motion by grading the displacement and stiffness of a segment to their applied manual force. Rating scales varied, but in one study an 11 point

scale was used.[106] This means that clinicians were asked to estimate which of 11 stress strain curves they perceived within a 2 to 2.8 mm sagittal translation displacement of a lumbar segment; a formidable and unrealistic task. It is probably not surprising that a systematic review based on many of these earlier studies found reliability of manual examination to be low[107] and thus questioned the continued use of manual examination in practice. In contrast, a more recent in vitro study of three manual mobilization techniques of the atlanto-axial joint found that both inter-observer and intra-observer reliability to produce similar motion with the techniques was high.[108] Thus more research asking different question, and using different designs and measures might throw a different light on manual examination or manually induced segmental movement.

It is often difficult to shape a clinical art into a quantifiable research question. Importantly other

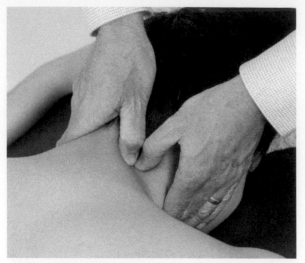

Fig. 9.12 ■ A unilateral posteroanterior glide (PA) is performed on C3–4. The PA glide can be regarded as a gentle provocation test that will elicit a reaction from the deep segmental muscles overlying the joint (multifidus) in response to the manual provocation. The extensor muscles overlying the facet joints are shifted medially so that the clinician can locate the thumbs as close as possible to the lamina of C3. The fingers and hands gently grip the side of C3 and the neck. The movement is produced by gentle elbow extension and flexion as direct force by the thumb will be painful. Pain produced by a clinician's thumbs in performance of the technique could result in false positive findings.

relevant questions of manual examination have been asked. A crucial question has been whether a patient's neck pain is associated with painful segmental dysfunction and whether clinicians can reliability detect this segmental dysfunction. In these respects, manual examination is proving to be an accurate and valuable method of examination.[109–114] Most studies have validated its accuracy against the accepted gold standard of diagnostic anaesthetic blocks. This judgement from manual examination requires essentially a yes/no decision based on a simultaneous, multifaceted (metacognitive) assessment of both the nature and amount of tissue resistance to the manually applied force, the perceived displacement and the degree of pain provocation.

Palpation or manual examination is a fundamental test in health care practice, whether it is to palpate an abdominal mass, to detect the tenderness and muscle guarding of acute appendicitis or to elicit painful cervical segmental dysfunction. Thus the questioned use of manual examination,[107] on the basis of some poorly conceived tissue compliance studies can in turn be questioned with the wisdom of hindsight. Nevertheless, claims of precision with these tests with respect to motion and tissue resistance to motion also need to be modified to be in line with the evidence. Manual examination is an important diagnostic test that adds to the understanding of the patient's neck pain condition.[115] In perspective, x-rays cannot reliably identify a symptomatic segment. This realizes the need and importance of a skilled manual examination to identify the presence (or absence) and location of symptomatic cervical segment(s) in a patient's neck pain or headache disorder. Judgement can also be made of the comparability of the joint signs to the level of reported pain when reasoning the relative contributions of peripheral and/or central mechanisms in a patient's neck pain presentation.

Instability tests

Craniocervical instability and loss of ligamentous integrity must be considered in patients who have either sustained head or neck trauma (motor vehicle crash, sporting injury, fall), have an inflammatory arthritis (such as rheumatoid arthritis and ankylosing spondylitis), an inherited condition such as Down syndrome or who have congenital anomalies in the upper cervical region.[116–118] Trauma from a motor vehicle crash may cause ligament injury[119,120] but the area of most controversy is the frequency of craniocervical ligament ruptures in the absence of a concurrent fracture or dislocation. Diagnosis is difficult. There is controversy about the relevance of MRI signal changes in alar and transverse ligaments as they pertain to structural damage[121] and reported pain and disability.[122] Without a gold standard radiological diagnosis, it is difficult to validate clinical tests. Thus it is not surprising that the outcomes of a systematic review of the diagnostic accuracy of upper cervical spine instability tests concluded that there was insufficient evidence to indicate that craniocervical ligament tests could accurately identify ligamentous instability.[123]

More recent work has investigated the content validity of several craniocervical ligaments tests on healthy young participants by determining if the tests displace relevant anatomic points consistent with the proposed mechanisms of the test. Measurements have been with MRI. These studies have confirmed the content validity of the clinical anterior shear (transverse ligament) and distraction (tectorial membrane) tests[124] as well as the side-bending (Fig. 9.13) and rotation stress tests for the alar ligaments.[125] The range of craniocervical rotation in the rotation stress test, should typically not be greater than 21 degrees in the presence of intact alar ligaments.[126] It is now necessary to determine if measuring displacement will have clinical utility in patients following neck trauma. Here in vivo variables such as muscle spasm may confound testing because these may occur, for example, with tests of the anterior cruciate ligaments of the knee.

Cervical segmental instability (C2–7) may be present as a result of trauma or it may be part of a degenerative process. Segmental instability is tested with an anteroposterior glide (Fig. 9.14). At this present time, it is unknown how much clinicians can rely on the outcomes of the cervical segmental stability tests or craniocervical ligament tests. In the clinical reasoning process, account is also taken of the history of onset and nature of symptoms. In a Delphi study, clinicians nominated a variety of symptoms that might arouse suspicion including a feeling of being unable to hold the head up, a desire for support either by a collar or hands, a feeling of instability or lack of control.[127] Protective muscle spasm would be expected. Thus a pattern of symptoms and signs is sought, rather than rely on any one test. Patients presenting with any neurological signs especially upper motor neuron signs, should be referred immediately for further medical investigations.

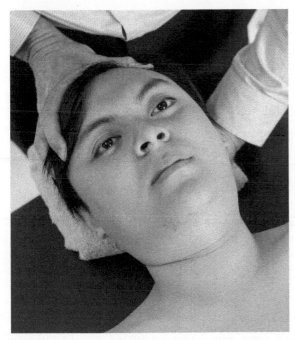

Fig. 9.13 ■ The lateral stress test for the alar ligaments. C2 is fixed between the clinician's thumb and index finger. The occiput and C1 are laterally flexed. There should be a solid end feel. The test is performed in neutral, slight flexion and extension to account for variation in ligament orientation. The rotational stress test may also be used for the alar ligaments. If the ligaments are partially or fully ruptured, some excess movement would be expected, but often muscle guarding may confound the tests. Nevertheless, there would be disturbed cervical afferentation and symptoms of pain and dizziness may be reproduced.

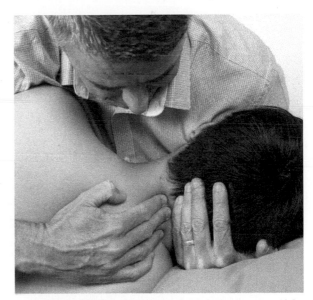

Fig. 9.14 ■ Manual test of sagittal glide. The test is used for the segments from C2-3 to C7-T1. The clinician stabilizes the caudal segment through placement of the fingers on either side of the spinous process. The head rests on the forearm and the hypothenar eminence and little finger grip the cephalad vertebra of the segment. The translation movement is performed by the arm and the clinician perceives any reduced tissue resistance to the movement and compares with adjacent segments. Symptoms may be reproduced.

ASSESSMENT OF THE NEUROMUSCULAR SYSTEM

In the initial assessment, attention is focused on testing the activation, coordination and endurance capacity of muscle groups. Tests are conducted under low-load conditions so that particular muscles can be targeted as much as possible. Tests against resistance necessarily recruit many muscles to resist the force. Furthermore, low-load tests can be performed without pain negating the effect of pain inhibition in the initial assessment. Tests of strength and higher-level endurance are conducted in subsequent assessments.

Scapular muscle tests

Scapular holding test (lower trapezius)

This test might be delayed if upper trapezius guarding has been observed in the postural assessment and the upper limb neurodynamic test has confirmed the presence of nerve tissue mechanosensitivity. The scapular holding test is a modified grade 3 test of the lower trapezius.[128] The modifications are that the arm is positioned by the side and the clinician places the scapula passively into a neutral position on the chest wall (Fig. 9.15). The patient is requested to hold this scapular position. Two aspects are assessed.

■ The pattern of muscle activity used to hold the scapular position. The clinician observes for activity in the lower trapezius together with "balanced" activity of other scapular muscles. Actions masking weakness of lower trapezius include dominant use of latissimus dorsi (arm and scapular depression), rhomboids or levator scapulae (downward rotation and elevation of the scapular border), infraspinatus/teres minor muscles (lifting and/or externally rotating the arm). Winging of the scapula indicates weakness of the serratus anterior.
■ The "holding capacity" of the lower trapezius (and serratus anterior). The low-load nature of this endurance test is akin to the muscle's functional role in holding the scapular position in upright postures. The patient is requested to hold the scapular position for approximately 5 seconds and the test is repeated up to 5 times or until the clinician has a good appreciation of the

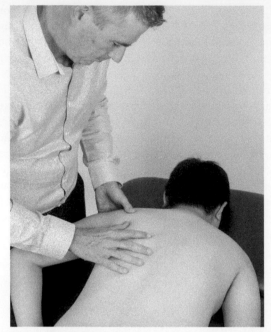

Fig. 9.15 ■ Scapular holding test. The clinician passively lifts the scapula onto the chest wall and requests the patient to hold the position. An analysis is made of the muscle strategy used to hold the position.

pattern of muscle use. Impaired holding capacity is observed when (1) the position cannot be held (i.e., the scapula slides towards an outer range position); (2) a "fatigue" tremor develops; or (3) the patient changes to another muscle strategy to hold the position (e.g., excessive use of latissimus dorsi).

Reassessment of cervical posteroanterior glides

Contraction of the scapular depressors in the scapular holding test induces reciprocal relaxation of the scapular elevators (e.g., levator scapulae, upper trapezius) and thus reduces muscle load on the cervical spine. This provides an opportunity to make a clinical assessment of the possible effect of reduced axioscapular muscle activity on segmental joint signs and pain. Following the manual examination of posteroanterior (PA) glides, the patient is asked to rate the pain provoked on the symptomatic segment. Immediately after the scapular holding test, the clinician again examines the PA glides on the same symptomatic segment and reassesses the pain rating. The response is interpreted in a similar way to the interpretation of posture correction.

The scapular holding test results in the following.

- A marked reduction in pain on PA provocation
  Interpretation: load from scapular elevator activity is a major contributor to segmental joint pain.
  Implication for management: train scapular muscles (trapezius, serratus anterior) and scapular posture to relieve unnecessary load. Training becomes a major feature of the intervention. The pattern fits for the role of poor scapular muscle control if both this test and the correction of scapular posture reduce pain. This response makes a convincing link between relief of pain and appropriate muscle control for patient motivation for exercise and training of posture.
- A slight reduction in pain on PA provocation
  Interpretation: load from scapular elevator activity is a part contributor to segmental joint pain.
  Implication for management: train scapular muscles (trapezius, serratus anterior) and scapular posture with the knowledge that the painful joint dysfunction will need to be addressed with other methods such as manipulative therapy and specific active segmental exercise.
- No reduction in pain on PA provocation
  Interpretation: load from scapular elevator activity has little or no direct role in the segmental joint pain.
  Implication for management: depending on the findings from other tests of scapular posture and movement control, findings suggest that other management is needed to address the painful joint dysfunction such as manipulative therapy and specific active segmental exercise.

This postfacilitation assessment of the PA provocative test can also be conducted after the craniocervical flexion test which reciprocally relaxes the cervical extensor muscles. Changes in pressure pain thresholds over the neck have been demonstrated after the muscle test.[129,130] The aim is to demonstrate how much segmental muscle spasm is potentially contributing to the joint pain and dysfunction.

Trapezius muscle tests

The scapular holding test emphasizes the lower portion of the trapezius muscle. The upper trapezius muscle is often a site of tenderness and feelings of "tightness" yet when a downwardly rotated scapular posture is observed, the upper trapezius is in a lengthened state. The upper trapezius is commonly weak and it has also been shown to be more fatigable in patients with neck pain.[131]

First impressions of trapezius muscle function were gained from the observation of posture and scapular motion during forward arm elevation. A better determination of trapezius function is gained from the control of the scapula in abduction. A test of resisted abduction in 110 degrees has been proposed as a better test of the tripartite trapezius muscle's ability to control upward scapular rotation, than separate tests of its three parts.[132] The upper trapezius can be formally tested with the classical test of a shoulder shrug. First the patient's capacity to shrug is determined by observing whether they can perform a correct upward rotation strategy of the scapula (i.e., activating upper trapezius), rather than a gross elevation of the scapula that encourages levator scapulae activity. The test is progressed from non-resisted to resisted with the use of arm position and load as indicated. Upper trapezius fatigability can be evaluated asking the patient to perform repeated shoulder abduction or shoulder shrugs.[131]

Serratus anterior test

Initial assessment of serratus anterior function was made from the observation of scapular posture and from the analysis of scapular control with light arm load and with arm elevation. The serratus anterior can be further tested with a classical muscle test of scapular protraction performed in lying or in sitting and in various positions of arm elevation. A closed chain test may be conducted, such as a push up from the wall or the more challenging position of four-point kneeling. Often the four-point kneeling or prone on elbows position is used with people with neck pain (as opposed to those with glenohumeral disorders). In these positions, the patient is encouraged to let their rib cage sink between their scapulae and then push through their arms to raise their rib cage back towards their scapulae, keeping the spine neutral (i.e., not flexing the thorax). This tests the capacity of the axioscapular muscles to fix the scapula to the chest wall in a neutral postural position under load. Substantial winging of the medial border of the scapula is an indication of poor axioscapular muscle control particularly of the serratus anterior muscle.

Axioscapular muscle length tests

Muscles with a tendency for overactivity or tightness include levator scapulae, suboccipital extensors, scalenes, pectoralis minor and major. Indications of overactivity are revealed in neck and scapular postures as well as muscle bulk. Observations are confirmed with formal muscle length tests.[133,134] We do not prioritize muscle length tests because our treatment philosophy is to train the impaired muscles or postures which underlie increased use of some muscles. For example, rather than stretch levator scapulae, we would prioritize training activity and control offered by the tripartite trapezius. Rather than stretch the suboccipital extensors, we train the deep cervical flexors and cervical posture. A notable exception is the pectoralis minor muscle where muscle stretching may be required to train scapular posture. Our approach is not to suggest that it is "wrong" to use muscle stretching in the management of a neck pain disorder, but often there is not a lasting effect of treatment unless the underlying impaired motor control is addressed. Muscle stretching is not indicated when muscle "shortness" is protective of nerve tissue mechanosensitivity (scalenes and upper trapezius in cases of neck and arm pain and suboccipital extensors muscles in cases of cervicogenic headache).

Craniocervical flexion test

The evidence indicates that poor activation and endurance of the deep cervical flexor muscles (longus capitis and longus colli) is common in people with acute and chronic neck pain regardless of the mechanisms of onset.[135–140] The deep cervical flexor muscles are tested in the craniocervical flexion test (CCFT).[141] The CCFT has content validity[54] and inter-therapist and intra-therapist reliability.[142–145] The test is low load and is performed in the initial assessment in patients with either acute or chronic neck pain conditions. The exception is when patients have signs of neural tissue mechanosensitivity. Before testing, the clinician screens for this occurrence (see Fig. 9.7A and B). The CCFT is delayed if neural tissue mechanosensitivity is present and instead, priority is given to nerve

tissue management. In the screening test, the clinician also assesses the range of craniocervical motion to gain a baseline for movement analysis during the CCFT.

Preparation for the test

The CCFT is performed in supine with the knees bent and the head and neck in a neutral position (no pillow) such that the line of the face is horizontal. When the patient's head is in slight extension (often associated with a thoracic or cervicothoracic kyphosis), layers of towel are placed under the head to gain a neutral position. Often layers of towel need to be placed behind the neck as well because a distance of no more than 0.5 to 1 cm is desirable between the supporting surface and the back of the neck. Too big a space encourages over inflation of the biofeedback's pressure pad which can force the neck into extension and invalidate the test. If the patient rests with the head in flexion, they are taught a neutral position by looking at a point on the ceiling slightly behind their head. They return to this position between each stage of the CCFT. The folded pad of the pressure biofeedback device (Stabilizer, Chattanooga, USA) is placed behind the neck so that it abuts the occiput. Patients (and clinicians) are unable to see or palpate the deep cervical flexors to know if they are contracting. This device guides the patient during the CCFT, by providing feedback on the target pressures to be achieved with each stage of the test. The air-filled pressure pad monitors the change in shape of the curve as it flattens with the contraction of the deep cervical flexors.[146] The pressure sensor is inflated to a baseline pressure of 20 mmHg, a standard pressure sufficient to fill the space between the testing surface and the neck. The air must be distributed throughout the pad and the pressure stabilized before testing commences (Fig. 9.16).

Craniocervical flexion is taught as an active assisted movement with instructions to feel the back of the head slide up the bed to nod the chin. Five, 2-mmHg progressive pressure increases are sequentially targeted from the baseline of 20 mmHg to a maximum of 30 mmHg. The movement should be performed gently and slowly, allowing a 2 to 3 second rest between stages. There is a learning effect, so the patient should practice the test once or twice before formal assessment.

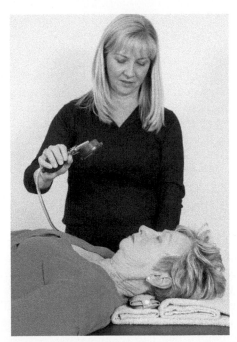

Fig. 9.16 ■ The craniocervical flexion test position. Folded towels may be used to position the head and neck in a neutral position. It is preferable to have no more than a 1-cm space between the back of the neck and the supporting surface. The pressure sensor is positioned behind the neck so that its edge abuts the occiput. Note the feedback is for the patient. The clinician must observe the pattern of movement and any substitution strategies during the test.

Formal test procedure

The formal test is conducted in two stages.[141]

Stage 1: Analysis of the range and quality of the five progressive stages of the craniocervical flexion.

Stage 2: Testing the isometric contraction of the deep cervical flexors.

Stage 1. The patient is requested to slowly feel the back of their head slide up the bed to nod their chin to reach the first target pressure of 22 mmHg. They hold the position for 2 or 3 seconds and then relax. This process is repeated through each of the four remaining stages of the test. The clinician analyzes the pattern and range of craniocervical flexion motion, observes the quality of the movement and observes or palpates for any excessive activity in the superficial flexors (SCM and scalenes). The motion of the head should be a rotation whose range increases proportionally through progressive stages of the test.[147]

Clinical measure: the stage of the test that the patient can achieve and momentarily hold with the correct craniocervical flexion movement and without excess SCM and scalene muscle activity is documented as the activation score. Expected scores in an asymptomatic population vary, but most achieve a score between 26 and 30 mm Hg. Persons with neck pain usually perform at the 22 to 24 mmHg levels.[138,144]

Several features indicate poor test performance.

- There is not a progressive increase in craniocervical flexion range of motion between stages. The patient attempts all stages of the test but uses a subtle head retraction action (i.e., pushes back on the pressure sensor) to attain the progressive pressure test increments.[54]
- The patient cannot perform all test stages regardless of their movement strategy.
- Movement is performed quickly to mask weakness.
- The clinician observes or palpates excessive activity in the SCM and scalene muscles. Some SCM and scalene muscle activity is normal especially in the latter stages of the CCFT but it is significantly less than that measured in people with neck pain.[54,137,138,140] Note there is an inverse relationship between activity in the SCM and the deep cervical flexors during the performance of the test, (i.e., the more activity in the SCM, the less activity in the deep cervical flexors).[148]
- If the patient is an upper costal breather, the test should be performed during slow expiration to minimize overactivity in the anterior scalene muscles.[149]
- The patient clenches their jaw to use the hyoid muscles to augment the contraction of the deep cervical flexor muscles. Correct the strategy by requesting the patient to adopt a resting position of the mandible during the test; ask them to lightly place their tongue on the roof of the mouth, position their lips together with their teeth slightly apart.
- On return from a test stage, the dial drops below 20 mmHg. (Check that the pressure in the pressure sensor was stabilized before testing). A true drop in pressure may indicate a deficit in proprioception,

with the patient overshooting the neutral head position on return from the movement.

- On return to the starting position, the dial may read a pressure greater than 20 mmHg. This usually reflects an inability to relax the muscles following a contraction. The muscles will relax, and the pressure will return to the baseline when the patient is asked to look at a spot on the ceiling behind their head.

Stage 2. This stage tests the endurance (or the tonic holding) of the deep cervical flexors. It can be conducted immediately after stage 1, but testing is delayed when substitution movements (e.g., head retraction) were dominant in stage 1 of the test. There is no purpose in testing the endurance of an incorrect muscle and movement strategy. In these cases, longus capitis and colli activation is trained first with the correct movement, and endurance is tested in a subsequent assessment.

In a research setting, the low-load endurance capacity of the deep cervical flexors is tested by determining the pressure level that the patient can hold steady for 10 seconds, with minimal activation of the SCM or anterior scalene muscles. The test is commenced at the lowest level (22 mmHg) and, if 10 repetitions of 10-second holds are achieved, the test is progressed to the next pressure target and so forth up to 30 mmHg or until the patient fails. In the clinical setting, this approach can be very time consuming and a short cut is used, which sacrifices a formal measure as might be required in research. The clinical testing starts at the 22 mmHg target but contractions are held for approximately 5 seconds and if after two to three repetitions, the patient is observed to be coping well, they relax for a few seconds and then attempt the next pressure level. The test is continued until the pressure level at which the patient fails is reached.

Clinical measure: the pressure level at which the patient fails. Training will begin at the pressure level below (e.g., if failed on 24 mmHg, training commences on 22 mmHg). Again, there is variability in performance between individuals, but most asymptomatic individuals can successfully perform repetitions of the test to at least 26 mmHg (if not 28 and 30 mmHg stages), whereas neck pain patients often do not achieve more than the first or the second levels of the test.[5,144,150]

Poor performance or failure is judged when the patient:

- cannot maintain craniocervical flexion in the test stage and reverts to a retraction strategy.
- cannot hold the pressure steady at the designated test level (the needle on the dial falls away even though the patient seems to be holding the head in a flexed position).
- cannot hold the position without overtly activating the superficial flexors.
- holds the position but with a jerky action, indicative of fatigue.

Cervical flexor strength and endurance

Tests of strength and endurance are performed as a progressive assessment in subsequent treatments, once the patient can control the craniocervical region in a head lift assessment. Early strength testing without adequate control may aggravate symptoms or conversely, pain inhibition may flaw test outcomes.

Neck flexor strength and endurance may be tested using dynamometry[151,152] but the most common test is a head lift test. This test has mainly been investigated as a strength test for the deep cervical flexors where an individual's ability to hold their head 2 cm off a supporting surface while controlling the chin position is timed. In this respect, the test has proven reliable.[153–156] Nevertheless, the SCM is the major flexor of the neck and the antigravity head lift is a test of the strength of all cervical flexors.

When considering endurance, the neck flexors have impaired capacity over a spectrum of contraction intensities. Poor endurance and fatigability occur at 50% and 20% to 25% of maximum voluntary capacity.[157,158] Thus endurance should not be tested in antigravity head lift tests only, but in positions where the effect of gravity and head load are reduced (e.g., various angles of reclined sitting).

Cervical extensor muscle tests

The cervical extensors weaken and may become more fatigable in association with neck pain (see Chapter 5). Factors that guide clinical testing is the emerging evidence that impairment is relatively more pronounced in the deeper extensor muscles of the cervical spine, such as semispinalis cervicis and multifidus[159–161] and that the suboccipital muscles frequently display atrophy or substantial fatty infiltrate in some people with WAD and older persons with headache.[159,162–165] Therefore assessment aims to bias these muscle groups.

The patient is positioned, as they personally tolerate initially, in one of three positions of decreasing gravitational load; either four-point kneeling (or alternatively prone with the head over the edge of the bed), prone on elbows or forward lean sitting propped on elbows. All cervical extensor muscles contribute to supporting the weight of the head against gravity. Tests are not specific to one muscle group but rather aim to target particular muscle groups.

Suboccipital muscles

Tests are conducted for the suboccipital extensors (rectus capitis major and minor) and for suboccipital rotators (obliquus capitis superior and inferior). The clinician gently stabilizes the C2 vertebra to assist in the localization of the movement to the upper cervical region.

For the rectus capitis major and minor muscles, the patient is asked raise and lower their chin to perform alternating small ranges of craniocervical extension and flexion (nodding action to say yes) while maintaining the cervical spine (C2–T1) in a neutral position (Fig. 9.17A). This is a familiar movement and usually the patient has no difficulty with it. Nevertheless, the movement is tested (and exercised) routinely based on the evidence of the morphological changes in the muscles in persons with neck pain disorders coupled with the knowledge of their major contribution to sensorimotor control (see Chapter 6).

The obliquus capitis superior and inferior are tested by asking the patient to perform small ranges of head rotation as if saying no (Fig. 9.17B). What is expected is a pure spin of the head on the neck (C1–2 rotation) with a range of no more than 30 to 40 degrees. The clinician must observe where motion is occurring. Often the motion occurs in the mid to lower cervical region rather than at C1–2, particularly in patients with upper cervical disorders. If this is the observation, then it is necessary to determine the origin of this altered movement pattern. To do this, the clinician now stabilizes C2 more firmly and asks the patient to again turn the head as if saying no. The patient may now be able to perform the C1–2 movement aided by the localizing input of the hand grip. Alternately, they cannot rotate their head to the desired ranges, and often they can

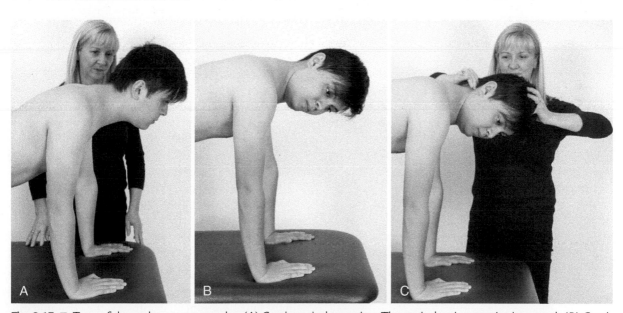

Fig. 9.17 ■ Tests of the neck extensor muscles. (A) Craniocervical extension. The cervical region remains in neutral. (B) Craniocervical rotation. Ensure that it is head rotation on the cervical spine (C1-2 rotation). Observe if movement is occurring in the mid cervical region which is an incorrect action. (C) C1-2 rotation is facilitated by stabilizing C1-2 and rotating the patient's head in an assisted active movement.

barely achieve any rotation. This may reflect C1–2 joint hypomobility or it may reflect poor proprioception and an inability to dissociate head from neck movement. This is easily differentiated by the clinician facilitating C1–2 rotation (Fig. 9.17C). There will be one of three results.

- Rotation range immediately begins to improve and approaches normal excursion. The reasoning is that joint hypomobility is not the issue, rather the patient has poor movement sense.
- Rotation range is blocked. This is often more movement to one side that the other and suggests C1–2 hypomobility. The finding should be consistent with the result of the cervical flexion rotation test.
- Facilitation improves the range of rotation but there is still less than acceptable range. There is a combination of problems; the patient has poor movement sense coupled with hypomobility at C1–2.

Cervical extensors

All cervical extensors will be recruited to support the weight of the head against gravity. The test nevertheless aims to bias the deeper cervical extensors (semispinalis cervicis and multifidus). The patient is requested to perform cervical extension while keeping the craniocervical region in a neutral position to place head extensor muscles such as splenius capitis and semispinalis capitis at a mechanical disadvantage. The axis of rotation passes through the C7 vertebra.

The craniocervical region is maintained in neutral during cervical extension by facilitating the position with an eye focus task. A pen or book is placed between the hands in the four-point kneeling position (or equivalent in other positions). The patient is asked to curl their neck down to look at their knees and then to curl it back as far as possible while keeping their eyes on the book/pen. In relation to instructions, the word "curl" is important to discourage a backward translation or retraction action (Fig. 9.18). Normally, the patient should be able to extend the neck to approximately 20 to 30 degrees. Poor performance in the test is indicated by the following:

- An inability to extend to 20 degrees; many neck pain patients cannot extend past the neutral

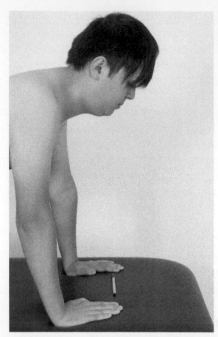

Fig. 9.18 ■ Cervical extension: the patient curls their head into extension while keeping their eyes on the book/pen (i.e., in a craniocervical neutral position). It is important to check that the patient can dissociate craniocervical extension from cervical extension and not allow the head extensors, such as splenius and semispinalis capitis, to contribute significantly to the extension movement.

position (also differentiate hypomobility in the cervicothoracic region limiting motion).
- The patient cannot dissociate head extension from neck extension, subtle extension of the cranium is observed, often in association with a visual outline of overactive splenius capitis and semispinalis capitis muscles.
- Fatigue. The patient reports they are tiring after a few repetitions. Alternately, the clinical observes an increasing lordosis develop in the upper cervical region as the cranial extensors begin to dominate the movement.

When active cervical extension is painful and limited, there can be a reluctance to test the cervical extensors in the initial assessment. Painful active extension should not deter testing because the loads and muscle actions are very different between the two tests. In testing positions for the cervical extensors, the compressive forces of head load and gravity are eliminated, and the movement is controlled by the extensor muscles. Patients usually find the test comfortable and they can stop short of pain if relevant.

Cervical extensor strength and endurance

Tests of strength and endurance are performed as a progressive assessment in subsequent treatments, once the patient can perform full range cervical extension with the craniocervical region maintained in a neutral position.

Neck extension strength may be tested with a dynamometer if available, or use may be made of a handheld dynamometer, which is a reliable method of measurement.[166] Endurance can be assessed using the modified Biering-Sorensen test,[167] and light weights may be added to the head to test endurance at different contraction intensities.

ASSESSMENT OF DISTURBANCES IN SENSORIMOTOR CONTROL

Assessments for impaired sensorimotor control are indicated when patients report dizziness, light headedness or feelings of unsteadiness in association with their neck pain. A legitimate argument could be raised to incorporate these tests routinely in all patients with neck pain because deficits in sensorimotor control have been found in those not complaining of these symptoms (see Chapter 6). However, these tests should be conducted routinely in patients with symptoms of dizziness/light headedness and in patients where the onset of neck pain is related to trauma. Sensorimotor testing should also be considered in patients not responding to management as expected.

Four sets of measures are undertaken; tests of cervical proprioception (joint position and movement sense), balance, oculomotor control and coordination. Differentiating whether an impairment is arising from a cervical or vestibular origin is always a challenge especially in patients with balance and eye movement control disturbances (see Chapter 10). Likewise, challenging is identifying the role of the cervical spine in altered sensorimotor control in patients who have sustained neck or head trauma such as a concussion or whiplash injury (see Chapter 10).

Cervical proprioception

Cervical position sense

Cervical position sense is commonly assessed in the clinical setting by measuring a person's ability to relocate their natural head posture while vision is occluded.[168] Joint position error is the angular difference between the starting natural head posture and that assumed following a neck movement. Errors are commonly measured following return from cervical extension, and rotation to the left and right, although return from flexion and lateral flexion can be assessed if time allows. As an extension of the test, cervical joint position sense can be assessed by measuring the accuracy in relocating selected points in range.[169]

Moderate deficits can be judged visually in the clinical situation, but joint position errors as little as 4 to 5 degrees[170,171] indicate a deficit in cervical joint position sense and are difficult to judge visually. A simple quantitative measure is preferable, and it becomes an outcome measure on which to reassess effects of management. A simple, reliable and valid measure involves the use of a target and a laser pointer mounted onto a lightweight headband.[168,172] Alternate measuring instruments include a gravity dependent goniometer,[173] or the use of a standard computer, webcam and free head tracking software.[174]

When the test is implemented using a laser and target, the patient sits comfortably such that the laser pointer is 90 cm away from a wall and the starting position is projected by the laser onto the wall (Fig. 9.19). The target is positioned so that the laser is in the centre of the target. The patient concentrates on the starting position, then closes their eyes. They actively move their head in a specified direction ([L] or [R] rotation or extension), then return to the starting position as accurately as possible. Six trials are optimal for research purposes,[175] but at least three consistent trials are considered satisfactory for clinical use. The participant's head is manually repositioned to the starting position between trials. No verbal feedback is provided, and the patient keeps the eyes closed between repetitions. Each return position is marked on the target. The difference between the starting and return points is measured in centimetres which can be converted to degrees.[172] In addition to the quantitative measure of cervical position sense, other signs of impaired cervical position sense

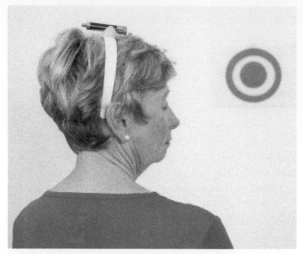

Fig. 9.19 ■ Head relocation accuracy: the laser pointer is placed on the head and the patient attempts to relocate the head as accurately as possible after performing a specific neck movement with the eyes closed.

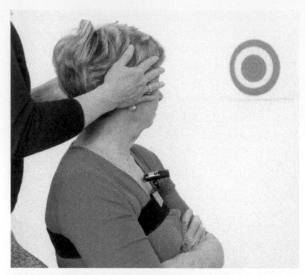

Fig. 9.20 ■ Trunk relocation accuracy: the laser is positioned on the sternum and the patient is asked to relocate the trunk back to the neutral position with the eyes closed. The examiner gently stabilizes the head throughout the test to prevent head motion.

may be observed including jerky movements, uncertainty or searching for the initial position, overshooting the initial position, reproduction of dizziness or there is a noticeable difference between movement patterns when performed with the eyes closed compared with eyes open.

An alternate test might be considered especially when aiming to differentiate vestibular and cervical causes of dizziness or light headedness. The laser is now attached to the sternum (Fig. 9.20), the head is held still (to neutralize a vestibular cause) and the patient rotates the trunk. Accuracy in trunk repositioning is used to measure joint position sense.[176,177]

Cervical movement sense

Cervical movement sense is tested by assessing the accuracy with which a patient can perform fine head and neck movements to trace intricate patterns such as a diagonal zigzag pattern. A pattern is placed on the wall 90 cm in front of the patient and it is traced using the laser method (Fig. 9.21). At present, a qualitative assessment is used to judge the accuracy of the motion, deviation from the target and the speed-accuracy trade-off. Work is currently underway to develop a quantitative method for this test. "The Fly" is a more sophisticated computerized method to measure accuracy of head and

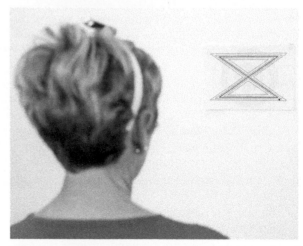

Fig. 9.21 ■ Movement sense: assessment of the quality of movement when the patient attempts to accurately move the laser on their head to trace the pattern ahead.

neck movement during unpredictable movements.[178] Applications using a smart phone to detect and compare neck motion will be a helpful clinical tool. A virtual reality device is also being researched for assessment of accuracy of head motion.[51]

Standing balance

The clinical examination of standing balance takes the patient through tasks that progressively challenge postural stability by altering foot position, visual input and the supporting surface. Balance in comfortable (Fig. 9.22) and subsequently narrow stance is assessed with the patient standing on a firm and then a soft surface such as a piece of 10 cm dense foam. The tests are performed with the eyes open and then closed. It is reasonable to expect that a person under the age of 60 years can maintain stability for up to 30 seconds in comfortable and narrow stance tests. Abnormal responses include large increases in sway, slower responses to correct sway or rigidity to prevent excessive sway as well as an inability to maintain balance. The test level and response are recorded. Research is continuing to develop ways to bias cervical proprioception in tests of balance.[179,180] Performance in normal stance is compared with stance when the head still faces forward but the trunk is rotated under the stationary head. Test results are encouraging for using torsion as a method to distinguish balance disturbances attributed to alterations of cervical afferent information from those of a vestibular cause.[179]

Patients aged under 45 years may require more challenging tasks to display balance deficits. To increase the challenge, balance can be tested in tandem and then single leg stance on a firm surface with eyes open and closed.[181] Patients with neck pain of either insidious or traumatic origin, and especially those complaining of dizziness or unsteadiness, have greater difficulty in completing the tandem stance tasks on a firm surface than asymptomatic persons.[181,182]

Consideration is also given to including dynamic tests such as the step test, timed 10 metre walk with head turns and tandem walk as required, for example, if the patient complains of dizziness when walking, loss of balance or falls (Fig. 9.23).[183,184] The Dynamic Gait Index[185] can be conducted in the clinical setting to provide measures of functional dynamic balance

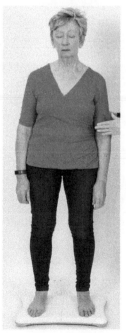

Fig. 9.22 ■ Balance in comfortable stance: balance with eyes closed is assessed with the head in neutral. Simple inexpensive devices such as the Wii board can be used to gain an objective measure of sway. A worsening of balance in the torsion (head still trunk rotated 45 degrees) compared with neutral head position may indicate a cervical cause of balance disturbances.

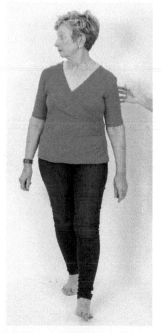

Fig. 9.23 ■ Walking with head turns: the quality and time to walk 10 metres when keeping the head still is compared with walking while moving the head in large range side-to-side or up-and-down movements.

especially in elders, where an increased risk of falls might be suspected.[186,187]

Oculomotor assessment

Oculomotor assessment incorporates qualitative assessment of the ability to (1) maintain gaze while moving the head and (2) eye follow while keeping the head still. These tests are not exclusive to, nor can they specifically differentiate, individuals with neck pain. They are often used in assessment of vestibular or central nervous system disorders. Nevertheless, some tests have been modified to bias a cervical component in attempts to determine the influence of the cervical region on the visual system. The routine tests are gaze stability and the smooth pursuit neck torsion test. They are performed with the patient sitting. Abnormal test responses include difficulty or inability to perform the task, reproduction of symptoms, jerky or non-fluent head or eye movements. In general, patients with neck related oculomotor disturbances do not present with nystagmus at rest or during these tests. Its presence is more indicative of vestibular pathology.

Gaze stability

Gaze stability is assessed by asking the patient to keep their eyes focused on a target while they actively move their head into flexion, extension and rotation to the left and right (Fig. 9.24). Pertinent findings are an inability to maintain focus on the target, awkward or reduced cervical motion (< 45 degrees despite having available movement without eye fixation) or reproduction of symptoms such as dizziness, blurring of vision or nausea. This test is performed relatively slowly rather than quickly to bias the cervical rather than vestibular afferents.

Eye follow: smooth pursuit neck torsion test

Eye follow is tested using the smooth pursuit neck torsion test.[188] In the test, eye follow is compared between the neutral head position and when the trunk is rotated on the head (neck torsion) so that input to the vestibular system is avoided. The patient is asked to keep the head still and follow, as closely as possible, a moving target (e.g. the clinician's index finger or a pen) with the eyes. The target is moved slowly side to side (20 degrees per second through a visual angle of 40 degrees). The test is first performed with the head and trunk in neutral

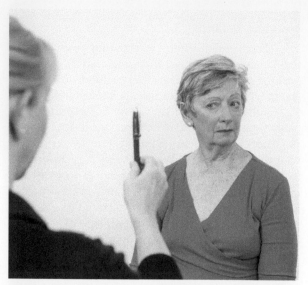

Fig. 9.24 ■ Gaze stability: the patient is asked to fixate on a point (e.g., pen) in front of them as they move their head as far as possible in each direction.

and then repeated with the neck torsioned to the left (left torsion) by rotating the trunk and shoulders 45 degrees to the right, keeping the head still. It is repeated with the trunk and shoulders rotated 45 degrees to the left (right torsion) again keeping the head still (Fig. 9.25A and B). Any difference is noted in smooth eye follow or symptom reproduction between the neutral and torsioned positions. Patients with neck pain are often unable to keep up with the target and display quick catch up eye movements (saccades) when the neck is in torsion, particularly when the target is crossing the midline. Table 9.2 lists possible outcomes of the test. Two points to note are that it can be normal to have saccadic eye movements at the extremes of the visual angle and with the change of movement direction.[189] An alternate cause is suspected when performance is poor when the head is in neutral and it is unchanged by adding neck torsion. Qualitative assessment of eye movement has acceptable validity and reliability,[190,191] but further accuracy is likely when patient symptoms are added to eye movement assessment.

Eye-head coordination; trunk-head coordination

Eye-head coordination is depicted in Fig. 9.26. The patient first moves the eyes to look at a target and

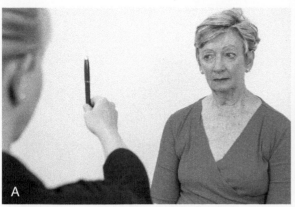
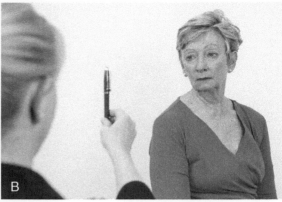

Fig. 9.25 ■ The smooth pursuit neck torsion test. (A) The patient follows a moving pen (40-degree angle, 20 degrees per second) with their eyes while keeping their head still. The clinician observes the pursuit of the eyes. (B) The pursuit of the eyes in neutral is compared with when the head is still and trunk turned to the left 45 degrees (right torsion). It is repeated on the other side. Increased catch up saccades in the torsion positions especially as they cross the midline and/or reproduction of symptoms in the torsion positions compared with the neutral position is a positive test.

TABLE 9.2

Rating scale smooth pursuit neck torsion test eye movements in neutral head position compared with torsion

Score	Rating definition
Negative 0	Smooth, precise eye movements in all positions
Negative 00	Catch up saccadic eye movements in the midline in all positions, but no change in eye movement in torsion versus neutral
Positive 1	Moderately positive, slight catch up saccades in the midline compared with neutral, can occur on either side
Positive 2	Strongly positive, many catch up saccadic eye movements in the midline when compared with neutral, can occur on either side

Adapted from Casa ED, Helbling JA, Meichtry A, et al. Head-eye movement control tests in patients with chronic neck pain; inter-observer reliability and discriminative validity. BMC Musculoskelet Disord 2014;15:16.

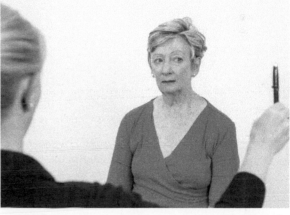

Fig. 9.26 ■ Eye-head coordination: the patient moves the eyes first to focus on a target 30 degrees away and then the head to the target ensuring the eyes keep focused on the target. This can be performed to the left, right and up and down.

then moves the head ensuring the eyes keep focused on the target. The eyes are then moved back to the centre, followed by the head. The test can be performed to left, right and up and down directions. Patients with neck pain are often unable to keep the head still while the eyes move or they lose focus during the head movements.[192,193] Eye and head movements can also be assessed by following a trunk or a hand movement.

Trunk-head coordination is assessed in standing. The patient holds the head still, eyes open looking straight ahead while rotating their trunk to the left and right (Fig. 9.27). Patients with neck pain often have difficulty keeping the head still while the trunk is moving or are unable to dissociate head and trunk movement. A positive test is an inability to fix the head and/or a decreased range of trunk movement. A laser mounted on the head can monitor any head motion.[194]

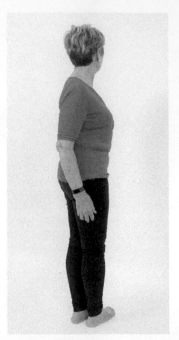

Fig. 9.27 ■ Trunk head coordination: the patient tries to hold the head still with the eyes open while rotating their trunk to the left and right.

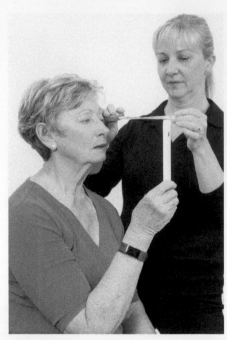

Fig. 9.28 ■ Near point convergence: the participant focuses on a small target at arm's length and slowly brings it toward the tip of their nose until they see two distinct images. The distance between the target and the tip of nose is measured and recorded (≥ 6 cm from the tip of the nose is considered abnormal).

Other causes of disturbances to the sensorimotor control system

Primary vestibular pathology may result from a whiplash injury, especially when it is associated with head trauma. Symptoms could be of vestibular origin in such patients or conversely, there is some evidence that the neck may influence vestibular function (see Chapter 6).[195] Disturbances of cervical sensory input may give rise to a mismatch of sensory input from the cervical and vestibular systems, which may contribute to asymmetry of the vestibulo-ocular reflex (VOR).[196] Some patients with neck pain who had previously normal vestibular function, could feasibly have an asymmetry of the VOR of a cervical origin.[197] Secondary vestibular influences on sensorimotor control may need to be considered in people with neck pain.

There is an overlap in responses between the vestibular and cervical musculoskeletal systems in a number of tests. In some patients, additional tests may be necessary to further examine vestibular function. A simple screening test, the vestibular oculomotor screening test (see Chapter 10) might be suitable in musculoskeletal practice.[198] It includes tests of saccadic and smooth pursuit eye movement, near point convergence (Fig. 9.28), gaze stability with fast head movements (180 beats per minute) and vision motion sensitivity (Fig. 9.29). An increase in symptoms of more than 2 points on an 11-point numerical rating scale is considered a positive response to either central or vestibular causes.

More specific tests of the VOR may be required such as head shaking nystagmus[183] or the head impulse test.[199] In cases where benign paroxysmal positional vertigo in the posterior canal is suspected, the Hallpike-Dix manoeuvre is the screening test.[183] For a more detailed review of vestibular evaluation, the clinician should consult texts designed specifically for that purpose.[183] Referral for a more thorough investigation of the vestibular or central nervous systems may be warranted where cervical causes of dizziness or disturbances in the sensorimotor system cannot be substantiated.

There are other causes of disturbances to sensorimotor control that could be concomitant with neck pain. These

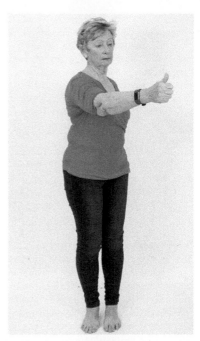

Fig. 9.29 ■ Visual motion sensitivity: the participant stands with feet shoulder width apart with the arm outstretched and focuses on their thumb while performing 5 repetitions of rotating the whole body (eyes, head and trunk) together through an 80-degree excursion to the right and left.

include medical conditions such as diabetes and merely the factor of ageing. Vestibular function deteriorates as a consequence of age.[200] In older patients, neck pain may magnify the degree of disturbances in sensorimotor control.[201] Such co-occurrences should not detract from the rehabilitation program but may influence speed of recovery or outcomes.

CONCLUSION

This chapter has provided a comprehensive set of tests for use in the clinical setting to detect impaired processes and function in patients presenting with neck pain disorders. Certainly not all tests are relevant for every patient and clinicians will need to prioritize examination procedures according to the patient's presentation. The physical examination provides a wealth of information. The clinician should be constantly reflecting on the patient's presenting complaint, testing if the pattern fits between complaints and physical findings and most importantly, using the examination findings to develop

with the patient, a relevant management approach. The management planning should address both the patient's current complaint and prevention of further episodes of neck pain, that is, restore function and not just provide pain relief. Likewise, a set of outcome measures informs on the effectiveness of the intervention as well as provides a set of incentives for the patient and clinician to achieve.

REFERENCES

1. Hengeveld E, Banks K. Maitland's vertebral manipulation: management of neuromusculoskeletal disorders. 8th ed. UK: Churchill Livingstone, Elsevier; 2013.
2. Abbott J, Schmitt J. Minimum important differences for the patient-specific functional scale, 4 region-specific outcome measures, and the numeric pain rating scale. J Orthop Sports Phys Ther 2014;44:560–4.
3. Westaway MD, Stratford PW, Blinkley JM. The patient-specific functional scale: validation of its use in persons with neck dysfunction. J Orthop Sports Phys Ther 1998;27:331–8.
4. Fisher A, Bacon C, Mannion V. The effect of cervical spine manipulation on postural sway in patients with non-specific neck pain. J Manipulative Physiol Ther 2015;38: 65–73.
5. Jull G, Trott P, Potter H, et al. A randomized controlled trial of exercise and manipulative therapy for cervicogenic headache. Spine 2002;27:1835–43.
6. Reid S, Callister R, Snodgrass S, et al. Manual therapy for cervicogenic dizziness: long-term outcomes of a randomised trial. Man Ther 2015;20:148–56.
7. Khayatzadeh S, Kalmanson O, Schuit D, et al. Cervical spine muscle-tendon unit length differences between neutral and forward head postures: biomechanical study using human cadaveric specimens. Phys Ther 2017;97:756–66.
8. Lau K, Cheung K, Chan K, et al. Relationships between sagittal postures of thoracic and cervical spine, presence of neck pain, neck pain severity and disability. Man Ther 2010;15: 457–62.
9. Quek J, Pua Y-H, Clark R, et al. Effects of thoracic kyphosis and forward head posture on cervical range of motion in older adults. Man Ther 2013;18:65–71.
10. De-la-Llave-Rincón A, Fernández-de-las-Peñas C, Palacios-Ceña D, et al. Increased forward head posture and restricted cervical range of motion in patients with carpal tunnel syndrome. J Orthop Sports Phys Ther 2009;39:658–64.
11. Oliveira A, Silva A. Neck muscle endurance and head posture: a comparison between adolescents with and without neck pain. Man Ther 2016;22:62–7.
12. Richards K, Beales D, Smith A, et al. Neck posture clusters and their association with biopsychosocial factors and neck pain in Australian adolescents. Phys Ther 2016;96:1576–87.
13. Yip C, Chiu T, Poon A. The relationship between head posture and severity and disability of patients with neck pain. Man Ther 2008;13:148–54.

14. ShaghayeghFard B, Ahmadi A, Maroufi N, et al. Evaluation of forward head posture in sitting and standing positions. Eur Spine J 2016;25:3577–82.

15. Falla D, Jull G, Russell T, et al. Effect of neck exercise on sitting posture in patients with chronic neck pain. Phys Ther 2007;87:408–17.

16. Nejati P, Lotfian S, Moezy A, et al. The study of correlation between forward head posture and neck pain in Iranian office workers. Int J Occup Med Environ Health 2015;28: 295–303.

17. Szeto G, Straker L, Raine S. A field comparison of neck and shoulder postures in symptomatic and asymptomatic office workers. Appl Ergon 2002;33:75–84.

18. Edmondston S, Sharp M, Symes A, et al. Changes in mechanical load and extensor muscle activity in the cervico-thoracic spine induced by sitting posture modification. Ergonomics 2011;54:179–86.

19. Xie Y, Szeto G, Dai J. Prevalence and risk factors associated with musculoskeletal complaints among users of mobile handheld devices: a systematic review. Appl Ergon 2017;59:132–42.

20. Vasavada A, Nevins D, Monda S, et al. Gravitational demand on the neck musculature during tablet computer use. Ergonomics 2015;58:990–1004.

21. Been E, Shefi S, Soudack M. Cervical lordosis: the effect of age and gender. Spine J 2017;17:880–8.

22. Grob D, Frauenfelder H, Mannion AF. The association between cervical spine curvature and neck pain. Eur Spine J 2007;16:669–78.

23. Caneiro J, O'Sullivan P, Burnett A, et al. The influence of different sitting postures on head/neck posture and muscle activity. Man Ther 2010;15:54–60.

24. Richardson C, Hodges P, Hides J. Therapeutic exercise for lumbopelvic stabilization: a motor control approach for the treatment and prevention of low back pain. 2nd ed. Edinburgh: Churchill Livingstone; 2004.

25. Sobush DC, Simoneau GG, Dietz KE, et al. The Lennie test for measuring scapular position in healthy young adult females: a reliability and validity study. J Orthop Sports Phys Ther 1996;23:39–50.

26. Dillen LV, McDonnell M, Susco T, et al. The immediate effect of passive scapular elevation on symptoms with active neck rotation in patients with neck pain. Clin J Pain 2007;23:641–7.

27. Ha S, Kwon O, Yi C, et al. Effects of passive correction of scapular position on pain, proprioception, and range of motion in neck-pain patients with bilateral scapular downward-rotation syndrome. Man Ther 2011;16:585–9.

28. McClure P, Michener L, Sennett B, et al. Direct 3-dimensional measurement of scapular kinematics during dynamic movements in vivo. J Shoulder Elbow Surg 2001;10:269–77.

29. Helgadottir H, Kristjansson E, Einarsson E, et al. Altered activity of the serratus anterior during unilateral arm elevation in patients with cervical disorders. J Electromyog Kinesiol 2011;21:947–53.

30. Armijo-Olivo S, Silvestre R, Fuentes J, et al. Electromyographic activity of the cervical flexor muscles in patients with temporomandibular disorders while performing the craniocervical flexion test: a cross-sectional study. Phys Ther 2011;91:1184–97.

31. Armijo-Olivo S, Silvestre R, Fuentes J, et al. Patients with temporomandibular disorders have increased fatigability of the cervical extensor muscles. Clin J Pain 2012;28:55–64.

32. Ballenberger N, Piekartz Hv, Danzeisen M, et al. Patterns of cervical and masticatory impairment in subgroups of people with temporomandibular disorders-an explorative approach based on factor analysis. Cranio 2017;20:1–11.

33. Grondin F, Hall T, Laurentjoye M, et al. Upper cervical range of motion is impaired in patients with temporomandibular disorders. Cranio 2015;33:91–9.

34. Piekartz H, Lüdtke K. Effect of treatment of temporomandibular disorders (TMD) in patients with cervicogenic headache: a single-blind, randomized controlled study. Cranio 2011;29:43–56.

35. Piekartz Hv, Pudelko A, Danzeisen M, et al. Do subjects with acute/subacute temporomandibular disorder have associated cervical impairments: a cross-sectional study. Man Ther 2016;26:208–15.

36. Norlander S, Gustavsson B, Lindell J, et al. Reduced mobility in the cervico-thoracic motion segment-a risk factor for musculoskeletal neck-shoulder pain: a two-year prospective follow-up study. Scand J Rehabil Med 1997;29:167–74.

37. Coombes B, Bisset L, Vicenzino B. Cervical dysfunction is evident in individuals with LE without obvious neck pain and may reflect central sensitization mechanisms. Further study of the nature of the relationship between cervical dysfunction and LE is required. J Manipulative Physiol Ther 2014;37: 79–86.

38. Fernández-de-Las-Peñas C, Cleland J, Palacios-Ceña M, et al. The effectiveness of manual therapy versus surgery on self-reported function, cervical range of motion, and pinch grip force in carpal tunnel syndrome: a randomized clinical trial. J Orthop Sports Phys Ther 2017;47:151–61.

39. Crawford H, Jull G. The influence of thoracic posture and movement on range of arm elevation. Physiother Theory Pract 1993;9:143–8.

40. Crosbie J, Kilbreath S, Hollmann L, et al. Scapulohumeral rhythm and associated spinal motion. Clin Biomech 2008;23: 184–92.

41. Stewart S, Jull G, Willems J, et al. An initial analysis of thoracic spine motion with unilateral arm elevation in the scapular plane. J Man Manipulative Ther 1995;3:15–21.

42. Theodoridis D, Ruston S. The effect of shoulder movements on thoracic spine 3D motion. Clin Biomech 2002;17: 418–21.

43. Grondin F, Hall T, von Piekartz H. Does altered mandibular position and dental occlusion influence upper cervical movement: a cross-sectional study in asymptomatic people. Musculoskelet Sci Pract 2017;27:85–90.

44. Snodgrass S, Cleland J, Haskins R, et al. The clinical utility of cervical range of motion in diagnosis, prognosis, and evaluating the effects of manipulation: a systematic review. Physiother 2014;100:290–304.

45. Waeyaert P, Jansen D, Bastiaansen M, et al. Three-dimensional cervical movement characteristics in healthy subjects and subgroups of chronic neck pain patients based on their pain location. Spine 2016;14:E908–14.

46. Edwards BC. Manual of combined movements. 2nd ed. Edinburgh: Churchill Livingstone; 1999.

47. Hall T, Briffa K, Hopper D, et al. Comparative analysis and diagnostic accuracy of the cervical flexion-rotation test. J Headache Pain 2010;11:391–7.

48. Schneider G, Jull G, Thomas K, et al. Derivation of a clinical decision guide in the diagnosis of cervical facet joint pain. Arch Phys Med Rehabil 2014;95:1695–701.

49. Röijezon U, Djupsjöbacka M, Björklund M, et al. Kinematics of fast cervical rotations in persons with chronic neck pain: a cross-sectional and reliability study. BMC Musculoskelet Disord 2010;11:222.

50. Sjölander P, Michaelson P, Jaricb S, et al. Sensorimotor disturbances in chronic neck pain-Range of motion, peak velocity, smoothness of movement, and repositioning acuity. Man Ther 2008;13:122–31.

51. Bahat HS, Chen X, Reznik D, et al. Interactive cervical motion kinematics: sensitivity, specificity and clinically significant values for identifying kinematic impairments in patients with chronic neck pain. Man Ther 2015;20:295–302.

52. Vasavada A, Li S, Delp S. Influence of muscle morphometry and moment arms on the moment - generating capacity of human neck muscles. Spine 1998;23:412–22.

53. López-de-Uralde-Villanueva I, Acuyo-Osorio M, Prieto-Aldana M, et al. Reliability and minimal detectable change of a modified passive neck flexion test in patients with chronic nonspecific neck pain and asymptomatic subjects. Musculoskelet Sci Pract 2017;28:10–17.

54. Falla DL, Jull GA, Hodges PW. Patients with neck pain demonstrate reduced electromyographic activity of the deep cervical flexor muscles during performance of the craniocervical flexion test. Spine 2004;29:2108–14.

55. Hall T, Robinson K, Fujinawa O, et al. Intertester reliability and diagnostic validity of the cervical flexion-rotation test. J Manipulative Physiol Ther 2008;31:293–300.

56. Tsang S, Szeto G, Lee R. Normal kinematics of the neck: the interplay between the cervical and thoracic spines. Man Ther 2013;18:431–7.

57. Bahat HS, Weiss P, Laufer Y. The effect of neck pain on cervical kinematics, as assessed in a virtual environment. Arch Phys Med Rehabil 2010;91:1884–90.

58. McCarthy C. Combined movement theory. UK: Churchill Livingstone, Elsevier; 2010.

59. Stamos I, Heneghan N, McCarthy C, et al. Inter-examiner reliability of active combined movements assessment of subjects with a history of mechanical neck problems. Man Ther 2012;17:438–44.

60. Clare H, Adams R, Maher C. Reliability of McKenzie classification of patients with cervical or lumbar pain. J Manipulative Physiol Ther 2005;28:122–7.

61. Takasaki H, Hall T, Oshiro S, et al. Normal kinematics of the upper cervical spine during the Flexion-Rotation Test - In vivo measurements using magnetic resonance imaging. Man Ther 2011;16:167–71.

62. Dvorak J, Dvorak V. Manual medicine. Diagnostics. Stuttgart, New York: Georg Thieme Verlag; 1984.

63. Hall T, Briffa K, Hopper D, et al. Long-term stability and minimal detectable change of the cervical flexion-rotation test. J Orthop Sports Phys Ther 2010;40:225–9.

64. Hall T, Briffa K, Hopper D, et al. The relationship between cervicogenic headache and impairment determined by the flexion-rotation test. J Manipulative Physiol Ther 2010;33:666–71.

65. Lemeunier N, da Silva-Oolup S, Chow N, et al. Reliability and validity of clinical tests to assess the anatomical integrity of the cervical spine in adults with neck pain and its associated disorders: part 1-A systematic review from the Cervical Assessment and Diagnosis Research Evaluation (CADRE) Collaboration. Eur Spine J 2017;26:2225–41.

66. Rubinstein S, Pool J, van Tulder M, et al. A systematic review of the diagnostic accuracy of provocative tests of the neck for diagnosing cervical radiculopathy. Eur Spine J 2007;16:307–19.

67. Thomas L. Cervical arterial dissection: an overview and implications for manipulative therapy practice. Man Ther 2016;21:2–9.

68. Mitchell J, Keene D, Dyson C, et al. Is cervical spine rotation, as used in the standard vertebrobasilar insufficiency test, associated with a measureable change in intracranial vertebral artery blood flow? Man Ther 2004;9:220–7.

69. Rushton A, Rivett D, Carlesso L, et al. International framework for the examination of the cervical region for cervical arterial dysfunction prior to orthopaedic manual therapy intervention. Man Ther 2014;19:222–8.

70. Sterling M, Jull G, Vicenzino B, et al. Sensory hypersensitivity occurs soon after whiplash injury and is associated with poor recovery. Pain 2003;104:509–17.

71. Chien A, Eliav E, Sterling M. Whiplash (grade II) and cervical radiculopathy share a similar sensory presentation: an investigation using quantitative sensory testing. Clin J Pain 2008;24:595–603.

72. Chua N, van Suijlekom H, Vissers K, et al. Differences in sensory processing between chronic cervical zygapophysial joint pain patients with and without cervicogenic headache. Cephalalgia 2011;31:953–63.

73. Jensen T, Baron R. Translation of symptoms and signs into mechanisms in neuropathic pain. Pain 2003;102:1–8.

74. Maxwell S, Sterling M. An investigation of the use of a numeric pain rating scale with ice application to the neck to determine cold hyperalgesia. Man Ther 2013;18:172–4.

75. Wainner R, Fritz J, Irrgang J, et al. Reliability and diagnostic accuracy of the clinical examination and patient self report measures for cervical radiculopathy. Spine 2003;28:52–62.

76. Jepsen J, Laursen L, Hagert C, et al. Diagnostic accuracy of the neurological upper limb examination I: inter-rater reproducibility of selected findings and patterns. BMC Neurol 2006;6:8.

77. Jepsen J, Laursen L, Hagert C, et al. Diagnostic accuracy of the neurological upper limb examination II: relation to symptoms of patterns of findings. BMC Neurol 2006;6:10.

78. Bennett M, Smith B, Torrance N, et al. The S-LANSS score for identifying pain of predominantly neuropathic origin: validation for use in clinical and postal research. J Pain 2005;6:149–58.

79. Krause S, Backonja M. Development of a neuropathic pain questionnaire. Clin J Pain 2003;19:306–14.

80. Lee M, McPhee R, Stringer M. An evidence-based approach to human dermatomes. Clin Anat 2008;21:363–73.

81. Schmid A, Brunner F, Luomajoki H, et al. Reliability of clinical tests to evaluate nerve function and mechanosensitivity of the upper limb peripheral nervous system. BMC Musculoskelet Disord 2009;21:11.

82. Apok V, Gurusinghe N, Mitchell J, et al. Dermatomes and dogma. Pract Neurol 2011;11:100–5.

83. Rolke R, Baron R, Maier C, et al. Quantitative sensory testing in the German Research Network on Neuropathic Pain (DFNS): standardized protocol and reference values. Pain 2006;123:231–43.

84. Nemani V, Kim H, Piyaskulkaew C, et al. Correlation of cord signal change with physical examination findings in patients with cervical myelopathy. Spine 2014;40:6–10.

85. Damodaran O, Rizk E, Rodriguez J, et al. Cranial nerve assessment: a concise guide to clinical examination. Clin Anat 2014;27:25–30.

86. Elvey R. Treatment of arm pain associated with abnormal brachial plexus tension. Aust J Physiother 1986;32:225–33.

87. Elvey R. Physical evaluation of the peripheral nervous system in disorders of pain and dysfunction. J Hand Ther 1997;10:122–9.

88. Hall T, Elvey R. Nerve trunk pain: physical diagnosis and treatment. Man Ther 1999;4:63–73.

89. Butler D. The sensitive nervous system. Adelaide: NOIgroup Publications; 2000.

90. Coppieters M, Kurz K, Mortensen T. The impact of neurodynamic testing on the perception of experimentally induced muscle pain. Man Ther 2005;10:52–60.

91. Maitland G. The slump test: examination and treatment. Aust J Physiother 1985;31:215–19.

92. Nee R, Jull G, Vicenzino B, et al. The validity of upper-limb neurodynamic tests for detecting peripheral neuropathic pain. J Orthop Sports Phys Ther 2012;42:413–24.

93. Coppieters M, Stappaerts K, Janssens K, et al. Reliability of detecting 'onset of pain' and 'submaximal pain' during neural provocation testing of the upper quadrant. Physiother Res Int 2002;7:146–56.

94. Coppieters M, Stappaerts K, Wouters L, et al. Aberrant protective force generation during neural provocation testing and the effect of treatment in patients with neurogenic cervicobrachial pain. J Manipulative Physiol Ther 2003;26:99–106.

95. Coppieters M, Stappaerts K, Staes F, et al. Shoulder girdle elevation during neurodynamic testing: an assessable sign? Man Ther 2001;6:88–96.

96. Sterling M, Treleaven J, Jull G. Responses to a clinical test of nerve tissue provocation in whiplash associated disorders. Man Ther 2002;7:89–94.

97. Zito G, Jull G, Story I. Clinical tests of musculoskeletal dysfunction in the diagnosis of cervicogenic headache. Man Ther 2006;11:118–29.

98. Enix D, Scali F, Pontell M. The cervical myodural bridge, a review of literature and clinical implications. J Can Chiropr Assoc 2014;58:184–92.

99. Hack GD, Koritzer RT, Robinson WL, et al. Anatomic relation between the rectus capitis posterior minor muscle and the dura mater. Spine 1995;20:2484–6.

100. Pontell M, Scali F, Enix D, et al. Histological examination of the human obliquus capitis inferior myodural bridge. Ann Anat 2013;195:522–6.

101. Jull G. Management of cervical headache. Man Ther 1997;2:182–90.

102. Kaltenborn F, Evjenth O, Kaltenborn TB, et al. Manual mobilization of the joints: the spine. vol. 2. 4th ed. Oslo: Norli; 2003.

103. Maitland GD, Hengeveld E, Banks K, et al. Maitland's vertebral manipulation. 7th ed. London: Butterworth; 2005.

104. Mulligan B. Manual therapy 'NAGS', 'SNAGS', 'MWMS'. 5th ed. Wellington: Plane View Press; 1995.

105. Hing W, Hall T, Rivett D, et al. The mulligan concept of manual therapy. Sydney: Churchill Livingstone, Elsevier; 2015.

106. Maher C, Adams R. Reliability of pain and resistance assessments in clinical manual lumbar spine examination. Phys Ther 1994;74:801–11.

107. van Trijffel E, Anderegg Q, Bossuyt P, et al. Inter-examiner reliability of passive assessment of intervertebral motion in the cervical and lumbar spine: a systematic review. Man Ther 2005;10:256–69.

108. Cattrysse E, Provyn S, Kool P, et al. Reproducibility of global three-dimensional motion during manual atlanto-axial rotation mobilization: an in vitro study. J Man Manip Ther 2010;18: 15–20.

109. Clec'h YL, Peterson C, Brunner F, et al. Cervical facet joint imaging-guided injections: a comparison of outcomes in patients referred based on imaging findings Vs palpation for pain. J Manipulative Physiol Ther 2016;39:480–6.

110. Hall T, Briffa K, Hopper D, et al. Reliability of manual examination and frequency of symptomatic cervical motion segment dysfunction in cervicogenic headache. Man Ther 2010;15: 542–6.

111. Jull G, Bogduk N, Marsland A. The accuracy of manual diagnosis for cervical zygapophysial joint pain syndromes. Med J Aust 1988;148:233–6.

112. Jull G, Zito G, Trott P, et al. Inter-examiner reliability to detect painful upper cervical joint dysfunction. Aust J Physiother 1997;43:125–9.

113. Phillips D, Twomey L. A comparison of manual diagnosis with a diagnosis established by a uni-level lumbar spinal block procedure. Man Ther 1996;1:82–7.

114. Schneider G, Jull G, Thomas K, et al. Intrarater and interrater reliability for select clinical tests in patients referred for diagnostic facet joint blocks in the cervical spine. Arch Phys Med Rehab 2013;94:1628–34.

115. Rabey M, Hall T, Hebron C, et al. Reconceptualising manual therapy skills in contemporary practice. Musculoskelet Sci Pract 2017;29:28–32.

116. Holden W, Taylor S, Stevens H, et al. Neck pain is a major clinical problem in ankylosing spondylitis, and impacts on driving and safety. Scand J Rheumatol 2005;34:159–60.

117. Kim D, Hilibrand A. Rheumatoid arthritis in the cervical spine. J Am Acad Orthop Surg 2005;13:463–74.

118. Mintken P, Metrick L, Flynn T. Upper cervical ligament testing in a patient with os odontoideum presenting with headaches. J Orthop Sports Phys Ther 2008;38:465–75.

119. Fice J, Cronin D. Investigation of whiplash injuries in the upper cervical spine using a detailed neck model. J Biomech 2012;45:1098–102.

120. Vetti N, Kråkenes J, Ask T, et al. Follow-up MR imaging of the alar and transverse ligaments after whiplash injury: a prospective controlled study. AJNR Am J Neuroradiol 2011;32:1836–41.

121. Li Q, Shen H, Li M. Magnetic resonance imaging signal changes of alar and transverse ligaments not correlated with whiplash-associated disorders: a meta-analysis of case-control studies. Eur Spine J 2013;22:14–20.

122. Myran R, Zwart J, Kvistad K, et al. Clinical characteristics, pain, and disability in relation to alar ligament MRI findings. Spine 2011;36:E862–7.

123. Hutting N, Scholten-Peeters G, Vijverman V, et al. Diagnostic accuracy of upper cervical spine instability tests: a systematic review. Phys Ther 2013;93:1686–95.

124. Osmotherly P, Rivett D, Rowe L. The anterior shear and distraction tests for craniocervical instability. An evaluation using magnetic resonance imaging. Man Ther 2012;17:416–21.

125. Osmotherly P, Rivett D, Rowe L. Construct validity of clinical tests for alar ligament integrity: an evaluation using magnetic resonance imaging. Phys Ther 2012;92:718–25.

126. Osmotherly P, Rivett D, Rowe L. Toward understanding normal craniocervical rotation occurring during the rotation stress test for the alar ligaments. Phys Ther 2013;93:986–92.

127. Cook C, Brismée J-M, Fleming R, et al. Identifiers suggestive of clinical cervical spine instability: a Delphi study of physical therapists. Phys Ther 2005;85:895–906.

128. Kendall F, McGeary E, Provance P. Muscles: testing and function. 4th ed. Baltimore: Williams and Wilkins; 1993.

129. Lluch E, Schomacher J, Gizzi L, et al. Immediate effects of active craniocervical flexion exercise versus passive mobilisation of the upper cervical spine on pain and performance on the craniocervical flexion test. Man Ther 2014;19:25–31.

130. O'Leary S, Falla D, Hodges PW, et al. Specific therapeutic exercise of the neck induces immediate local hypoalgesia. J Pain 2007;8:832–9.

131. Falla D, Farina D. Muscle fiber conduction velocity of the upper trapezius muscle during dynamic contraction of the upper limb in patients with chronic neck pain. Pain 2005;116: 138–45.

132. Cibulka M, Weissenborn D, Donham M, et al. A new manual muscle test for assessing the entire trapezius muscle. Physiother Theory Pract 2013;29:242–8.

133. Evjenth O, Hamberg J. Muscle stretching in manual therapy. Alfta: Alfta Rehab Forlag; 1984.

134. Janda V. Muscles and motor control in cervicogenic disorders: assessment and management. In: Grant R, editor. Physical therapy of the cervical and thoracic spine. 2nd ed. New York: Churchill Livingstone; 1994. p. 195–216.

135. Chiu T, Law E, Chiu T. Performance of the craniocervical flexion test in subjects with and without chronic neck pain. J Orthop Sports Phys Ther 2005;35:567–71.

136. Johnston V, Jull G, Souvlis T, et al. Neck movement and muscle activity characteristics in office workers with neck pain. Spine 2008;33:555–63.

137. Jull G, Amiri M, Bullock-Saxton J, et al. Cervical musculoskeletal impairment in frequent intermittent headache. Part 1: subjects with single headaches. Cephalalgia 2007;27:793–802.

138. Jull G, Kristjansson E, Dall'Alba P. Impairment in the cervical flexors: a comparison of whiplash and insidious onset neck pain patients. Man Ther 2004;9:89–94.

139. Steinmetz A, Claus A, Hodges P, et al. Neck muscle function in violinists/violists with and without neck pain. Clin Rheumatol 2016;35:1045–51.

140. Sterling M, Jull G, Vicenzino B, et al. Development of motor system dysfunction following whiplash injury. Pain 2003;103:65–73.

141. Jull G, O'Leary S, Falla D. Clinical assessment of the deep cervical flexor muscles: the craniocervical flexion test. J Manipulative Physiol Ther 2008;31:525–33.

142. Arumugam A, Mani R, Raja K. Interrater reliability of the craniocervical flexion test in asymptomatic individuals–a cross-sectional study. J Manipulative Physiol Ther 2011;34:247–53.

143. James G, Doe T. The craniocervical flexion test: intra-tester reliability in asymptomatic subjects. Physiother Res Int 2010;15:144–9.

144. Jull G, Barrett C, Magee R, et al. Further clinical clarification of the muscle dysfunction in cervical headache. Cephalalgia 1999;19:179–85.

145. Juul T, Langberg H, Enoch F, et al. The intra- and inter-rater reliability of five clinical muscle performance tests in patients with and without neck pain. BMC Musculoskelet Disord 2013;3:339.

146. Mayoux-Benhamou MA, Revel M, Vallee C, et al. Longus colli has a postural function on cervical curvature. Surg Radiol Anat 1994;16:367–71.

147. Falla DL, Campbell CD, Fagan AE, et al. Relationship between craniocervical flexion range of motion and pressure change during the craniocervical flexion test. Man Ther 2003;8:92–6.

148. Jull G, Falla D. Does increased activity of the superficial neck flexor muscles during performance of the craniocervical flexion test reflect reduced activation of the deep flexor muscles in people with neck pain? Man Ther 2016;25:43–7.

149. Cagnie B, Danneels L, Cools A, et al. The influence of breathing type, expiration and cervical posture on the performance of the craniocervical flexion test in healthy subjects. Man Ther 2008;13:232–8.

150. Jull GA. Deep cervical neck flexor dysfunction in whiplash. J Musculoskel Pain 2000;8:143–54.

151. O'Leary S, Falla D, Jull G, et al. Muscle specificity in tests of cervical flexor muscle performance. J Electromyogr Kinesiol 2007;17:35–40.

152. O'Leary S, Vicenzino B, Jull G. A new method of isometric dynamometry for the cranio-cervical flexors. Phys Ther 2005;85:556–64.

153. Domenech M, Sizer P, Dedrick G, et al. The deep neck flexor endurance test: normative data scores in healthy adults. PM R 2011;3:105–10.

154. Grimmer K. Measuring the endurance capacity of the cervical short flexor muscle group. Aust J Physiother 1994;40: 251–4.

155. Jarman N, Brooks T, James C, et al. Deep neck flexor endurance in the adolescent and young adult: normative data and associated attributes. PM R 2017;9:969–75.

156. Kumbhare D, Balsor B, Parkinson W, et al. Measurement of cervical flexor endurance following whiplash. Disabil Rehabil 2005;27:801–7.

157. Falla D, Rainoldi A, Merletti R, et al. Myoelectric manifestations of sternocleidomastoid and anterior scalene muscle fatigue in chronic neck pain patients. Clin Neurophysiol 2003;114:488–95.

158. O'Leary S, Jull G, Kim M, et al. Cranio-cervical flexor muscle impairment at maximal, moderate, and low loads is a feature of neck pain. Man Ther 2007;12:34–9.

159. Elliott J, Pedler A, Jull G, et al. Differential changes in muscle composition exist in traumatic and non-traumatic neck pain. Spine 2014;39:39–47.

160. O'Leary S, Cagnie B, Reeve A, et al. Is there altered activity of the extensor muscles in chronic mechanical neck pain? A functional magnetic resonance imaging study. Arch Phys Med Rehabil 2011;92:929–34.

161. Schomacher J, Erlenwein J, Dieterich A, et al. Can neck exercises enhance the activation of the semispinalis cervicis relative to the splenius capitis at specific spinal levels? Man Ther 2015;20:694–702.

162. Elliott J, Jull G, Noteboom J, et al. Fatty infiltration in the cervical extensor muscles in persistent whiplash associated disorders (WAD): an MRI analysis. Spine 2006;31:E847–55.

163. Elliott J, Pedler A, Kenardy J, et al. The temporal development of fatty infiltrates in the neck muscles following whiplash injury: an association with pain and posttraumatic stress. PLoS ONE 2011;6:e21194.

164. McPartland JM, Brodeur RR, Hallgren RC. Chronic neck pain, standing balance, and suboccipital muscle atrophy - a pilot study. J Manipulative Physiol Ther 1997;20:24–9.

165. Uthaikhup S, Assapun J, Kothan S, et al. Structural changes of the cervical muscles in elder women with cervicogenic headache. Musculoskelet Sci Pract 2017;29:1–6.

166. Geary K, Green B, Delahunt E. Intrarater reliability of neck strength measurement of rugby union players using a handheld dynamometer. J Manipulative Physiol Ther 2013;36:444–9.

167. Lee H, Nicholson L, Adams R. Neck muscle endurance, self-report, and range of motion data from subjects with treated and untreated neck pain. J Manipulative Physiol Ther 2005;28:25–32.

168. Revel M, Andre-Deshays C, Minguet M. Cervicocephalic kinesthetic sensibility in patients with cervical pain. Arch Phys Med Rehabil 1991;72:288–91.

169. Loudon JK, Ruhl M, Field E. Ability to reproduce head position after whiplash injury. Spine 1997;22:865–8.

170. Kristjansson E, Dall'Alba P, Jull G. A study of five cervicocephalic relocation tests in three different subject groups. Clin Rehabil 2003;17:768–74.

171. Treleaven J, Jull G, Sterling M. Dizziness and unsteadiness following whiplash injury - characteristic features and relationship to cervical joint position error. J Rehab Med 2003;35: 36–43.

172. Roren A, Mayoux-Benhamou M, Fayad F, et al. Comparison of visual and ultrasound based techniques to measure head repositioning in healthy and neck-pain subjects. Man Ther 2009;14:270–7.

173. Treleaven J. Dizziness, unsteadiness, visual disturbances, and sensorimotor control in traumatic neck pain. J Orthop Sports Phys Ther 2017;47:492–502.

174. Basteris A, Pedler A, Sterling M. Evaluating the neck joint position sense error with a standard computer and a webcam. Man Ther 2016;26:231–4.

175. Swait G, Rushton A, Miall C, et al. Evaluation of cervical proprioceptive function. Spine 2007;32:E692–701.

176. Chen X, Treleaven J. The effect of neck torsion on joint position error in subjects with chronic neck pain. Man Ther 2013;18:562–7.

177. Hides J, Smith MF, Mendis M, et al. A prospective investigation of changes in the sensorimotor system following sports concussion. An exploratory study. Musculoskelet Sci Pract 2017;29: 7–19.

178. Kristjansson E, Oddsdottir G. "The Fly": a new clinical assessment and treatment method for deficits of movement control in the cervical spine: reliability and validity. Spine 2010;35:E1298–305.

179. Williams K, Tarmizi A, Treleaven J. Use of neck torsion as a specific test of neck related postural instability. Musculoskelet Sci Pract 2017;29:115–19.

180. Yu L, Stokell R, Treleaven J. The effect of neck torsion on postural stability in subjects with persistent whiplash. Man Ther 2011;16:339–43.

181. Treleaven J, Jull G, LowChoy N. Standing balance in chronic whiplash- Comparison between subjects with and without dizziness. J Rehab Med 2005;37:219–23.

182. Field S, Treleaven J, Jull G. Standing balance: a comparison between idiopathic and whiplash-induced neck pain. Man Ther 2008;13:183–91.

183. Herdman S, Clendaniel R. Vestibular rehabilitation. 4th ed. Philadelphia FA: Davis Company; 2014.

184. Stokell R, Yu A, Williams K, et al. Dynamic and functional balance tasks in subjects with persistent whiplash: a pilot trial. Man Ther 2011;16:394–8.

185. Shumway-Cook A, Baldwin M, Polissar N, et al. Predicting the probability for falls in community-dwelling older adults. Phys Ther 1997;77:812–19.

186. Quek J, Brauer S, Clark R, et al. New insights into neck-pain-related postural control using measures of signal frequency and complexity in older adults. Gait Posture 2014;39:1069–73.

187. Quek J, Treleaven J, Clark R, et al. Towards understanding factors underpinning postural instability in older adults with neck pain. Gait Posture 2018;60:93–8.

188. Tjell C, Rosenhall U. Smooth pursuit neck torsion test: a specific test for cervical dizziness. Amer J Otol 1998;19:76–81.

189. Treleaven J, Jull G, LowChoy N. Smooth pursuit neck torsion test in whiplash associated disorders- Relationship to self reports of neck pain and disability, dizziness and anxiety. J Rehab Med 2005;37:219–23.

190. Daley L, Giffard P, Thomas L, et al. Validity of clinical measures of smooth pursuit eye movement control in patients with idiopathic neck pain. Musculoskel Sci Prac 2018;33:18–23.

191. Casa ED, Helbling JA, Meichtry A, et al. Head-eye movement control tests in patients with chronic neck pain; inter-observer

reliability and discriminative validity. BMC Musculoskelet Disord 2014;15:16.

192. Grip H, Jull G, Treleaven J. Head eye co-ordination and gaze stability using simultaneous measurement of eye in head and head in space movements -potential for use in subjects with a whiplash injury. J Clin Monit Comput 2009;23:31–40.

193. Treleaven J, Jull G, Grip H. Head eye co-ordination and gaze stability in subjects with persistent whiplash associated disorders. Man Ther 2011;16:252–7.

194. Treleaven J, Takasaki H, Grip H. Trunk head co-ordination in neck pain; 2012. IFOMPT; Quebec Canada.

195. Hikosaka O, Maeda M. Cervical effects on abducens motoneurons and their interaction with vestibulo-ocular reflex. Exp Brain Res 1973;18:512–1530.

196. Fischer A, Verhagen W, Huygen P. Whiplash injury. A clinical review with emphasis on neurootological aspects. Clin Otolaryngol 1997;22:192–201.

197. Padoan S, Karlberg M, Fransson P, et al. Passive sustained turning of the head induces asymmetric gain of the vestibulo-ocular reflex in healthy subjects. Acta Otolaryngol 1998;118:778–82.

198. Mucha A, Collins M, Elbin R, et al. A brief vestibular/ocular motor screening (voms) assessment to evaluate concussions preliminary findings. Am J Sports Med 2014;42:2479–86.

199. Halmagyi G, Curthoys I. Clinical testing of otolith function. Ann NY Acad Sci 1999;871:195–204.

200. Speers R, Ashton-Miller J, Schultz A, et al. Age differences in abilities to perform tandem stand and walk tasks of graded difficulty. Gait Posture 1998;7:207–13.

201. Poole E, Treleaven J, Jull G. The influence of neck pain on balance and gait parameters in community-dwelling elders. Man Ther 2008;13:317–24.

10

THE DIFFERENTIAL DIAGNOSIS OF SYMPTOMS AND SIGNS OF SENSORIMOTOR CONTROL DISTURBANCES

■ ■ ■ ■ ■ ■ ■ ■ ■ ■ ■ ■ ■ ■ ■ ■ ■ ■ ■ ■

The proprioceptive, visual and vestibular systems together provide input into the sensorimotor system for control of head and eye movement and postural stability. They interact closely in function and dysfunction. Cervical proprioceptors have reflex connections to both the vestibular and visual systems. They can influence the function of these systems and can also partially compensate for any deficits. Changes in cervical somatosensory information (Chapter 6) can influence the control, interaction and tuning of afferent input. This, in turn, may cause secondary adaptive responses in the visual or vestibular systems.[1–4] Likewise, both visual and vestibular deficits can impact on the cervical spine and cause altered head and neck positioning or increased muscle activity. A primary vestibular problem is often associated with a neck complaint[5,6] and altered vision can directly influence cervical musculature.[7,8] Thus there are many interactions and variables to appreciate to effectively clinically reason in differential diagnosis.

Signs and symptoms of altered sensorimotor control may be caused by a primary cervical, visual or vestibular problem, which may or may not cause secondary changes in the other systems. Further, increased reliance on the cervical spine may be required in circumstances where visual or vestibular input is impaired. If the cervical system subsequently becomes unreliable, this could lead to further amplification of symptoms stemming from visual or vestibular dysfunction. A mixed presentation may occur with coexisting visual, vestibular and cervical causes of sensorimotor disturbances (e.g., a postconcussion syndrome; age changes in the elderly). Certain medications and emotions such as anxiety can perpetuate or cause disturbances via several mechanisms.[9,10] Postconcussion, altered autonomic nervous system function and its control of cerebral blood flow can also exacerbate symptoms.[11] Consequently, it can be difficult to determine the precise causes of sensorimotor control disturbances. Nevertheless, it is essential to be aware of all possible common causes of dizziness, visual disturbances, tinnitus, altered head and eye movement control and postural instability, and be able to determine; (1) when a cervical cause or component is present or not; (2) when treatment directed towards the cervical spine is indicated; and (3) when referral is required for specialist assessment and investigations.

DIFFERENTIAL DIAGNOSIS OF DIZZINESS

Cervical dizziness attributed to altered cervical afferent input is often described as unsteadiness or light headedness. It is common in neck disorders especially in persons with persistent whiplash-associated disorders (WAD)[12] and cervicogenic headache.[13] Yet altered cervical afferent input is not the only possible cause of dizziness or light-headedness. The relationship between the cervical spine and dizziness has, and still is, a source of controversy. There are few reliable clinical tests to differentiate cervical from other causes of dizziness and some neurologists reject a possible cervical aetiology of symptoms.[14–16] Nevertheless, there is sufficient experimental and clinical evidence to support a cervical cause.[12,17–20] For instance, a cervical cause is supported when people with neck pain and dizziness have greater deficits in specific tests of cervical sensorimotor control compared with people without dizziness.[12,21–23] A cervical cause is also supported when symptoms improve with treatments directed specifically towards the cervical spine.[18,24–27]

A cervical disorder is more readily accepted as the cause of dizziness when neck pain is of an idiopathic origin. This is in contrast with dizziness associated with trauma such as a whiplash injury where other causes of dizziness are possible (e.g., an associated vestibular injury). It has also been proposed that dizziness and unsteadiness associated with WAD are side effects of medication or anxiety caused by either ongoing pain or financial gain.[28] Our research counters this view. We have found no difference between patients with chronic WAD with and without dizziness in medication intake, anxiety levels or compensation status. Neither do these features influence measures of sensorimotor control.[12,21,22,29] Other causes of dizziness must always be considered, but in the absence of traumatic brain injury following a whiplash injury, dizziness is most commonly caused by altered cervical afferent input.[12,30–35]

Conditions that must be considered in the differential diagnosis of dizziness include: central vestibular causes (vertebrobasilar insufficiency, cervical arterial dissection, vestibular migraine and mild brain injury/concussion) and peripheral vestibular disorders (e.g., benign paroxysmal positional vertigo [BPPV], labyrinthine concussion, or otolith disorders). The clinician should be cognizant of all causes to facilitate differentiation of dizziness in the patient presenting with neck pain.

Central vestibular disorders

Central vestibular disorders relate to any central nervous system (CNS) cause of vertigo. The most likely central vestibular causes to present to a musculoskeletal clinician are those secondary to cervical vascular disorders (vertebrobasilar insufficiency [VBI], or cervical artery dissection [CAD]), mild brain injury/concussion or vestibular migraine.

Cervical vascular disorders

Vascular supply to the vestibular system depends on arteries that originate from the basilar artery, which has supply from the vertebral arteries. Central vertigo and other neurological symptoms, arising from vascular compromise, are common to both VBI and CAD because the arteries also supply other cerebral structures including the vestibular system.[36] The reader is directed to a review by Thomas[37] on cervical arterial dysfunction.

VBI is more common in elderly patients who have degenerative musculoskeletal and peripheral or cardiovascular changes that may impact on blood flow in the cervical arteries. Abnormal vertebral artery blood flow and subsequent dizziness can also occur following a whiplash injury.[38,39] Although VBI can cause dizziness, its importance and frequency as a cause of dizziness in neck pain disorders has probably been overestimated because of concerns with the use of high velocity manipulative thrust procedures. Nevertheless due care is needed even with the use of low velocity manipulative therapy techniques in the management of older patients.[40,41] Patients with VBI may report transient vertigo and neurological symptoms that can be reproduced with sustained neck positioning and do not abate when the position is held. There may be a latent effect where symptoms are experienced soon after the head is returned to the neutral position.[42–44] However, other studies have found that dizziness is uncommon even in the presence of vertebral artery blood flow abnormalities. Nevertheless, caution is always warranted, especially in patients who develop symptoms with VBI testing because of a potential risk of a cerebrovascular incident.

CAD is a tear or haematoma in the wall of the artery. CAD accounts for 10% to 25% of ischaemic stroke in the young to middle-aged population. It can occur spontaneously, but commonly follows minor neck or head trauma.[45] The most common initial symptoms are unilateral neck pain or headache. Thus a person with impending CAD could inadvertently present to a musculoskeletal clinician for treatment.[37] Those in early stage CAD must be identified so that they can be referred for vital medical management, avoiding unnecessary and potentially harmful treatment. CAD can be confirmed with medical imaging such as magnetic resonance angiography or computed tomography angiography.[37,46] Risk factors for CAD include: genetic predisposition or history of migraine;[47] recent infection and even very minor head or neck trauma such as jerky head movements or heavy lifting.[48] Although rare, an ischaemic event and CAD soon after a whiplash injury has been reported in a few isolated cases.[42] However, generally damage to the vertebral artery is thought to be rare in the absence of a fracture or dislocation,[49,50] and if it occurs, it may be asymptomatic owing to collateral artery compensation.

Thomas et al.[51,52] suggests that CAD be suspected particularly in persons under the age of 55 years, who present with moderate to severe, new or unusual unilateral neck pain and/or headache associated with any unexplained transient or ongoing specific neurological dysfunction including dizziness within the last five weeks. Neurological signs and symptoms relevant to the area of the brain supplied by the cervical vertebral arteries, such as Horner syndrome, tinnitus, facial pain, vertigo and/or ataxia, should be considered but may not present initially.[53] Other risk factors, such as recent minor neck or head trauma and infection, must be noted. Work is currently underway to develop and test a clinical prediction tool to assist primary care providers in early diagnosis of CAD.

Minor brain injury

Dizziness from central vestibular dysfunction can result from a minor brain injury sustained from a direct blow to the head in a motor vehicle crash or a blunt injury trauma to the head or neck from a sports injury or other causes. Brain injury should be considered especially with reports of amnesia or head trauma.[54,55] Minor brain injury or concussion is an occasional cause of dizziness postwhiplash, but is a more common cause in contact sports injuries. However, a cervical cause of dizziness is also relatively common after blunt head trauma[20] and the role of cervical trauma in concussion incidents is being investigated as a primary cause of dizziness and other symptoms.[56-61]

Vestibular migraine

Vestibular migraine is a common cause of central vestibular vertigo with a population incidence of 1%. It occurs predominantly in middle-aged females.[62] It is characterized by episodic vertigo lasting several minutes to days. It can be associated with migraine headaches and, during an attack, clinical signs of central vestibular dysfunction may be apparent. There are usually no signs of abnormal vestibular function between attacks.[63] Preattack auras (reversible neurological symptoms) and postdromal fatigue can occur.[64,65] The precise cause is unknown, but there are suggestions

that in some cases it is triggered by neck injury and pain.[62,66]

Peripheral vestibular lesions

In cases of neck trauma, injurious forces can shear the delicate structures of the peripheral vestibular system which can result in vertigo attributable to either benign BPPV, labyrinthine concussion or otolith disorders.[20] Trauma can also rupture the otic capsule window resulting in a perilymph fistula.[67] In cases of nontraumatic neck pain, the main considerations in differential diagnosis are Ménière disease, labyrinth infections, vestibular neuronitis, acoustic neuromas and BPPV.[36]

There is considerable controversy regarding the frequency of peripheral vestibular versus cervical causes of dizziness in the whiplash injured patient, although there is a greater likelihood of a vestibular cause (35%) when there has been a mild head injury.[20,67,68] At one extreme, many consider vestibular disorders to be the primary cause of dizziness, although these reports are based largely on clinical patterns rather than tests of the vestibular system.[32,69,70] Other studies, which have screened with vestibular tests, report variable proportions.[20] Hinoki et al.[71] and Fischer et al.[1] reported normal vestibular test results in most of their whiplash cohorts, although many participants had some vestibular hyperactivity reasoned to result from limited neck movement and pain, with subsequent vestibulo-ocular reflex enhancement. Injuries induced by axial rotation as against linear acceleration in the crash may result in different types of neuro-otological injury.[72] The clinician should seek details of the injuring mechanism in the patient interview and choose tests accordingly to differentiate possible causes of the disturbances.

Benign paroxysmal positional vertigo

BPPV is the most common cause of peripheral vestibular vertigo. Symptoms are usually sudden-onset, short-duration vertigo, often accompanied by nausea and vomiting. Symptoms follow movements such as rolling over in bed and tilting the head back and are the result of otolith debris moving into the semicircular canal. The posterior canal is most commonly involved, but it can occur in the other canals.[68] Symptoms and signs of BPPV can cease either spontaneously or after otolith repositioning manoeuvers, but they can reappear.[73]

Possible causes are trauma, infection, degeneration or idiopathic.

Perilymph fistula

A perilymph fistula is an abnormal opening in the inner ear. Symptoms such as dizziness, vertigo, imbalance, nausea, tinnitus or fullness of the ear are reproduced with changes in ear pressure that occur with for instance, coughing, sneezing and loud noises.[74,75]

Ménière disease

Ménière disease is a disorder of the inner ear that can cause episodes of vertigo. The symptoms are variable but the most common are severe attacks of spontaneous rotational vertigo, that last from 20 minutes to several hours. They can be accompanied by tinnitus and hearing loss.[76]

Labyrinthitis and vestibular neuronitis

Labyrinthitis and vestibular neuronitis are characterized by acute, sustained vertigo with associated nausea and vomiting, which is aggravated with any position change. The patient may be forced to stay in bed for several days.[36] Patients may present to musculoskeletal clinicians in the subacute phase with dizziness, neck pain and stiffness resulting from attempts to limit head movement to avoid symptom exacerbation.

Acoustic neuroma

An acoustic neuroma is a slow growing benign tumour on the eighth (vestibulocochlear) cranial nerve and thus can cause both hearing and balance deficits. Symptoms such as tinnitus, true hearing loss, vertigo, imbalance and fullness in the ear are common.[36]

DIFFERENTIAL DIAGNOSIS OF OTHER SYMPTOMS

After dizziness, the most common sensorimotor symptoms associated with neck pain are visual disturbances[77] and tinnitus[78,79] but other symptoms such as subjective hearing loss and fullness in the ear can also occur. Similar to dizziness, there can be several causes of these symptoms. They can have peripheral and central vestibular causes and can also be caused by altered cervical input. Differential diagnosis of these symptoms takes on a similar process to that used for dizziness.

Specific unique aspects to consider for both visual symptoms and tinnitus will now be explored.

Visual system disturbances

After neck or head trauma, any dysfunctions in functionally related structures in the visual pathway can cause a variety of visual symptoms such as blurred or double vision, photophobia, difficulty with focusing, reading and tracking objects. Deficits can include strabismus (crossed eyes), convergence and/or accommodation insufficiency and oculomotor, binocular or visual spatial dysfunction. Collectively, these signs and symptoms are termed *posttrauma vision syndrome*.[80,81] Disturbance to the optokinetic reflex can also occur and has been noted as a specific finding after concussion.[82]

The role of the visual system should be considered in development or persistence of neck pain or discomfort. Unfavourable, challenging or demanding visual tasks or visual dysfunction may influence cervical posture, movement and muscle activity. Some direct relationships have been observed between unfavourable visual conditions and neck muscle activity which were independent of postural changes. This is thought to reflect a possible interaction between the visual system, sympathetic nervous system and the head-stabilizing muscles.[83] Visual ergonomics may be a potential driver of symptoms in some patients.[7,83–85]

Tinnitus

Tinnitus is associated with peripheral vestibular disorders such as Ménière disease, perilymph fistula[74] or labyrinthine concussion[86] or central vestibular disorders such as vestibular migraine.[62] Tinnitus can also result from abnormal cervical afferent input known as cervicogenic somatic tinnitus (CST). Specifically CST is characterized by severe subjective tinnitus with associated neck complaints in the absence of objective hearing deficits.[87] There is a high prevalence of tinnitus in temporomandibular dysfunction, which too may be associated with neck, head and face pain.[88]

CLINICAL EXAMINATION

The diagnosis should establish a correlation between symptoms such as dizziness, visual disturbances and tinnitus and signs of cervical spine dysfunction. Diagnosis is based on the patient's history, the clinical assessment of cervical musculoskeletal and sensorimotor impairments and, if required, the use of oculomotor, vestibular functional tests and a neurological examination to exclude vestibular and or visual disorders.[89] At present the primary criterion to confirm cervicogenic dizziness is exclusion of other pathologies. Nevertheless, a cluster of tests is emerging that may be useful for diagnosing cervical-related causes to assist differential diagnosis. This is especially important for patients with coexisting pathology.

History and interview

The clinician seeks a pattern to link symptoms to likely causes. The type of symptoms (dizziness or unsteadiness, tinnitus or visual complaints), the temporal relationship with neck pain, their frequency and duration and triggering factors help to distinguish cervical sensorimotor disturbances from other causes. However, the picture can be clouded in subacute vestibular conditions when compensatory adaptations have already been made and reports of unsteadiness or imbalance rather than vertigo become the main complaint.[90] Some patients report neck pain or stiffness as a consequence of adaptations to limit head movements to minimize dizziness or vertigo symptoms.[6] In this latter case, the dizziness is caused by a primary vestibular pathology and a cervical musculoskeletal problem is a secondary comorbidity.

Symptom differentiation

Table 10.1 presents a summary of the characteristic features of dizziness of various origins to consider in differential diagnosis.

Cervical dizziness is usually described as episodic unsteadiness or light headedness[91,92] but not true vertigo (environment and self-spinning), which is more characteristic of vestibular pathology.[93] Peripheral vestibular causes, apart from vestibular neuritis and Ménière disease, are often of short duration. They can be accompanied by hearing loss and tinnitus, but do not present with neurological signs. This is different to central vestibular complaints where vertigo duration can be longer and is usually associated with neurological signs such as cranial nerve impairments, ataxia and coordination difficulties.[94]

Visual complaints such as blurred vision, sensitivity to light, visual fatigue and difficulty judging distances are common in cervical disorders.[77,95] They probably reflect disturbances in the cervico-ocular reflexes and the close links between the eye and neck musculature.[33] Complaints of double vision or spots and words moving are common in visual system disorders but are uncommon in cervical disorders. Tinnitus, fullness in the ear and subjective hearing complaints may be associated with cervical disorders[79,87] but are more common in peripheral vestibular disorders.

The behaviour of symptoms assists differential diagnosis. Symptoms of cervical sensorimotor origin are usually exacerbated by specific neck movements or positions rather than whole body movement (vestibular), coughing (increased intracranial pressure) or anxiety.[96] Symptoms should co-vary with neck pain and there should be a close temporal relationship with onset of pain or injury. Accordingly, relief of symptoms should occur with relief of neck pain.[89,91] Thus symptom description, temporal pattern and aggravating factors are the foundation for differential diagnosis.[12,90,97–99] Recently, the combination of three questions on the dizziness handicap inventory (i.e., the combination of answering yes to: "Does looking up or does moving your head quickly increase your symptoms?" and answering no to: "Are you afraid to leave your house because of symptoms?") were shown to be useful to diagnose cervicogenic dizziness.[96] However, symptoms alone cannot be used to determine the diagnosis. This is illustrated in studies of dizziness postconcussion, where symptoms could not confirm or dismiss a cervical component. Rather, physical signs of musculoskeletal impairment, particularly the identification of upper cervical joint signs with manual examination, were most useful to indicate cervical involvement.[100–103]

Physical assessment

Cervical musculoskeletal examination

The clinician seeks a pattern of cervical musculoskeletal dysfunction (e.g., reduced range of motion, painful cervical joint dysfunction plus altered neuromuscular control) in conjunction with cervical related sensorimotor signs and symptoms to confirm a cervical origin of symptoms.[104,105] The presence of these cervical musculoskeletal impairments, especially involving the upper cervical spine, were central to patients whose main complaint was cervicogenic dizziness[26,103] and in patients with concussion who responded positively to treatment of the cervical region.[101]

TABLE 10.1

Characteristic features of dizziness of different origins

Type	Cervical	Vertebral artery	BPPV	Perilymph fistula	Peripheral vestibular	Central vestibular	Psychologic	Visual	Vestibular migraine
Description	Unsteady Light-headed	Faint Vertigo Dizziness	Vertigo	Vertigo Imbalance Motion intolerant	Vertigo Unsteady Motion intolerant	Imbalance Motion intolerant	Float/rocking Fullness in head	Light sensitive Objects move	Vertigo Unsteady
Frequency	Episodic	Episodic	Discreet attacks	Episodic Constant	Episodic vertigo Constant unsteady	Varies	Varies	Varies	Recurrent attacks
Duration	Mins-hours	Several secs	Secs	Constant	Secs to minutes	Varies	Varies	Varies	5 mins to 72h
Aggravate	Neck pain/ movement	Sustained neck extension or rotation	Rolling in bed Looking up Lying down	Visual challenges Increased ICC Loud noises	Head positions or movement	Spontaneous or provoked	Stress Anxiety Hyperventilation	Reading Visual stimuli Eye movements	Physical activity Stress Diet Lack of sleep Menstruation
Relieve	Decreased neck pain	Neck back to neutral	Subsides if stay in provoking position		Head/body still	Varies	Relaxation	Rest	Medication

Associated symptoms	Blurred vision Photosensitive Visual fatigue Nausea Tinnitus	Dizziness Dysarthria Dysphagia Diplopia Drop attacks Nystagmus Numbness Nausea	Nausea Vomiting	Unilateral tinnitus Aural pressure Hearing loss	Nausea Vomiting Hearing loss Tinnitus Ear fullness	Nausea Imbalance CNS signs Double vision Visual field shift	Lump throat Heart palpitations Tight chest	Other visual symptoms Double vision, Fatigue Headache	Moderate to severe headache Photo, phono sensitivity Nausea / vomiting Motion sensitivity Visual Aura
Suggested cause	Abnormal cervical afferent input	Vertebral artery dissection/ insufficiency	Debris in endolymph	Leak of perilymph fluid	Vascular injuries Fractures Trauma Acoustic neuroma	Brain stem Cerebellum	Anxiety Stress	Ambient visual system dysfunction	? Vasospasm in the brain
Main signs	Cervical MsK JPE >4.5 degrees CECNT SPNT Cervical torsion Trunk head coordination Absence other findings	VBI tests? ? Positive selected cranial nerve tests coordination tests	Positive Hallpike Dix or head roll	Positive pressure	Head impulse Head shake DVA En-bloc movements	Spontaneous or gaze evoked nystagmus [a]Oculomotor deficits or exacerbation of symptoms (VOMS) Ataxia	Nil	Midline shift NPC Accommodation Oculomotor Eye malalignment	Normal vestibular tests between attacks

[a]Oculomotor- smooth pursuit, saccades, skew deviation, near point convergence.
CECNT, Comfortable stance eyes closed neck torsion; CNS, central nervous system; DVA, dynamic visual acuity; H, hours; ICC, inter-cranial pressure; JPE, joint position error; Mins, minutes; MsK, musculoskeletal; NPC, near point convergence; SPNT, smooth pursuit neck torsion; VBI, vertebrobasilar insufficiency; VOMS, vestibular oculomotor screening.

Cervical sensorimotor examination

At present, the consensus is that tests to identify vestibular or CNS dysfunction have stronger clinical utility than tests for cervical causes of dizziness and sensorimotor control disturbances.[106] Nevertheless, some tests designed to support a cervical aetiology may help differential diagnosis, recognizing that a cluster of tests is more likely to be discriminatory than individual tests.[103] For example, in a study comparing patients with cervicogenic dizziness and BPPV, the combination of a cervical joint position error of greater than 4.5 degrees in at least one movement direction, abnormal responses to the cervical torsion test and the smooth pursuit neck torsion test collectively, were specific to cervicogenic dizziness.[103]

Not one sensorimotor test alone can confirm the diagnosis. Rather clinical reasoning towards differential diagnosis is based on findings of a cluster of sensorimotor tests, together with the patient's symptomatic reports and the presence of cervical musculoskeletal impairments. Sensorimotor tests with most discriminating potential, based on both laboratory and clinical studies, include cervical joint position tests and tests where neck torsion is incorporated.[103]

Neck torsion versus en-bloc trunk torsion

Neck torsion refers to movement of the neck via rotation of the trunk on a stable head. Its purpose is to selectively stimulate the cervical rather than the vestibular afferents. This is different to en-bloc tests, where there is simultaneous trunk and head rotation (no relative neck rotation) such that the vestibular rather than the cervical afferents are stimulated. When symptoms are reproduced with en-bloc rather than neck torsion movements, it suggests a vestibular rather than a cervical cause and vice versa.[36] Several studies investigating smooth eye pursuit,[21,33] balance[107] and joint position error (JPE) have incorporated neck torsion into tests to support a cervical cause of sensorimotor deficits.

The difference in performance when the head is in neutral compared with the torsion position is used to make decisions in tests of smooth pursuit eye movement and balance. Impaired cervical afferentation is indicated when there is a decrease in the ability to eye follow smoothly or an increase in postural sway occurs when the tests are performed in neck torsion compared with neutral positions. These changes observed with neck torsion in patients with neck pain disorders are not seen in healthy controls or in patients with brain injury or peripheral vestibular pathology.[21,33,108] A recent study also demonstrated that near point visual convergence was altered in persons with idiopathic neck pain when tested in torsion compared with the neutral position supporting its potential use in differential diagnosis.[109]

In researching the test of JPE, we developed a modified test where the head was held still and the patient repositioned the trunk to neutral (the laser pointer was attached to the chest rather than the head).[110] Patients with neck pain had significantly greater errors in almost all the "JPE torsion tests" when compared with healthy controls. The JPE torsion test may be more appropriate than the conventional JPE test when trying to differentiate altered cervical afferentation from vestibular dysfunction in people with chronic neck pain and dizziness, but this hypothesis needs further exploration.[111]

Another test using similar methodology is the cervical torsion test. In this test, similar to the torsion tests above, the head is held still, and the patient rotates the trunk to the left, then returns to neutral, then rotates the trunk to the right, and finally returns to neutral. This test was found to be one of a cluster of useful discriminating tests for cervicogenic dizziness.[103] Each position is sustained for 30 seconds and nystagmus of greater than 2 degrees in any of the end range or neutral positions is considered a positive test.[103] L'Heureux-Lebeau and colleagues[103] demonstrated a positive test in 52% of patients with cervicogenic dizziness compared with 8% in patients with diagnosed BPPV. In similar tests, where observation rather than measurement of nystagmus was used, 64% of whiplash patients demonstrated nystagmus.[112] However, up to 50% of subjects with no cervical pathology showed some observable nystagmus with this test[113] possibly from elicitation of the normal cervico-ocular reflex.[89] Thus more research is required to determine the real value of this test.

Vestibular and visual tests

More specific tests are required when vestibular or visual deficits are suspected in patients with neck trauma or when complaints are more indicative of these pathologies. The reader is again referred to Table 10.1 for a potential schema for differential diagnosis, possible symptom and physical test findings.

Recently a clinical vestibular oculomotor screening test (VOMS) was developed as a postconcussion test.[114] It uses exacerbation of symptoms (headache, fogginess, dizziness and nausea) following each of the clinical tests of saccades, smooth pursuit, gaze stability, near point convergence and vision motion sensitivity, to screen for both peripheral and central vestibular signs and visual system impairment. Another study used a similar approach with the addition of the response to an optokinetic reflex (OKR) stimulus.[82]

VOMS, OKR and positional BPPV tests are relatively quick and easy for clinicians to institute and can be good screening tests to assist differential diagnosis and direct management. Nevertheless, in patients in whom symptoms cannot be explained using these measures, referral to a vestibular physiotherapist or a behavioural optometrist or vision therapist may be warranted for a more thorough investigation of the vestibular, CNS, or visual systems using specialized equipment. Appropriate medical referral for further diagnostic workup and management may be required in some cases.

In benign cases where a cervical component is suspected, even in the presence of vestibular pathology, a closely monitored trial of treatment directed towards the cervical spine is warranted. Vestibular rehabilitation is often compromized when there is a cervical component and thus treatment directed towards the cervical spine in the first instance is recommended. In contrast, in circumstances where the visual system is the main driver of the patient's complaints, visual problems may need to be addressed first to allow gains to be maintained with cervical management.

CONCLUSION

Diagnosis of a cervical cause of symptoms of sensorimotor control disturbances is based on a combination of tests rather than any single test. The clinical reasoning considers the patient's symptomatic reports and history in combination with results from the physical examination of the cervical musculoskeletal system and tests for cervical sensorimotor control. Tests of vestibular and visual function may also be required as directed by the examination findings.

REFERENCES

1. Fischer A, Huygen PLM, Folgering HT, et al. Vestibular hyperreactivity and hyperventilation after whiplash injury. J Neurol Sci 1995;132(1):35–43.
2. Fischer A, Verhagen WIM, Huygen PLM. Whiplash injury. A clinical review with emphasis on neuro-otological aspects. Clin Otolaryngol 1997;22:192–201.
3. Hikosaka O, Maeda M. Cervical effects on abducens motoneurons and their interaction with vestibulo-ocular reflex. Exp Brain Res 1973;18:512–30.
4. Solarino B, Coppola F, Di Vella G, et al. Vestibular evoked myogenic potentials (vemps) in whiplash injury: a prospective study. Acta Otolaryngol 2009;129:976–81.
5. Bjorne A, Berven A, Agerberg G. Cervical signs and symptoms in patients with Meniere's disease: a controlled study. Cranio 1998;16:194–202.
6. Asama Y, Goto F, Tsutsumi T, et al. Objective evaluation of neck muscle tension and static balance in patients with chronic dizziness. Acta Otolaryngol 2012;132:1168–71.
7. Richter HO. Neck pain brought into focus. Work 2014;47:413–18.
8. Richter HO, Zetterlund C, Lundqvist LO. Eye-neck interactions triggered by visually deficient computer work. Work 2011;39:67–78.
9. Furman JM, Jacob RG. A clinical taxonomy of dizziness and anxiety in the otoneurological setting. J Anxiety Disord 2001;15:9–26.
10. Passatore M, Roatta S. Influence of sympathetic nervous system on sensorimotor function: whiplash associated disorders (WAD) as a model. Eur J Appl Physiol 2006;98:423–49.
11. Leddy JJ, Willer B. Use of graded exercise testing in concussion and return-to-activity management. Curr Sports Med Rep 2013;12:370–6.
12. Treleaven J, Jull G, Sterling M. Dizziness and unsteadiness following whiplash injury: characteristic features and relationship with cervical joint position error. J Rehabil Med 2003;35:36–43.
13. Jull G, Stanton W. Predictors of responsiveness to physiotherapy treatment of cervicogenic headache. Cephalalgia 2005;25:101–8.
14. Brandt T. Cervical vertigo-reality or fiction? Audiol Neurootol 1996;1:187–96.
15. Yacovino DA, Hain TC. Clinical characteristics of cervicogenic-related dizziness and vertigo. Semin Neurol 2013;33:244–55.
16. van Leeuwen RB, van der Zaag-Loonen H. Dizziness and neck pain: a correct diagnosis is required before consulting a physiotherapist. Acta Neurol Belg 2017;117:241–4.
17. Reid SA, Rivett DA. Manual therapy treatment of cervicogenic dizziness: a systematic review. Man Ther 2005;10:4–13.
18. Heikkila H, Johansson M, Wenngren BI. Effects of acupuncture, cervical manipulation and NSAID therapy on dizziness and impaired head repositioning of suspected cervical origin: a pilot study. Man Ther 2000;5:151–7.
19. Humphreys BK, Bolton J, Peterson C, et al. A cross-sectional study of the association between pain and disability in neck pain patients with dizziness of suspected cervical origin. J Whiplash Relat Disord 2003;1:63–73.
20. Ernst A, Basta D, Seidl RO, et al. Management of posttraumatic vertigo. Otolaryngol Head Neck Surg 2005;132:554–8.

21. Treleaven J, Jull G, Low Choy N. Smooth pursuit neck torsion test in whiplash associated disorders - relationship to self reports of neck pain and disability, dizziness and anxiety. J Rehabil Med 2005;37:219–23.

22. Treleaven J, Jull G, Low Choy N. Standing balance in persistent wad - comparison between subjects with and without dizziness. J Rehabil Med 2005;37:224–9.

23. Tjell C, Tenenbaum A, Sandström S. Smooth pursuit neck torsion test - a specific test for whiplash associated disorders? J Whiplash Relat Disord 2003;1:9–24.

24. Karlberg M, Magnusson M, Malmstrom EM, et al. Postural and symptomatic improvement after physiotherapy in patients with dizziness of suspected cervical origin. Arch Phys Med Rchabil 1996;77:874–82.

25. Galm R, Rittmeister M, Schmitt E. Vertigo in patients with cervical spine dysfunction. Eur Spine J 1998;7:55–8.

26. Reid SA, Callister R, Snodgrass SJ, et al. Manual therapy for cervicogenic dizziness: long-term outcomes of a randomised trial. Man Ther 2015;20:148–56.

27. Reid SA, Rivett DA, Katekar MG, et al. Comparison of Mulligan sustained natural apophyseal glides and Maitland mobilizations for treatment of cervicogenic dizziness: a randomized controlled trial. Phys Ther 2014;94:466–76.

28. Ferrari R, Russell AS. Development of persistent neurologic symptoms in patients with simple neck sprain. Arthritis Care Res 1999;12:70–6.

29. Treleaven J, Jull G, LowChoy N. The relationship of cervical joint position error to balance and eye movement disturbances in persistent whiplash. Man Ther 2006;11:99–106.

30. Hildingsson C, Wenngren BI, Toolanen G. Eye motility dysfunction after soft-tissue injury of the cervical-spine - a controlled, prospective-study of 38 patients. Acta Orthop Scand 1993;64:129–32.

31. Gimse R, Bjorgen IA, Tjell C, et al. Reduced cognitive functions in a group of whiplash patients with demonstrated disturbances in the posture control system. J Clin Exp Neuropsychol 1997;19:838–49.

32. Rubin AM, Woolley SM, Dailey VM, et al. Postural stability following mild head or whiplash injuries. Am J Otol 1995;16:216–21.

33. Tjell C, Rosenhall U. Smooth pursuit neck torsion test: a specific test for cervical dizziness. Am J Otol 1998;19:76–81.

34. Heikkila H, Astrom PG. Cervicocephalic kinesthetic sensibility in patients with whiplash injury. Scand J Rehabil Med 1996;28:133–8.

35. Treleaven J. Dizziness handicap inventory (DHI). Aust J Physiother 2006;52:67.

36. Herdman S, Clendaniel RA. Vestibular rehabilitation. 4th ed. Philadelphia: Davis Company; 2014.

37. Thomas LC. Cervical arterial dissection: an overview and implications for manipulative therapy practice. Man Ther 2016;21:2–9.

38. Panjabi MM, Cholewicki J, Nibu K, et al. Mechanism of whiplash injury. Clin Biomech (Bristol, Avon) 1998;13:239–49.

39. Endo K, Ichimaru K, Komagata M, et al. Cervical vertigo and dizziness after whiplash injury. Eur Spine J 2006;15:886–90.

40. Cagnie B, Barbaix E, Vinck E, et al. Atherosclerosis in the vertebral artery: an intrinsic risk factor in the use of spinal manipulation? Surg Radiol Anat 2006;28:129–34.

41. Cagnie B, Barbaix E, Vinck E, et al. Extrinsic risk factors for compromised blood flow in the vertebral artery: anatomical observations of the transverse foramina from C3 to C7. Surg Radiol Anat 2005;27:312–16.

42. Michaud TC. Uneventful upper cervical manipulation in the presence of a damaged vertebral artery. J Manipulative Physiol Ther 2002;25:472–83.

43. Arnold C, Bourassa R, Langer T, Stoneham G. Doppler studies evaluating the effect of a physical therapy screening protocol on vertebral artery blood flow. Man Ther 2004;9:13–21.

44. Thompson L, Rivett D, Bolton P, editors. Changes in vertebral artery blood flow during neck rotation. Musculoskeletal Physiotherapy Australia 13th Biennial conference. Sydney Australia: 2003.

45. Robertson JJ, Koyfman A. Cervical artery dissections: a review. J Emerg Med 2016;51:508–17.

46. Sheikh HU. Headache in intracranial and cervical artery dissections. Curr Pain Headache Rep 2016;20:8.

47. Mawet J, Debette S, Bousser MG, et al. The link between migraine, reversible cerebral vasoconstriction syndrome and cervical artery dissection. Headache 2016;56:645–56.

48. Thomas LC, Rivett DA, Attia JR, et al. Risk factors and clinical features of craniocervical arterial dissection. Man Ther 2011;16:351–6.

49. Kloen P, Patterson JD, Wintman BI, et al. Closed cervical spine trauma associated with bilateral vertebral artery injuries. Arch Orthop Trauma Surg 1999;119:478–81.

50. Biffl WL, Moore EE, Elliott JP, et al. The devastating potential of blunt vertebral arterial injuries. Ann Surg 2000;231:672–81.

51. Thomas LC. Cervical arterial dissection: an overview and implications for manipulative therapy practice. Man Ther 2016;21:2–9.

52. Thomas LC, Rivett DA, Attia JR, et al. Risk factors and clinical presentation of cervical arterial dissection: preliminary results of a prospective case-control study. J Orthop Sports Phys Ther 2015;45:503–11.

53. Fukuhara K, Ogata T, Ouma S, et al. Impact of initial symptoms for accurate diagnosis of vertebral artery dissection. Int J Stroke 2015;10:30–3.

54. Taylor AE, Cox CA, Mailis A. Persistent neuropsychological deficits following whiplash: evidence for chronic mild traumatic brain injury? Arch Phys Med Rehabil 1996;77:529–35.

55. Wenngren B, Pettersson K, Lowenhielm G, et al. Eye motility and auditory brainstem response dysfunction after whiplash injury. Acta Orthop Scand 2002;122:276–83.

56. Ellis MJ, Leddy JJ, Willer B. Physiological, vestibulo-ocular and cervicogenic post-concussion disorders: an evidence-based classification system with directions for treatment. Brain Inj 2015;29:238–48.

57. Marshall CM, Vernon H, Leddy JJ, et al. The role of the cervical spine in post-concussion syndrome. Phys Sportsmed 2015;43:274–84.

58. Schneider K, Meeuwisse WH, Nettel-Aguirre A, et al. Cervicovestibular physiotherapy in the treatment of individuals with persistent symptoms following sport related concussion: a randomised controlled trial. Br J Sports Med 2013;47:e1.

59. Schneider KJ. Sport-related concussion: optimizing treatment through evidence-informed practice. J Orthop Sports Phys Ther 2016;46:613–16.

60. Schneider KJ, Meeuwisse WH, Kang J, et al. Preseason reports of neck pain, dizziness, and headache as risk factors for concussion in male youth ice hockey players. Clin J Sport Med 2013;23:267–72.

61. Schneider KJ, Meeuwisse WH, Nettel-Aguirre A, et al. Cervicovestibular rehabilitation in sport-related concussion: a randomised controlled trial. Br J Sports Med 2014;48:1294–8.

62. Morganti LO, Salmito MC, Duarte JA, et al. Vestibular migraine: clinical and epidemiological aspects. Braz J Otorhinolaryngol 2016;82:397–402.

63. Lee JW, Jung JY, Chung YS, et al. Clinical manifestation and prognosis of vestibular migraine according to the vestibular function test results. Korean J Audiol 2013;17:18–22.

64. O'Connell Ferster AP, Priesol AJ, et al. The clinical manifestations of vestibular migraine: a review. Auris Nasus Larynx 2017;44:249–52.

65. Zhang YX, Kong QT, Chen JJ, et al. International Classification of Headache Disorders 3rd edn Beta-based field testing of vestibular migraine in China: demographic, clinical characteristics, audiometric findings and diagnosis statues. Cephalalgia 2016;36:240–8.

66. Lempert T, Olesen J, Furman J, et al. Vestibular migraine: diagnostic criteria. J Vestib Res 2012;22:167–72.

67. Grimm RJ. Inner ear injuries in whiplash. J Whiplash Relat Disord 2002;1:65–75.

68. Dispenza F, De Stefano A, Mathur N, et al. Benign paroxysmal positional vertigo following whiplash injury: a myth or a reality? Am J Otolaryngol 2011;32:376–80.

69. Toglia JU. Acute flexion-extension injury of neck - electronystagmographic study of 309 patients. Neurology 1976;26:808–14.

70. Chester JB. Whiplash, postural control, and the inner-ear. Spine 1991;16:716–20.

71. Hinoki M. Vertigo due to whiplash injury: a neuro-otological approach. Acta Otolaryngol 1975;419:9–29.

72. Geiger G, Aliyev RM. Whiplash injury as a function of the accident mechanism neuro-otological differential diagnostic findings. Unfallchirurg 2012;115:629–34.

73. Bhattacharyya N, Gubbels SP, Schwartz SR, et al. Clinical practice guideline: benign paroxysmal positional vertigo (update). Otolaryngol Head Neck Surg 2017;156:S1–47.

74. Fitzgerald DC. Persistent dizziness following head trauma and perilymphatic fistula. Arch Phys Med Rehabil 1995;76:1017–20.

75. Grimm RJ, Hemenway WG, Febray PR, et al. The perilymph fistula syndrome defined in mild head trauma. Acta Otolaryngol Suppl 1989;464:221–5.

76. Neff BA, Staab JP, Eggers SD, et al. Auditory and vestibular symptoms and chronic subjective dizziness in patients with Ménière's disease, vestibular migraine, and Ménière's disease with concomitant vestibular migraine. Otol Neurotol 2012;33:1235–44.

77. Treleaven J, Takasaki H. Characteristics of visual disturbances reported by subjects with neck pain. Man Ther 2014;19:203–7.

78. Michiels S, Hallemans A, Van de Heyning P, et al. Measurement of cervical sensorimotor control: the reliability of a continuous linear movement test. Man Ther 2014;19:399–404.

79. Peng BG, Pang XD, Yang H. Chronic neck pain and episodic vertigo and tinnitus. Pain Med 2015;16:200–2.

80. Hunt AW, Mah K, Reed N, et al. Oculomotor-based vision assessment in mild traumatic brain injury: a systematic review. J Head Trauma Rehabil 2016;31:252–61.

81. Padula WV, Argyris S. Post trauma vision syndrome and visual midline shift syndrome. Neurorehabilitation 1996;6:165–71.

82. McDevitt J, Appiah-Kubi KO, Tierney R, et al. Vestibular and oculomotor assessments may increase accuracy of subacute concussion assessment. Int J Sports Med 2016;37:738–47.

83. Mork R, Bruenech JR, Thorud HMS. Effect of direct glare on orbicularis oculi and trapezius during computer reading. Optom Vis Sci 2016;93:738–49.

84. Richter HO, Banziger T, Abdi S, et al. Stabilization of gaze: a relationship between ciliary muscle contraction and trapezius muscle activity. Vision Res 2010;50:2559–69.

85. Thorud HMS, Helland M, Aaras A, et al. Eye-related pain induced by visually demanding computer work. Optom Vis Sci 2012;89:E452–64.

86. Choi MS, Shin SO, Yeon JY, et al. Clinical characteristics of labyrinthine concussion. Korean J Audiol 2013;17:13–17.

87. Michiels S, Van de Heyning P, Truijen S, et al. Does multi-modal cervical physical therapy improve tinnitus in patients with cervicogenic somatic tinnitus? Man Ther 2016;26:125–31.

88. Buergers R, Kleinjung T, Behr M, et al. Is there a link between tinnitus and temporomandibular disorders? J Prosthet Dent 2014;111:222–7.

89. Wrisley DM, Sparto PJ, Whitney SL, Furman J. Cervicogenic dizziness: a review of diagnosis and treatment. J Orthop Sports Phys Ther 2000;30:755–66.

90. Treleaven J, LowChoy N, Darnell R, et al. Comparison of sensorimotor disturbance between subjects with persistent whiplash-associated disorder and subjects with vestibular pathology associated with acoustic neuroma. Arch Phys Med Rehabil 2008;89:522–30.

91. Bracher ES, Almeida CI, Almeida RR, et al. A combined approach for the treatment of cervical vertigo. J Manipulative Physiol Ther 2000;23:96–100.

92. Karlberg M, Persson L, Magnusson M. Impaired postural control in patients with cervico-brachial pain. Acta Otolaryngol Suppl 1995;440–2.

93. Baloh R, Halmagyi G. Disorders of the vestibular system. New York: Oxford University Press; 1996.

94. Alpini D, Ciavarro GL, Andreoni G, et al. Evaluation of head-to-trunk control in whiplash patients using digital craniocorpography during a stepping test. Gait Posture 2005;22:308–16.

95. Hülse M, Holzl M. Vestibulospinal reflexes in patients with cervical disequilibrium ("the cervical staggering"). HNO 2000;48:295–301.

96. Reid SA, Callister R, Katekar MG, et al. Utility of a brief assessment tool developed from the dizziness handicap inventory to screen for cervicogenic dizziness: a case control study. Musculoskelet Sci Pract 2017;30:42–8.

97. Imai T, Higashi-Shingai K, Takimoto Y, et al. New scoring system of an interview for the diagnosis of benign paroxysmal positional vertigo. Acta Otolaryngol 2016;136:283–8.

98. Cohen JM, Bigal ME, Newman LC. Migraine and vestibular symptoms-identifying clinical features that predict "vestibular migraine. Headache 2011;51:1393–7.

99. Cohen JM, Newman LC, Bigal ME. Classifying vestibular migraine: demographics, associated features, and triggers. Cephalalgia 2009;29:162 3.

100. Leddy JJ, Baker JG, Merchant A, et al. Brain or strain? Symptoms alone do not distinguish physiologic concussion from cervical/vestibular injury. Clin J Sport Med 2015;25:237–42.

101. Kennedy E, Quinn D, Tumilty S, et al. Clinical characteristics and outcomes of treatment of the cervical spine in patients with persistent post-concussion symptoms: a retrospective analysis. Musculoskelet Sci Pract 2017;29:91–8.

102. Reid SA, Callister R, Katekar MG, et al. Effects of cervical spine manual therapy on range of motion, head repositioning, and balance in participants with cervicogenic dizziness: a randomized controlled trial. Arch Phys Med Rehabil 2014;95:1603–12.

103. L'Heureux-Lebeau B, Godbout A, Berbiche D, et al. Evaluation of paraclinical tests in the diagnosis of cervicogenic dizziness. Otol Neurotol 2014;35:1858–65.

104. Malmstrom EM, Karlberg M, Melander A, et al. Cervicogenic dizziness - musculoskeletal findings before and after treatment and long-term outcome. Disabil Rehabil 2007;29:1193–205.

105. Jull GA, O'Leary SP, Falla DL. Clinical assessment of the deep cervical flexor muscles: the craniocervical flexion test. J Manipulative Physiol Ther 2008;31:525–33.

106. Reneker JC, Moughiman MC, Cook CE. The diagnostic utility of clinical tests for differentiating between cervicogenic and other causes of dizziness after a sports-related concussion: an international delphi study. J Sci Med Sport 2015;18:366–72.

107. Yu LJ, Stokell R, Treleaven J. The effect of neck torsion on postural stability in subjects with persistent whiplash. Man Ther 2011;16:339–43.

108. Williams K, Tarmizi A, Treleaven J. Use of neck torsion as a specific test of neck related postural instability. Musculoskelet Sci Pract 2017;29:115–19.

109. Giffard P, Daly L, Treleaven J. Influence of neck torsion on near point convergence in subjects with idiopathic neck pain. Musculoskelet Sci Pract 2017;32:51–6.

110. Chen X, Treleaven J. The effect of neck torsion on joint position error in subjects with chronic neck pain. Man Ther 2013;18:562–7.

111. Chen XQ, Treleaven J. The effect of neck torsion on joint position error in subjects with chronic neck pain. Man Ther 2013;18:562–7.

112. Oosterveld WJ, Kortschot HW, Kingma GG, et al. Electronystagmographic findings following cervical whiplash injuries. Acta Otolaryngol 1991;111:201–5.

113. Norre ME. Cervical vertigo. Diagnostic and semiological problem with special emphasis upon "cervical nystagmus". Acta Otorhinolaryngol Belg 1987;41:436–52.

114. Mucha A, Collins MW, Elbin RJ, et al. A brief vestibular/ocular motor screening (voms) assessment to evaluate concussions preliminary findings. Am J Sports Med 2014;42:2479–86.

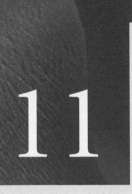

11

HEADACHE: THE DIFFERENTIAL DIAGNOSIS OF CERVICAL MUSCULOSKELETAL CAUSES OR CONTRIBUTORS

Headache is a common disorder that does not discriminate on the basis of age, gender or sociodemographic parameters.[1] Headache comes at high personal, social and financial costs.[1-3] Historically, physiotherapists have long had an interest in cervicogenic headache, a headache secondary to a cervical musculoskeletal disorder.[4] In recent years, there has been increasing interest in the primary headaches, migraine and tension-type headache (TTH) because neck pain is frequent in these headaches with as many as 60% to 80% of people with migraine and TTH reporting neck pain with their headache.[5-8] Neck pain is so frequent that some suggest that future Global Burden of Disease studies group neck pain with headache rather than with low-back pain[1] because aetiologically, the thought is that much neck pain is secondary to headache.[3] Furthermore, manual therapy to the cervical spine (manipulation, mobilization, massage) appears to be the most common non-medical treatment used for the management of common recurrent headaches such as migraine, TTH and cervicogenic headache either on a practitioner-prescribed or self-prescribed basis.[9] Thus there appears to be an assumption that headache-associated neck pain and cervical musculoskeletal dysfunction are automatically related.

It goes without saying that treatment should match the condition, for example, triptans are indicated for migraine but not for cervicogenic headache. Likewise, treating the neck with methods such as cervical manipulation and mobilization is indicated for cervicogenic headache. Yet are these methods always indicated when neck pain accompanies primary headaches such as

migraine and TTH? This chapter focuses on the critical question of differential diagnosis of cervical musculoskeletal causes or contributors to various headache forms that underpins the relevance or not of local neck treatments such as manipulative therapy and specific therapeutic exercise in the management of various headache types.

NECK PAIN AND HEADACHE

Neck pain is a frequent symptom of headache. The critical question is: "Does the presence of neck pain with headache implicate a cervical musculoskeletal cause?" It is invalid to assume that the site of pain always overlies its source, for example, intense forearm pain may be a symptom of a centrally located cervical radiculopathy, anterior knee pain may have its origin in the hip. Similarly, headache-related neck pain may have a local or remote source.

The mechanism underlying the relationship between head and neck pain involves convergence between cervical and trigeminal afferents in the trigeminocervical nucleus in the brainstem. Nociceptive afferents from the upper three cervical nerves (C1, C2, C3) converge onto common second-order neurons that also receive afferents from the trigeminal nerve.[10] The pathway is bidirectional. It not only explains how nociception from the upper three cervical segments can refer pain into the frontal region of the head, but also in the presence of central sensitization and increased excitability to converging synaptic inputs, how nociception from trigeminal afferents can refer pain into the neck.[11-13]

Migraine is a primary headache. It is a neurobiological disorder that is not fully understood, but the role of the trigeminovascular system, sensitization of pain pathways, the central nervous system (CNS) and neurotransmission are all considered in possible mechanisms. Neck pain is common and palpation of the neck may produce headache.[14] There are reports of findings of cervical musculoskeletal dysfunction in persons with migraine,[15,16] but equally, there is evidence that the neck pain is part of migraine symptomology and not a symptom of local neck dysfunction. When the neck pain associated with the migraine responds to acute triptan therapy,[17] it implies that the pains share an underlying pathophysiology rather than having separate causes. There is a body of research suggesting that migraine-associated neck pain is a biomarker for central sensitization[18] because neck pain and migraine are often tightly linked. For example, neck pain intensity is related to migraine severity, neck pain and nausea increase with the increasing migraine severity,[6] neck pain is predictive of migraine-related disability and the higher the neck pain, the more treatment resistant is the migraine.[19] Migraineurs may not automatically relate neck pain to the beginning of a headache attack,[20] which often delays them taking medication.[21] It was shown that migraines were better managed when medications were taken at the first sign of neck pain.[18]

Thus neck pain may be part of the migraine symptom complex, without any necessary contribution from local cervical musculoskeletal disorders. Certainly this would fit with the results of several studies, which have not found cervical musculoskeletal impairment in persons with migraine.[22–29] It would also fit with the evidence that manipulative therapy and other local treatments directed towards the neck do not make substantive changes to headache frequency or intensity or to the course of migraine.[30–32]

Nevertheless, the prevalence of neck pain and disability appears to increase with migraine chronicity.[6,33] The classification of chronic migraine in the current International Headache Classification (ICHD III)[34] may also present confusion in terms of the relationship between cervical musculoskeletal dysfunction and migraine. Chronic migraine is defined as "headache occurring on 15 or more days per month for more than 3 months, which has the features of migraine headache on at least 8 days per month" (ICHD III p650). This means that a person diagnosed with chronic migraine could have eight migraines and seven or more cervicogenic headaches per month, which could account for any cervical musculoskeletal signs associated with chronic migraine. There is already well-recognized symptomatic overlap between migraine and cervicogenic headache, which could add to diagnostic confusion.[35] Thus there needs to be care in history taking to tease out potentially different headache types, otherwise there could be flawed conclusions about the role of cervical musculoskeletal dysfunction in migraine.

The same questions present about the role of neck pain and cervical musculoskeletal dysfunction in TTH. The pathogenesis of TTH is still uncertain. Even though TTH is classified as a primary headache in the ICHD III, both central and peripheral mechanisms may be at play, suggesting that it may be a primary or secondary headache or both.[34] TTH, with the potential diversity in causes or contributors, presents the greatest challenge in differential diagnosis. Some associate TTH with the same cervical musculoskeletal dysfunction that classifies cervicogenic headache,[36] others regard the presence of trigger points in neck muscles as an indication of cervical musculoskeletal dysfunction,[37] whereas others find no association between cervical musculoskeletal dysfunction and TTH.[26,29] Similar to migraine, TTH when classified as chronic (> 15 headache days per month) requires that only eight headaches fulfil the TTH criteria,[34] meaning that chronic TTH can potentially be a mix of headaches. There is some evidence that manipulative therapy and other physical therapies may be helpful for TTH,[38,39] but in many studies, it is difficult to know if the headaches, albeit named TTH, were clearly TTH when responding to therapies that have proven efficacious for cervicogenic headache. The potential heterogeneity in causes and contributors to TTH indicate the need for a skilled clinical examination of the cervical region to determine the role or not of cervical musculoskeletal dysfunction in an individual's TTH presentation.

Neck pain is a critical feature of cervicogenic headache and is a classification criterion.[34,40] In contrast to most other headache forms, neck pain is a main feature of cervicogenic headache. Characteristically, pain begins in the neck and once it builds up, the headache begins.[41] The neck pain is directly associated with cervical musculoskeletal dysfunction. Restricted neck motion and symptomatic upper cervical joint dysfunction (relief of pain by anaesthetic joint blocks or blocks of the medial branch of the dorsal ramus) are classification criteria. Cervicogenic headache is classified as a secondary headache, directly attributable to cervical musculoskeletal dysfunction where traditional treatments for cervical musculoskeletal dysfunction have proven helpful.[39,42–45]

It would be simple if cervical musculoskeletal dysfunction was related to one headache type, cervicogenic headache, but it is far from straightforward. The role of cervical musculoskeletal dysfunction in migraine and TTH as a causative, contributing or comorbid factor is still to be determined. Cervical musculoskeletal dysfunction may also contribute to other headache types, such as headaches associated with craniomandibular dysfunction and concussion[46–48] and is a frequent comorbid feature of headache in older persons.[8] Mixed headaches are common. Patients may suffer two different headache types concurrently as indicated in the definitions of chronic migraine and TTH. The role of neck pain is probably more complex than a simple neck-headache relationship. The Norwegian longitudinal population-based cohort study found a bidirectional relationship between the development of chronic musculoskeletal complaints (cervical, lumbar, extremity pain) and the development of chronic daily headache. Persons who developed chronic musculoskeletal complaints were almost twice as likely to develop chronic headaches and vice versa.[49] The authors summarized that either shared underlying mechanisms via CNS sensitization, psychological predisposition, reduced pain coping skills or shared genetic susceptibility could underlie these relationships.

Neck pain associated with headache may have a local or remote source. This behoves the clinician to undertake an effective clinical examination of the headache patient. It is important to listen to the description of the history, onset, temporal pattern and behaviour of headache and determine whether the story matches the classification criteria for a particular headache type or has aberrant features which might suggest mixed or other headache types. From the perspective of any associated neck pain, a skilled physical examination of the cervical region is necessary to determine the presence or not and comparability of any cervical musculoskeletal dysfunction.

WHAT DEFINES CERVICAL MUSCULOSKELETAL DYSFUNCTION?

There is little consistency in the headache literature as to which cervical musculoskeletal impairments are measured and which need to be present to conclude that cervical musculoskeletal dysfunction has a causative, contributory or comorbid role in a particular headache type.

The history of cervicogenic headache has witnessed several proposed causes. Early candidates were: irritation of the cervical sympathetic nerve running along the vertebral artery or cervical migraine (since disproven);[50] cervical discal disorders; and disorders of the cervical nerve roots.[51–54] Work from the 1960s onwards confirmed that the most common source is referred pain from the upper cervical joints (C0–3) with C1–2 and C2–3 articulations probably the more common sites.[55–58] Other segments are not excluded. Reports of headache relief with surgery to lower segments are not uncommon.[59] Radiological imaging of painful upper cervical joints, especially in younger to middle age usually does not demonstrate any relevant pathological change. However, osteoarthritis was evident radiologically in late middle-aged to older-aged persons with cervicogenic headache using bone single-photon emission computed tomography/computed tomography.[60] In advanced osteoarthritis, C2 spondylitic radiculopathy was reported as the lesion causing cervicogenic headache.[61]

Any structure innervated by the upper three cervical nerves is capable of referring pain into the head via common neurons in the trigeminocervical nucleus. Nevertheless as per the classification criteria for cervicogenic headache,[34,40] articular dysfunction and movement impairments are fundamental to defining cervicogenic headache or a cervical role in headache. Painful joint dysfunction does not occur in isolation and will always be associated with changes in the neuromuscular system. The nervous system and sensorimotor system may also contribute to the pain syndrome. The question is: "Which impairments are fundamental to define a cervical musculoskeletal cause or contributor to headache?"

Articular system

Reduced cervical motion and relief of headache with anaesthetic cervical joint or nerve blocks are classification criteria for cervicogenic headache,[34,40] and most studies investigating cervical musculoskeletal impairments in headache include measures of cervical range of movement.[15,23,26,29,62,63] Reduced motion is consistently found in cervicogenic headache cohorts of all ages and the cervical flexion rotation test has proven validity to identify headaches associated with C1–2 dysfunction.[8,26,28,29,63–66]

The second criterion for diagnosis of cervicogenic headache is the presence of upper cervical joint dysfunction. Radiological imaging is often not informative but manual examination is a safe clinical alternative. Manual examination has not been without its controversies, but when the question and clinical decision is simply to nominate whether or not a person has symptomatic upper cervical joint dysfunction, it is proving to be a valid and valuable examination technique.[26,28,66–71] It is worthy of note that reproduction of headache by palpating a cervical structure whether bone or muscle is not necessarily a positive sign of a cervical cause.[14] The CNS is sensitized in both migraine and TTH, and a peripheral nociceptive stimulus into a sensitized system can be expected to aggravate headache. Neck tenderness alone is non-discriminative and cannot be regarded as a positive joint sign for cervicogenic headache. Rather joint dysfunction is present when the clinician detects with manual examination, altered segmental motion, altered resistance to the induced motion and pain is reproduced. Manual handling must be skilful. Thumb and finger contact must never elicit discomfort or pain, it will confound interpretation. Poor manual skills can result in false positive findings.

Neuromuscular system

Changes in muscle function occur in reaction to painful joint dysfunction and include changes in motor control and reduced strength and endurance. Changes documented to date specifically in cervicogenic headache include: an altered pattern of flexor muscle activity (reduced activation of the deep cervical flexors and heightened activity in the superficial flexors) as measured in the craniocervical flexion test (CCFT); and reduced strength and endurance of the craniocervical flexors, the cervical flexors and cervical extensors.[22,24,26,28,72] Migraine cohorts have not demonstrated the altered pattern of muscle activity in the CCFT,[26,28,73] or demonstrated reduced strength in the craniocervical flexors,[24] cervical flexors and extensors.[26,74] One study reported

differences in the CCFT in migraine patients compared with controls, but the mean value recorded for the CCFT (26 mmHg) was within values for pain-free individuals.[16] Changes in muscle function have, in the main, not been demonstrated in TTH.[22,26,73] One small study of TTH revealed that 4 out of 10 subjects had poor performance in the CCFT.[75] Reduced neck extensor strength but not flexor strength was demonstrated in one study of migraine[76] and one of TTH.[77] Reduced extensor strength, without any deficit strength or endurance in the flexors, is not a typical finding of a cervical musculoskeletal disorder. These findings might reflect pain inhibition with the application of resistance during the test procedure because both headaches are associated with considerable pericranial tenderness.

Muscle trigger points have been regarded by some as primary cervical musculoskeletal dysfunction.[37,78,79] However, trigger points can be present in migraine and TTH as well as in non-musculoskeletal conditions such as cancer pain, visceral pain and chronic prostatitis.[62,78,80–85] Perhaps they are better considered as a secondary reaction in muscles to a pain state of various origins. The presence of trigger points does not determine or differentiate a cervicogenic headache. In relation to headache, most research into trigger points has been conducted with TTH.

It is not surprising that changes in neck muscle activity are observed in migraine cohorts.[76,82,86] This is likely to be a reaction to pain rather than a reaction to primary cervical musculoskeletal dysfunction, given the evidence, on balance, of the lack of cervical musculoskeletal dysfunction in migraine. It is possible that these instances of general muscle tension underlie feelings of neck stiffness that may accompany headache, although a biomechanical study of stiffness characteristics of the upper cervical spine in rotation revealed no differences between persons with migraine, TTH and controls.[87]

Posture

Static postures, in particular, angles representing a forward head posture (FHP) have been measured as an indication of the presence of cervical musculoskeletal dysfunction. The literature is divided on the relevance of this measure to neck pain disorders because studies are divided on a relationship between the static FHP and neck pain disorders, including cervicogenic headache.[28,72,88] The FHP is not a feature of migraine[15,28,79] but has been found in some groups of chronic TTH, and lesser so in episodic TTH, yet the FHP has not related to headache frequency, intensity or duration.[62,75,78,89] As a static FHP is not always associated with a cervical musculoskeletal disorder, it is not a measure to define a cervical musculoskeletal cause or contributor to headache. Nevertheless, evidence is mounting for a relationship between assuming a FHP while working and neck pain,[90–92] but this functional posture has not been examined in migraine, TTH or indeed cervicogenic headache.

Neural system

There are anatomic links between the deep cervical muscles and spinal dura mater[93] and movements of the upper cervical spine and suboccipital muscles can move the spinal dura mater in this region. The spinal dura in this region is innervated by the upper three cervical nerves. If it becomes irritated and sensitive to movement (e.g., from neighbouring joint inflammation) or has reduced extensibility, it is capable of contributing to, or causing headache as a "cervicogenic source". There has been little research into nerve tissue mechanosensitivity in cervicogenic headache or indeed in other headache types.[28,44,94,95] Preliminary evidence suggests that nerve tissue mechanosensitivity may contribute to a cervicogenic headache in, at most, 8% to 10% of cases.[28,44] Although important to recognize in those cases, the low incidence of nerve tissue mechanosensitivity cannot serve as a feature to define a cervical cause or contributor to headache.

Sensorimotor dysfunction

Sensorimotor control and differentiation of sensorimotor disturbances such as proprioception and balance deficits are considered in detail in Chapters 6 and 10. Sensorimotor dysfunction is certainly not uncommon in cervical spine disorders, especially when the symptoms of dizziness and unsteadiness are present. In one trial of cervicogenic headache, about 30% of participants reported light headedness/dizziness.[44] However, sensorimotor disturbances are not unique to cervical musculoskeletal causes. They can be a feature of post-concussion headache[96] and migraine, particularly vestibular migraine where a recent study estimated that 21% of a migraine cohort had vestibular migraine.[97,98] Findings of sensorimotor disturbances are disparate in

TTH,[99–101] but there is very little research in this field. Symptoms and disturbances in sensorimotor control are not unique to cervicogenic headache and therefore cannot serve as a feature to differentiate a cervical cause. Nevertheless, there is every possibility that measures to differentiate cervical-related sensorimotor control disturbances may emerge in the future.

Cervical musculoskeletal dysfunction defined

We return to the question of which cervical musculoskeletal impairments need to be present to indicate a cervical musculoskeletal cause or role in headache. Population-based findings of reduced cervical motion or muscle strength are characteristic of cervicogenic headache but are not helpful in differential diagnosis of the individual patient. Each measure has age and gender effects and with the exception of the flexion rotation test,[25] there are no cut-off values for ranges of cervical movement or strength to suggest what is "normal" or dysfunctional. In practice, the clinician does not make a decision based on one feature. Rather clinical reasoning decisions are based on a pattern of dysfunction. Musculoskeletal features consistently present in cervicogenic headache populations are reduced range of movement, upper cervical joint dysfunction and impaired neuromuscular function, both in the CCFT as well as cervical flexor and extensor muscle strength. Indeed, it is these features in combination that have been shown to be highly specific and sensitive to differentiate a cervical musculoskeletal source of headache, (i.e., distinguish cervicogenic headache from migraine and TTH).[22,26]

The presence collectively of reduced cervical motion (either in single planes, or specific test movement combinations e.g., the flexion rotation test,[25,63] the extension rotation test[11]), upper cervical joint dysfunction and poor cervical muscle function is a fundamental signature of cervical musculoskeletal dysfunction. This pattern should be present if the neck pain associated with headache is to be attributed to a cervical musculoskeletal cause.

CERVICAL MUSCULOSKELETAL DYSFUNCTION IN HEADACHE: CLINICAL DECISIONS

Cervical musculoskeletal disorders are the primary cause of cervicogenic headache. Yet cervical musculoskeletal dysfunction may be present in other headache types: headaches associated with craniomandibular dysfunction, headaches associated with concussion, mixed headaches and chronic migraine or TTH which, by definition, can include a second headache type which could be cervicogenic.

The clinical examination, headache history and behaviour as well as the physical examination assumes considerable importance in differential diagnosis. The decisions required from a cervical musculoskeletal perspective are first, whether or not there is a pattern of cervical musculoskeletal dysfunction (reduced motion, painful upper cervical joint dysfunction, and impaired neuromuscular function). When the pattern is not present, any neck pain is more probably part of the headache symptom complex. If the pattern of cervical musculoskeletal dysfunction is present, then the decisions are whether (1) it has a primary causative role (the pattern of headache history, symptoms and magnitude of dysfunction match a cervicogenic headache classification); (2) a contributing role (e.g., the magnitude of cervical musculoskeletal dysfunction does not

match the history of headache intensity and frequency); or (3) a comorbid role (i.e., the behaviour of neck pain and associated cervical musculoskeletal dysfunction is not consistently related to the headache) (Fig. 11.1). Treatment decisions and expectations of outcomes are based on these decisions.

CONCLUSION

Neck pain commonly accompanies headache. It is fundamental to know whether such neck pain is related to a local cervical musculoskeletal cause or whether it is part of the headache symptom complex, if understanding is to be progressed of the role of cervical musculoskeletal disorders in cervicogenic and other headache types and to offer patients appropriate treatment.

Cervical musculoskeletal disorders are clearly linked to cervicogenic headache (or a neck-related headache as an alternate term) but the literature is divided about any link between cervical musculoskeletal dysfunction and migraine and TTH in a causative role. Several aspects probably underlie this uncertainty, including the

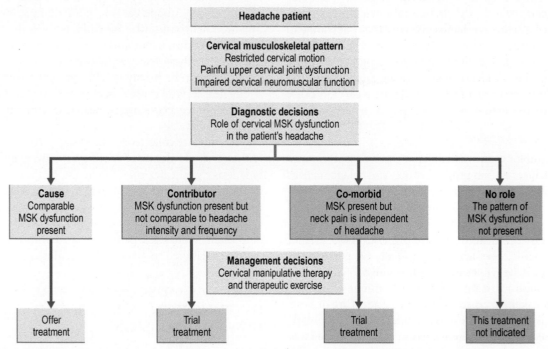

Fig. 11.1 ■ Clinical reasoning on the role of cervical musculoskeletal dysfunction in a patient's headache to inform treatment planning. *MSK*, Musculoskeletal.

relevance of single signs. Another problem in today's literature is that inclusion criteria for headache cohorts are often described as "according to the ICHD III classification criteria" or "as diagnosed by a neurologist", but no detail of the headache characteristics are provided to ensure "pureness" of the classification in the population studied.[102] Thus when a study reports reduced cervical motion in migraine or TTH, there is uncertainty about the result knowing that there can be confusion in diagnosis between migraine without aura and cervicogenic headache[20,35] and that chronic migraine or TTH can include seven or more headache days per month of a second headache type.[34] Thus two important criteria for future studies investigating cervical musculoskeletal dysfunction in different headache types are confirmation of the population studied and whether all of the key determinants of cervical musculoskeletal function were present, (i.e., the pattern of reduced range of movement, upper cervical joint dysfunction and impaired neuromuscular function).

These recommendations also apply to inclusion criteria for clinical trials. Management methods of cervical manipulative therapy and specific exercise have been used successfully to treat cervicogenic headache. These methods can also be helpful when cervical musculoskeletal dysfunction is an apparent "contributor" to headache.[103] Yet to use these methods to treat headache-associated neck pain that is not related to a local joint and neuromuscular dysfunction lacks rationale and potentially detracts from evidence of their effectiveness. This is not to suggest that persons with migraine and TTH without any cervical joint or neuromuscular dysfunction cannot gain some benefit from some forms of hands on treatment to the neck, instruction in relaxation, pain coping skills and lifestyle advice as part of multiprofessional management, but this management approach has a different rationale.

More research and critical thinking in clinical practice is required to better understand the role of cervical musculoskeletal dysfunction in various headache types. Future clinical trials are required to evaluate the benefits of management methods for the cervical spine when they are knowingly directed towards a proposed causative, contributing or comorbid role of cervical musculoskeletal dysfunction if the true benefits of treating the neck in headache are to be understood.

REFERENCES

1. Vos T, Barber R, Bell B, et al. Global, regional, and national incidence, prevalence, and years lived with disability for 301 acute and chronic diseases and injuries in 188 countries, 1990-2013: a systematic analysis for the Global Burden of Disease Study 2013. Lancet 2015;386:743–800.
2. Linde M, Gustavsson A, Stovner L, et al. The cost of headache disorders in Europe: the Eurolight project. Eur J Neurol 2012;19:703–11.
3. Steiner T, Stovner L, Vos T. GBD 2015: migraine is the third cause of disability in under 50s. J Headache Pain 2016;17:104.
4. Sjaastad O, Saunte C, Hovdahl H, et al. "Cervicogenic" headache. An hypothesis. Cephalalgia 1983;3:249–56.
5. Ashina S, Bendtsen L, Lyngberg A, et al. Prevalence of neck pain in migraine and tension-type headache: a population study. Cephalalgia 2015;35:211–19.
6. Calhoun A, Ford S, Millen C, et al. The prevalence of neck pain in migraine. Headache 2010;50:1273–7.
7. Landgraf M, Kries Rv, Heinen F, et al. Self-reported neck and shoulder pain in adolescents is associated with episodic and chronic migraine. Cephalalgia 2016;36:807–11.
8. Uthaikhup S, Sterling M, Jull G. Cervical musculoskeletal impairment is common in elders with headache. Man Ther 2009;14:636–41.
9. Moore C, Sibbritt D, Adams J. A critical review of manual therapy use for headache disorders: prevalence, profiles, motivations, communication and self-reported effectiveness. BMC Neurol 2017;17:61.
10. Bogduk N, Govind J. Cervicogenic headache: an assessment of the evidence on clinical diagnosis, invasive tests, and treatment. Lancet Neurol 2009;8:959–68.
11. Bartsch T. Migraine and the neck: new insights from basic data. Curr Pain Headache Rep 2005;9:191–6.
12. Bartsch T, Goadsby P. The trigeminocervical complex and migraine: current concepts and synthesis. Curr Pain Headache Rep 2003;7:371–6.
13. Bartsch T, Goadsby PJ. Anatomy and physiology of pain referral patterns in primary and cervicogenic headache disorders. Headache Curr 2005;2:42–8.
14. Watson D, Drummond P. Head pain referral during examination of the neck in migraine and tension-type headache. Headache 2012;52:1226–35.
15. Ferracini G, Florencio L, Dach F, et al. Musculoskeletal disorders of the upper cervical spine in women with episodic or chronic migraine. Eur J Phys Rehabil Med 2017;53:342–50.
16. Luedtke K, Stark W, May A. Musculoskeletal dysfunction in migraine patients. Cephalalgia 2018;38:865–75.
17. Kaniecki R. Migraine and tension-type headache: an assessment of challenges in diagnosis. Neurology 2002;58:S15–20.
18. Calhoun A, Ford S. Double-blind, placebo-controlled, crossover study of early-intervention with sumatriptan 85/naproxen sodium 500 in (truly) episodic migraine: what's neck pain got to do with it? Postgrad Med 2014;126:86–90.
19. Ford S, Calhoun A, Kahn K, et al. Predictors of disability in migraineurs referred to a tertiary clinic: neck pain, headache characteristics, and coping behaviors. Headache 2008;48:523–8.

20. Viana M, Sances G, Terrazzino S, et al. When cervical pain is actually migraine: an observational study in 207 patients. Cephalalgia 2018;38:383–8.

21. Calhoun A, Ford S, Pruitt A. Presence of neck pain may delay migraine treatment. Postgrad Med 2011;123:163–8.

22. Amiri M, Jull G, Bullock-Saxton J, et al. Cervical musculoskeletal impairment in frequent intermittent headache. Part 2: subjects with multiple headaches. Cephalalgia 2007;27:891–8.

23. Bevilaqua-Grossi D, Pegoretti K, Goncalves M, et al. Cervical mobility in women with migraine. Headache 2009;49:726–31.

24. Dumas JP, Arsenault AB, Boudreau G, et al. Physical impairments in cervicogenic headache: traumatic vs. non-traumatic onset. Cephalalgia 2001;21:884–93.

25. Hall T, Briffa K, Hopper D, et al. Comparative analysis and diagnostic accuracy of the cervical flexion-rotation test. J Headache Pain 2010;11:391–7.

26. Jull G, Amiri M, Bullock-Saxton J, et al. Cervical musculoskeletal impairment in frequent intermittent headache. Part 1: subjects with single headaches. Cephalalgia 2007;27:793–802.

27. Robertson BA, Morris M. The role of cervical dysfunction in migraine: a systematic review. Cephalalgia 2008;28:474–83.

28. Zito G, Jull G, Story I. Clinical tests of musculoskeletal dysfunction in the diagnosis of cervicogenic headache. Man Ther 2006;11:118–29.

29. Zwart JA. Neck mobility in different headache disorders. Headache 1997;37:6–11.

30. Bevilaqua-Grossi D, Gonçalves M, Carvalho G, et al. Additional effects of a physical therapy protocol on headache frequency, pressure pain threshold, and improvement perception in patients with migraine and associated neck pain: a randomized controlled trial. Arch Phys Med Rehabil 2016;97:866–74.

31. Chaibi A, Tuchin P, Russell M. Manual therapies for migraine: a systematic review. J Headache Pain 2011;12:127–33.

32. Chaibi A, Benth J, Tuchin P, et al. Chiropractic spinal manipulative therapy for migraine: a three-armed, single-blinded, placebo, randomized controlled trial. Eur J Neurol 2017;24:143–53.

33. Florencio L, Chaves T, Carvalho G, et al. Neck pain disability is related to the frequency of migraine attacks: a cross-sectional study. Headache 2014;54:1203–10.

34. Headache Classification Subcommittee of the International Headache Society. The International Classification of Headache Disorders 3rd Edn. Cephalalgia 2013;33:629–808.

35. Yi X, Cook A, Hamill-Ruth R, et al. Cervicogenic headache in patients with presumed migraine: missed diagnosis or misdiagnosis? J Pain 2005;6:700–3.

36. Castien R, Blankenstein A, Windt Dvd, et al. The working mechanism of manual therapy in participants with chronic tension-type headache. J Orthop Sports Phys Ther 2013;43:693–9.

37. Abboud J, Marchand A, Sorra K, et al. Musculoskeletal physical outcome measures in individuals with tension-type headache: a scoping review. Cephalalgia 2013;33:1319–36.

38. Chaibi A, Russell M. Manual therapies for primary chronic headaches: a systematic review of randomized controlled trials. J Headache Pain 2014;15:67.

39. Varatharajan S, Ferguson B, Chrobak K, et al. Are non-invasive interventions effective for the management of headaches associated with neck pain? An update of the Bone and Joint Decade Task Force on Neck Pain and Its Associated Disorders by the Ontario Protocol for Traffic Injury Management (OPTIMa) Collaboration. Eur Spine J 2016;25:1971–99.

40. Sjaastad O, Fredriksen TA, Pfaffenrath V. Cervicogenic headache: diagnostic criteria. The Cervicogenic Headache International Study Group. Headache 1998;38:442–5.

41. Sjaastad O, Fredriksen TA, Sand T. The localisation of the initial pain of attack: a comparison between classic migraine and cervicogenic headache. Funct Neurol 1989;4:73–8.

42. Chaibi A, Russell M. Manual therapies for cervicogenic headache: a systematic review. J Headache Pain 2012;13:351–9.

43. Hall T, Chan HT, Christensen L, et al. Efficacy of a C1-C2 self-sustained natural apophyseal glide (SNAG) in the management of cervicogenic headache. J Orthop Sports Phys Ther 2007;37:100–7.

44. Jull G, Trott P, Potter H, et al. A randomized controlled trial of exercise and manipulative therapy for cervicogenic headache. Spine 2002;27:1835–43.

45. Ylinen J, Nikander R, Nykänen M, et al. Effect of neck exercises on cervicogenic headache: a randomised controlled trial. J Rehabil Med 2010;42:344–9.

46. Finkel A, Ivins B, Yerry J, et al. Which matters more? A retrospective cohort study of headache characteristics and diagnosis type in soldiers with mTBI/Concussion. Headache 2017;57:719–28.

47. Kennedy E, Quinn D, Tumilty S, et al. Clinical characteristics and outcomes of treatment of the cervical spine in patients with persistent post-concussion symptoms: a retrospective analysis. Musculoskelet Sci Pract 2017;29:91–8.

48. von Piekartz H, Pudelko A, Danzeisen M, et al. Do subjects with acute/subacute temporomandibular disorder have associated cervical impairments: a cross-sectional study. Man Ther 2016;26:208–15.

49. Hagen K, Linde M, Steiner T, et al. The bidirectional relationship between headache and chronic musculoskeletal complaints: an 11-year follow-up in the Nord-Trøndelag Health Study (HUNT). Eur J Neurol 2012;19:1447–54.

50. Bogduk N, Lambert G, Duckworth J. The anatomy and physiology of the vertebral nerve in relation to cervical migraine. Cephalalgia 1981;1:11–24.

51. Barré M. Sur un syndrome sympatique cervical posterieur et sa cause frequente: l'arthrite cervicale. Rev Neurol 1926;33:1246–8.

52. Bärtschi-Rochaix W. Migraine cervicale, das encephale syndrome nach Halswirbeltrauma. Bern: Huber; 1949.

53. Hunter C, Mayfield F. Role of the upper cervical roots in the production of pain in the head. Am J Surg 1949;48:743–51.

54. Raney A, Raney R. Headache: a common symptom of cervical disc lesions. Report of cases. Arch Neurol Psychiatr 1948;59:603–21.

55. Bogduk N, Marsland A. On the concept of third occipital headache. J Neurol Neurosurg Psychiatry 1986;49:775–80.

56. Bogduk N, Marsland A. The cervical zygapophysial joints as a source of neck pain. Spine 1988;13:610–17.

57. Ehni G, Benner B. Occipital neuralgia and C_1-C_2 arthrosis. New Engl J Med 1984;310:127.

58. Trevor-Jones R. Osteoarthritis of the paravertebral joints of the second and third cervical vertebrae as a cause of occipital headache. S Afr Med J 1964;38:392–4.

59. Liu J, Cadena G, Panchal R, et al. Relief of cervicogenic headaches after single-level and multilevel anterior cervical diskectomy: a 5-year post hoc analysis. Global Spine J 2016;6:563–70.

60. Russo V, Duits A, Dhawan R, et al. Joint arthropathy at the craniovertebral junction. Scintigraphic patterns on bone SPECT/CT. Br J Neurosurg 2017;31:45–9.

61. Fujiwara Y, Izumi B, Fujiwara M, et al. C2 spondylotic radiculopathy: the nerve root impingement mechanism investigated by para-sagittal CT/MRI, dynamic rotational CT, intraoperative microscopic findings, and treated by microscopic posterior foraminotomy. Eur Spine J 2017;26:1073–81.

62. Fernández-de-Las-Peñas C, Cuadrado M, Pareja J. Myofascial trigger points, neck mobility, and forward head posture in episodic tension-type headache. Headache 2007;47:662–72.

63. Hall T, Robinson K, Fujinawa O, et al. Intertester reliability and diagnostic validity of the cervical flexion-rotation test. J Manipulative Physiol Ther 2008;31:293–300.

64. Budelmann K, Piekartz Hv, Hall T. Is there a difference in head posture and cervical spine movement in children with and without pediatric headache? Eur J Pediatr 2013;172:1349–56.

65. Hall T, Briffa K, Hopper D, et al. The relationship between cervicogenic headache and impairment determined by the flexion-rotation test. J Manipulative Physiol Ther 2010;33:666–71.

66. Rubio-Ochoa J, Benítez-Martínez J, Lluch E, et al. Physical examination tests for screening and diagnosis of cervicogenic headache: a systematic review. Man Ther 2016;21:35–40.

67. Gijsberts TJ, Duquet W, Stoekart R, et al. Pain-provocation tests for C0-4 as a tool in the diagnosis of cervicogenic headache. Cephalalgia 1999;19:436.

68. Hall T, Briffa K, Hopper D, et al. Reliability of manual examination and frequency of symptomatic cervical motion segment dysfunction in cervicogenic headache. Man Ther 2010;15:542–6.

69. Howard P, Behrns W, Martino M, et al. Manual examination in the diagnosis of cervicogenic headache: a systematic literature review. J Man Manip Ther 2015;23:210–18.

70. Jull G, Bogduk N, Marsland A. The accuracy of manual diagnosis for cervical zygapophysial joint pain syndromes. Med J Aust 1988;148:233–6.

71. Schneider G, Jull G, Thomas K, et al. Derivation of a clinical decision guide in the diagnosis of cervical facet joint pain. Arch Phys Med Rehabil 2014;95:1695–701.

72. Watson DH, Trott PH. Cervical headache: an investigation of natural head posture and upper cervical flexor muscle performance. Cephalalgia 1993;13:272–84.

73. Wanderley D, Filho AM, Neto JC, et al. Analysis of dimensions, activation and median frequency of cervical flexor muscles in young women with migraine or tension-type headache. Braz J Phys Ther 2015;19:243–50.

74. Horwitz S, Stewart A. An exploratory study to determine the relationship between cervical dysfunction and perimenstrual migraines. Physiother Can 2015;67:30–8.

75. Fernandez-de-las-Penas C, Perez-de-Heredia M, Molero-Sanchez A, et al. Performance of the craniocervical flexion test, forward head posture, and headache clinical parameters in patients with chronic tension-type headache: a pilot study. J Orthop Sports Phys Ther 2007;37:33–9.

76. Florencio L, Oliveira Ad, Carvalho G, et al. Cervical muscle strength and muscle coactivation during isometric contractions in patients with migraine: a cross-sectional study. Headache 2015;55:1312–22.

77. Madsen B, Søgaard K, Andersen L, et al. Neck and shoulder muscle strength in patients with tension-type headache: a case-control study. Cephalalgia 2016;36:29–36.

78. Sohn J, Choi H, Lee S, et al. Differences in cervical musculoskeletal impairment between episodic and chronic tension-type headache. Cephalalgia 2010;30:1514–23.

79. Tali D, Menahem I, Vered E, et al. Upper cervical mobility, posture and myofascial trigger points in subjects with episodic migraine: case-control study. J Bodyw Mov Ther 2014;18:569–75.

80. Anderson R, Sawyer T, Wise D, et al. Painful myofascial trigger points and pain sites in men with chronic prostatitis/chronic pelvic pain syndrome. J Urol 2009;182:2753–8.

81. Ferracini G, Florencio F, Dach F, et al. Myofascial trigger points and migraine-related disability in women with episodic and chronic migraine. Clin J Pain 2017;33:109–15.

82. Florencio L, Ferracini G, Chaves T, et al. Active trigger points in the cervical musculature determine the altered activation of superficial neck and extensor muscles in women with migraine. Clin J Pain 2017;33:238–45.

83. Hasuo H, Ishihara T, Kanbara K, et al. Myofacial trigger points in advanced cancer patients. Indian J Palliat Care 2016; 22:80–4.

84. Huang Q, Liu L. Wet needling of myofascial trigger points in abdominal muscles for treatment of primary dysmenorrhoea. Acupunct Med 2014;32:346–9.

85. Palacios-Ceña M, Castaldo M, Wang K, et al. Relationship of active trigger points with related disability and anxiety in people with tension-type headache. Medicine (Baltimore) 2017;96:e6548.

86. Florencio L, Oliveira A, Lemos T, et al. Patients with chronic, but not episodic, migraine display altered activity of their neck extensor muscles. J Electromyogr Kinesiol 2016;30:66–72.

87. Dugailly P, Decuyper A, Salem W, et al. Analysis of the upper cervical spine stiffness during axial rotation: a comparative study among patients with tension-type headache or migraine and asymptomatic subjects. Clin Biomech 2017;42:128–33.

88. Farmer P, Snodgrass S, Buxton A, et al. An investigation of cervical spinal posture in cervicogenic headache. Phys Ther 2015;95:212–22.

89. Fernández-de-las-Peñas C, Alonso-Blanco C, Cuadrado M, et al. Neck mobility and forward head posture are not related to headache parameters in chronic tension-type headache. Cephalalgia 2007;27:158–64.

90. Falla D, Jull G, Russell T, et al. Effect of neck exercise on sitting posture in patients with chronic neck pain. Phys Ther 2007;87:408–17.

91. Mingels S, Dankaerts W, Etten Lv, et al. Comparative analysis of head-tilt and forward head position during laptop use between females with postural induced headache and healthy controls. J Bodyw Mov Ther 2016;20:533–41.

92. Szeto G, Straker L, Raine S. A field comparison of neck and shoulder postures in symptomatic and asymptomatic office workers. Appl Erg 2002;33:75–84.

93. Palomeque-Del-Cerro L, Arráez-Aybar L, Rodríguez-Blanco C, et al. A systematic review of the soft-tissue connections between neck muscles and dura mater: the myodural bridge. Spine 2017;42:49–54.

94. Piekartz Hv, Schouten S, Aufdemkampe G. Neurodynamic responses in children with migraine or cervicogenic headache versus a control group. A comparative study. Man Ther 2007;12:153–60.

95. Rumore AJ. Slump examination and treatment in a patient suffering headache. Aust J Physiother 1989;35:262–3.

96. Schneider K, Meeuwisse W, Nettel-Aguirre A, et al. Cervicovestibular rehabilitation in sport-related concussion: a randomised controlled trial. Br J Sports Med 2014;48:1294–8.

97. Carvalho G, Bonato P, Florencio L, et al. Balance impairments in different subgroups of patients with migraine. Headache 2017;57:363–74.

98. Yollu U, Uluduz D, Yilmaz M, et al. Vestibular migraine screening in a migraine-diagnosed patient population, and assessment of vestibulocochlear function. Clin Otolaryngol 2017;42:225–33.

99. Giacomini P, Alessandrini M, Evangelista M, et al. Impaired postural control in patients affected by tension-type headache. Eur J Pain 2004;8:579–83.

100. Ishizaki K, Mori N, Takeshima T, et al. Static stabilometry in patients with migraine and tension-type headache during a headache-free period. Psychiatry Clin Neurosci 2002;56:85–90.

101. Marchand A, Cantin V, Murphy B, et al. Is performance in goal oriented head movements altered in patients with tension type headache? BMC Musculoskelet Disord 2014;15:179.

102. Aguila M, Rebbeck T, Mendoza K, et al. Definitions and participant characteristics of frequent recurrent headache types in clinical trials: a systematic review. Cephalalgia 2018;38:786–93.

103. Uthaikhup S, Assapun J, Watcharasaksilp K, et al. Effectiveness of physiotherapy for seniors with recurrent headaches associated with neck pain and dysfunction: a randomized controlled trial. Spine J 2017;17:46–55.

Section 4

CLINICAL MANAGEMENT

This section discusses the management of patients with neck pain disorders. The various components of an intervention are discussed in separate chapters but all features are considered concurrently in clinical practice. Communication and education occur continually throughout treatment. Physical treatments for pain management and relief of other associated symptoms are applied in an integrated manner together with exercise programs to rehabilitate the various impairments in neuromuscular and sensorimotor function. The importance of self-management strategies is highlighted and comprehensive programs are developed and progressed throughout the management period.

As mentioned, topics have been considered separately in sequential chapters, for ease and clarity of presentation of information. Therefore Chapter 18 presents a series of case examples to demonstrate the clinical reasoning process and the necessary multimodal management approach for patients with cervical spine disorders.

12 PRINCIPLES OF MANAGEMENT

Management programs are based on a comprehensive clinical reasoning process to interpret and apply the detailed information gained about the patient and their neck pain disorder in the patient interview and physical examination. The principles of management revolve around patient-centred care in which the patient receives relevant information and contributes to decisions about their care.[1] Good management relies on an effective therapeutic relationship between the patient and clinician, which is based on good communication where the patient is assured that their concerns are being heard and understood.

Management programs are developed within the framework of the biopsychosocial model. The model itself does not provide any specific guidance as to which interventions should be implemented. Rather it encourages consideration of biological, behavioural/psychological and social aspects of a patient's presentation both in management and in evaluating outcomes. The relative contributions of the three domains of the model are very fluid, and they will not stay constant. They vary between patients and within a patient as they progress through their rehabilitation.

Pain is commonly the primary reason that a patient seeks help for a neck disorder. As is well appreciated, pain is a multidimensional sensory and emotional experience, and the management of pain is a major multidisciplinary field of practice and research. Pain can be managed with pharmacotherapies, physical therapies as well as various psychological and cognitively based behavioural therapies. In a patient-centred approach to managing people with neck pain, often some components of many of these therapies will be used, albeit in differing proportions depending on the individual patient's needs. We focus in this text on the management of pain with physical therapies with attendant education, self-management programs and patient empowerment. Yet management programs must not focus on pain relief only. Pain relief is very important to the patient, but the real burden for the person and society in general, lies not in a single episode of neck pain but in its recurrent or persistent nature and consequent years lived with a disability.[2] Management programs must change as treatment goals change from pain relief, to restoration of full function, to prevention of recurrent episodes. All management programs must have a focus on rehabilitation.

The principles of management incorporate:

- A patient-centred approach featuring clear communication, the provision of relevant information and a diagnosis, and inclusion of the patient in decision making.
- The development of collaborative intervention strategies from a physiotherapy perspective, which will help the patient reduce neck pain and disability and promote optimal function and participation.
- The use of a combination of approaches which may include education on a variety of topics, manual therapies, various exercise strategies, self-management strategies and work and lifestyle advice.

■ Strategies to enhance coping or other personal skills to assist patients to (1) manage their neck in both pain and nonpainful states and (2) comply with home exercise and self-management programs, which support and enhance treatment gains.

■ Strategies to fulfil aims of preventing further recurrent episodes of and slowing disease progression: (1) provision of a simple long-term preventative regime for patients to continue; (2) help patients to problem solve to adjust leisure or work practices to care for their neck.

■ A self-management program for the patient to use if, in the future, the neck pain disorder appears to be returning.

SELECTION OF MANAGEMENT STRATEGIES

Selection of management strategies is guided by the clinical reasoning process throughout the patient interview and physical examination. The clinical reasoning process around selection of management strategies is guided by the principles of evidence-based practice (EBP), integration of best available research evidence, clinical expertise, and patient values and circumstances.[3] Clinical practice guidelines (CPGs) are a primary tool of EBP. Other tools that might inform the clinical reasoning process are subordinate to CPGs. These include clinical prediction rules and subgrouping, which are tools that attempt to match specific interventions or management approaches to particular patient presentations.

Clinical practice guidelines

CPGs are built on the outcomes of systematic reviews and where possible, meta-analyses of the research evidence. They are developed by a panel of multidisciplinary experts who produce recommendations that aim to optimize patient care. Recommendations are variously provided on: assessment, particularly to identify "red flags" or risks of harm, contraindications to particular treatments; prognostic indicators for a good, fair, poor or delayed recovery; treatment methods with evidence of effectiveness for different stages of various neck pain disorders; recommendations on actions that should be taken if the patient is not responding to treatment; and recommendations for outcome

measures.[4,5] Contemporary guideline development may also include aspects that patients have nominated as important from their experiences and needs.[6] This fulfils the ideology of EBP.[3] In one CPG for the management of whiplash-associated disorders (WAD),[6] patient input was sought and their recommendations were that guidelines be mindful of terminology used both for the persons who sustained the injury and in describing the injury (e.g., calling whiplash a minor injury was distressing). They also recommended that an emphasis be placed on partnerships and shared decision making between patient and health care provider; that the emotional distress of being in a car crash be recognized and actively managed when necessary, and that the injured persons be repeatedly oriented to the health care system and insurance industry about which many were nonfamiliar. Such recommendations provide sound advice to clinicians.

One set of CPGs have been developed for specific categories of neck pain disorders namely; WAD, cervical radiculopathy and insidious onset neck pain.[4,5,7,8] Within these disorder categories, treatment guidelines are provided for subclassifications of whiplash—WAD grades I–III,[9] and neck-associated disorders—NAD I–III.[10] Differentiation is also made for the acute/subacute or persistent stages of neck pain disorders for management recommendations. Another recently updated CPG classified neck pain disorders on the basis of categories within the International Classification of Diseases (ICD) together with the relevant impairment-based category for neck pain according to the International Classification of Functioning, Disability, and Health (ICF).[11] Four classifications were derived and treatment recommendations were provided for: neck pain with mobility deficits; neck pain with headaches; neck pain with movement coordination impairments; and neck pain with radiating pain.

CPGs direct the use of treatments that have evidence of effectiveness and discourage use of treatments with no evidence of effect or evidence of harm based on the available evidence. For example, for neck pain of 3 months or less, based on the evidence, a multimodal program inclusive of structured patient education in combination with range of motion exercises and mobilization or manipulation is recommended. Clinicians are advised not to use structured education alone, strain-counterstrain techniques, collars or electrotherapy modalities because there is no evidence of effectiveness for these methods.[4]

CPGs, as the name implies, are guidelines to the prescription of best evidence-based treatment. They do not inform on the precise technique of treatment, combination of techniques or dosage that may be best for the individual patient. This relies on the clinician's reasoning based on the findings of the patient interview and physical examination. CPGs have other limitations. For example, as explored in Chapter 5, evidence indicates that neck pain is associated with considerable change in neuromuscular function, yet a guideline for neck pain of 3months or less did not include any recommendation for exercise to address this muscle dysfunction.[4] This runs counter to any principles of rehabilitation for musculoskeletal disorders. Although there is evidence of effectiveness of exercise in the management of neck pain disorders,[12] randomized controlled trials (RCT) of exercise are yet to be conducted in this acute/subacute group with idiopathic neck pain. Thus there is no evidence for exercise for this neck pain category that the guideline can use in recommendations. Recommendations are made on the available evidence. This deficit not only points out the urgent need for clinical trials of exercise in this specific patient group but also highlights the limitations of evidence-based guidelines. CPGs point the way, but patient management must still be informed by the clinician's reasoning and a research informed physical examination and management approach.

Clinical prediction rules

Clinical prediction rules (CPRs) are developed for diagnostic, prognostic and prescriptive purposes. For interventions, a CPR guides prescription of a certain treatment technique. There is considerable heterogeneity in the presentation of patients with neck pain disorders. Likewise, there is no universal response to any one treatment. Thus CPRs attempt to better match patients to treatments. They are based on historical and physical characteristics that predict patients' responses to that treatment and are usually derived from an RCT. Several prescriptive CPRs have been developed to direct treatments for neck disorders. As examples, CPRs have been developed to identify patients with neck pain who may respond to neck manipulation,[13,14] to thoracic spine manipulation,[15] to traction and exercise,[16] and for patients with neck and arm pain, to neural tissue mobilization.[17]

Although in principle a valuable prescriptive tool, CPRs are failing in the validation process. In other words, the technique or treatment designated by the CPR is not producing a superior effect against a comparison treatment when tested prospectively in a new clinical trial using a new group of patients. This failure is not limited to techniques for neck pain but is occurring for CPRs for the lumbar spine and other regions.[18–22] Reasons proposed for the apparent failure of many prescriptive CPRs include, for instance, vastly inadequate sample sizes and considerable statistical methodological limitations in the original derivations of the rules.[23,24] Thus at present, the use of CPRs does not have strong scientific support, but further research with stringent scientific methodology might change this state. Therefore CPRs could be used to direct a certain management technique(s), but at present there is no evidence that the technique(s) would result in a superior outcome to another treatment method.

CPRs in principle may assist in the initial prescription of a treatment or treatment technique, but they cannot act as a stand-alone tool. CPRs offer no guidance on the progression of the technique/treatment nor on any other treatment that might be required for rehabilitation of the patient's neck pain disorder. Furthermore, they provide no alternative for the neck pain patient whose presentation does not fit the rule, nor any alternative if the prescribed treatment technique proves not to be efficacious. Thus even if valid CPRs become available, they will always be a secondary supplementary tool to the primary tool of the clinical reasoning process in patient assessment and management.

Subgrouping

Subgrouping is another method to try to deal with the heterogeneity in neck pain disorders to better match treatments to individuals. Subgrouping has gained greater attention for low-back pain. For cervical spine disorders, there are essentially two physiotherapy-based subgrouping systems to guide management. One subgroups patients on ICD and ICF criteria based on the patient's clinical presentation, that is, neck pain with mobility deficits; neck pain with headaches; neck pain with movement coordination impairments; and neck pain with radiating pain.[11,25] A treatment approach is proposed for each classification derived from available evidence. The other system subgroups patients based on a particular management approach—Mechanical Diagnosis and Therapy (MDT). In this system, the pain response to repeated movement is assessed and patients are classified into one of four basic syndromes: posture, dysfunction, reducible derangement, irreducible derangement or "other" category.[26,27] The category directs which movement or postural strategy will be used in management.

Subgrouping can assist in selecting a treatment technique or proposing a management regime that might be suitable for a particular patient but they have limitations. For example, the four subgroups based on ICD and ICF criteria[11] describe four different, very legitimate symptom sets, but it is easy to think of numerous patient presentations outside these four descriptions. Similarly, the MDT classification provides no guidance if patient's fall into the "other" category. It is easy to be critical, but it is probably an impossible task to create subgroups that could cover all possible presentations of neck pain disorders.[28] In addition, current subgrouping schemes are quite narrow in their focus and do not consider, for example, pain mechanisms that may influence management approaches. There is an emphasis on dealing with the presenting complaint but not on a full rehabilitation program, which aims to reduce recurrence of the disorder. The schemes do not position themselves in the biopsychosocial context of neck pain disorders. These limitations do not dismiss the usefulness of these classifications systems in contributing to management decisions, but as with CPRs, they best operate as a secondary supplementary tool to the primary tool of the clinical reasoning process in patient assessment and management.

SELECTION OF INTERVENTIONS

It is now well appreciated that there is no single modality "magic bullet" that has the answer for the management of patients with neck pain disorders. No one modality or approach can improve all dimensions of a neck disorder. Evidence from systematic reviews and uptake in CPGs supports the prescription of multimodal management.[4,5,29] Selection of specific interventions as

a manual/manipulative therapy, exercise or sensorimotor training will be discussed in the relevant chapters. Here broader issues behind recommendations for selection of interventions are considered.

Recommendations for an intervention or management approach in a CPG are guided by the cumulative evidence of effectiveness from a number of RCTs. A factor governing the strength of the recommendation for an intervention is the quality of the RCTs. The quality of the RCTs is assessed in terms of methodological excellence, for example, concealed randomization; blinding of assessors, patients' therapists; intention-to treat statistical analysis. However, there is not a formal evaluation of the suitability of the many clinical aspects of the RCT, such as the population studied, the intervention chosen or the primary outcome measure. Quality in these aspects could be argued to be equally as important as methodological excellence in gauging the strength of the evidence for a particular intervention.

The problem of heterogeneity in presentations within populations with neck pain disorders is well appreciated as is the false expectation that all patients will respond in a similar manner to an intervention. Inclusion criteria in RCTs, such as individuals with non-specific neck pain of 3 months' duration or more and between the ages of 18 and 65 years stand to recruit many different presentations of neck pain disorders. An intervention may have excellent results for one patient but is ineffective in another patient. The washout consequence of diverse results from a heterogeneous population is agreed to be one of the possible reasons for small to, at best, moderate effect sizes gained by most if not all potentially beneficial treatments for neck pain. Thus it is essential that as homogeneous a population as possible is recruited into future RCTs. Nevertheless, even though they continue to be the mainstay to produce evidence, RCTs cannot replicate the varying characteristics of individual patient encounters in clinical practice. With the current situation, clinicians must be aware that an overall small effect size in an RCT does not mean that an intervention might not have a large effect for a particular patient presentation.

It is not only necessary to recruit a homogeneous population into an RCT, but the population needs to have "the condition" for which the intervention is suitable, if a judgement of the efficacy of an intervention is to be made. For example, cervical manipulative therapy added to medication was shown to add no substantive benefit on migraine frequency over medication alone in patient management.[30] This finding cannot reflect adversely on the effectiveness of manipulative therapy. Rather it could be argued that it is an expected finding because there is no substantive evidence that migraine is associated with cervical musculoskeletal dysfunction (see Chapter 11). Similarly, a study tested a contention that psychological and social factors play a major role in the transition from acute to chronic neck pain. The researchers proposed that a behavioural graded activity program would be at least as effective as a program of advice, manipulative therapy and exercise.[31] The behavioural program was found to have no superior effect on future pain and disability at 12 months and it afforded no significant change in psychological variables. However, most participants recruited into the RCT in this transition phase did not have abnormal psychological features. Initial baseline scores for psychological features for the majority of participants were very low, so the possibility for change was marginal at best. Thus possessing "the condition" for which the intervention is suited is critical if any judgement is to be made about an intervention. As an example, there is growing interest in the contribution to neck pain of adverse scapular posture associated with poor muscle control. There is very preliminary evidence (case study) of effectiveness of a scapular retraining program.[32] The next step is to test the training program in an RCT. Considering participant selection, a major inclusion criteria (i.e., those potentially suited to the intervention) would be individuals who firstly, demonstrated altered scapular posture and secondly, whose pain and neck movement improved markedly when the scapula was positioned into a neutral posture (see Chapter 9). If this response was not achieved in a screening process for the trial, then training scapular posture is unlikely to be a successful intervention and such participants should not be included in this first RCT. An intervention can only be appraised when it is used for patients for whom it is indicated.

Another aspect to consider in judging the effectiveness of an intervention, is the "suitability" of the primary outcome measure on which it was judged. The primary outcome of most RCTs for the management of neck pain disorders is a pain rating, a score from a pain and disability questionnaire, or a patient's global perceived effect of treatment. This reflects an outcome relevant to the patient, which is correct, but it can be questioned if pain relief is the only expectation of an intervention and the only criterion on which an intervention is to be judged. Considering exercise, if an exercise intervention is prescribed for relief of neck pain, then it does not appear to matter what exercise mode (e.g., motor relearning or strengthening) is prescribed.[33,34] However pain is not the appropriate outcome measure if the intent of the exercise program is to optimize the function of the neck muscles for activities of daily living, work or sport. Muscle function measures are required as the primary outcomes. Of interest, when return of normal muscle control is the outcome, then it does matter what exercises are prescribed. As discussed in Chapter 5, exercise modes to train muscle coordination and restore direction specificity are different to those required to improve endurance or muscle strength. The primary outcome should also direct the dosage or training period required. Should there be an assumption that the training period will be the same when the intent is to modulate pain versus strengthening muscles? The effect of an intervention must be judged on an outcome relevant to its primary intent, not as currently, principally on pain relief.

CONCLUSION

The principles of management incorporate a patient-centred approach and development of collaborative intervention strategies for neck pain disorders. Multimodal management based on the individual patient's presentation and needs is the key in rehabilitation. A rehabilitation program should address the problems associated with the immediate episode of neck pain as well as establish a self-management regime towards prevention of recurrent episodes. The patient must have the knowledge and understanding to empower them to self-manage their neck pain. Selection of management strategies is guided by the principles of EBP. Nevertheless, clinical reasoning throughout the patient examination is the overarching process. The clinical reasoning process encourages and has the necessary flexibility in thought for interpretation of all information about the patient to guide the selection of appropriate individualized management strategies.

REFERENCES

1. Committee on Quality of Health Care in America. Institute of Medicine. Crossing the quality chasm: a new health system for the 21st Century. Washington, DC: National Academy Press; 2001.

2. GBD 2015 Disease and Injury Incidence and Prevalence Collaborators. Global, regional, and national incidence, prevalence, and years lived with disability for 310 diseases and injuries, 1990-2015: a systematic analysis for the Global Burden of Disease Study 2015. Lancet 2016;388:1545–602.

3. Sackett D, Richardson W, Rosenberg W, et al. Evidence-based medicine. How to practice and teach EBM. London: Churchill Livingstone; 1997.

4. Côté P, Wong J, Sutton D, et al. Management of neck pain and associated disorders: a clinical practice guideline from the Ontario Protocol for Traffic Injury Management (OPTIMa) Collaboration. Eur Spine J 2016;25:2000–22.

5. Motor Accident Authority NSW. Guidelines for the management of acute whiplash disorders for health professionals. Secondary guidelines for the management of acute whiplash disorders for health professionals 2014. maa.nsw.gov.au.

6. Lindsay G, Mior S, Côté P, et al. Patients' experiences with vehicle collision to inform the development of clinical practice guidelines: a narrative inquiry. J Manipulative Physiol Ther 2016;39: 218–28.

7. Kjaer P, Kongsted A, Hartvigsen J, et al. National clinical guidelines for non-surgical treatment of patients with recent onset neck pain or cervical radiculopathy. Eur Spine J 2017;26(9): 2242–57.

8. Wong J, Côté P, Shearer H, et al. Clinical practice guidelines for the management of conditions related to traffic collisions: a systematic review by the OPTIMa Collaboration. Disabil Rehabil 2015;37:471–89.

9. Spitzer WO, Skovron ML, Salmi LR, et al. Scientific monograph of the Quebec Task Force on whiplash-associated disorders: redefining "Whiplash" and its management. Spine 1995;20(8S): 1–73.

10. Guzman J, Hurwitz EL, Carroll LJ, et al. A new conceptual model of neck pain - Linking onset, course, and care: the Bone and Joint Decade 2000-2010 Task Force on Neck Pain and its Associated Disorders. Spine 2008;33:S14–23.

11. Blanpied P, Gross A, Elliott J, et al. Neck pain: revision 2017. J Orthop Sports Phys Ther 2017;47:A1–83.

12. Gross A, Paquin J, Dupont G, et al. Exercises for mechanical neck disorders: a Cochrane review update. Man Ther 2016;24: 25–45.

13. Puentedura E, Cleland J, Landers M, et al. Development of a clinical prediction rule to identify patients with neck pain likely to benefit from thrust joint manipulation to the cervical spine. J Orthop Sports Phys Ther 2012;42:577–92.

14. Tseng Y-L, Wang W, Chen W-Y, et al. Predictors for the immediate responders to cervical manipulation in patients with neck pain. Man Ther 2006;11:306–15.

15. Cleland J, Childs J, Fritz J, et al. Development of a clinical prediction rule for guiding treatment of a subgroup of patients with neck pain: use of thoracic spine manipulation, exercise, and patient education. Phys Ther 2007;87: 9–23.

16. Raney N, Petersen E, Smith T, et al. Development of a clinical prediction rule to identify patients with neck pain likely to benefit from cervical traction and exercise. Eur Spine J 2009;18: 382–9.

17. Nee R, Vicenzino B, Jull GA, et al. Baseline characteristics of patients with nerve-related neck and arm pain predict the likely response to neural tissue management. J Orthop Sports Phys Ther 2013;43:379–91.

18. Cleland J, Mintken P, Carpenter K, et al. Examination of a clinical prediction rule to identify patients with neck pain likely to benefit from thoracic spine thrust manipulation and a general cervical range of motion exercise: multi-center randomized clinical trial. Phys Ther 2010;90:1239–50.

19. Fernández-de-Las-Peñas C, Cleland J, Salom-Moreno J, et al. Prediction of outcome in women with carpal tunnel syndrome who receive manual physical therapy interventions: a validation study. J Orthop Sports Phys Ther 2016;46:443–51.

20. Hancock M, Maher C, Latimer J, et al. Independent evaluation of a clinical prediction rule for spinal manipulative therapy: a randomised controlled trial. Eur Spine J 2008;17: 936–43.

21. Learman K, Showalter C, O'Halloran B, et al. No differences in outcomes in people with low back pain who met the clinical prediction rule for lumbar spine manipulation when a pragmatic non-thrust manipulation was used as the comparator. Physiother Can 2014;66:359–66.

22. Mintken P, McDevitt A, Michener L, et al. Examination of the validity of a clinical prediction rule to identify patients with shoulder pain likely to benefit from cervicothoracic manipulation. J Orthop Sports Phys Ther 2017;47:133–49.

23. Haskins R, Cook C. Enthusiasm for prescriptive clinical prediction rules (eg, back pain and more): a quick word of caution. Br J Sports Med 2016;50:960–1.

24. Kent P, Boyle E, Keating J, et al. Four hundred or more participants needed for stable contingency table estimates of clinical prediction rule performance. J Clin Epidemiol 2017;82:137–48.

25. Childs J, Fritz J, Piva S, et al. Proposal of a classification system for patients with neck pain. J Orthop Sports Phys Ther 2004;34:686–96.

26. Clare H, Adams R, Maher C. Reliability of McKenzie classification of patients with cervical or lumbar pain. J Manipulative Physiol Ther 2005;28:122–7.

27. Hefford C. McKenzie classification of mechanical spinal pain: profile of syndromes and directions of preference. Man Ther 2008;13:75–81.

28. Jull G. Management of cervical spine disorders: where to now? J Orthop Sports Phys Ther 2012;42:A3–7.

29. Miller J, Gross A, D'Sylva J, et al. Manual therapy and exercise for neck pain: a systematic review. Man Ther 2010;15: 334–54.

30. Bevilaqua-Grossi D, Gonçalves M, Carvalho G, et al. Additional effects of a physical therapy protocol on headache frequency, pressure pain threshold, and improvement perception in patients

with migraine and associated neck pain: a randomized controlled trial. Arch Phys Med Rehabil 2016;97:866–74.

31. Pool J, Ostelo R, Knol D, et al. Is a behavioral graded activity program more effective than manual therapy in patients with subacute neck pain? Results of a randomized clinical trial. Spine 2010;35:1017–24.

32. McDonnell M, Sahrmann S, Dillen LV. A specific exercise program and modification of postural alignment for treatment of

cervicogenic headache: a case report. J Orthop Sports Phys Ther 2005;35:3–15.

33. Jull G, Trott P, Potter H, et al. A randomized controlled trial of exercise and manipulative therapy for cervicogenic headache. Spine 2002;27:1835–43.

34. Ylinen J, Nikander R, Nykänen M, et al. Effect of neck exercises on cervicogenic headache: a randomised controlled trial. J Rehabil Med 2010;42:344–9.

13

COMMUNICATION, EDUCATION AND SELF-MANAGEMENT

■ ■

This chapter considers three interrelated topics all of which are integral to good patient management. There has long been interest in the art and science of communication. A growing body of research points to the positive impacts of good communication and the negative impacts of poor communication on patient outcomes.[1,2] Good communication is central to patient-centred practice and intimately linked to effective education. Good communication and effective education can facilitate patient empowerment, which stands to enhance compliance in self-management strategies both throughout the treatment period as well as in efforts towards secondary or tertiary prevention.

COMMUNICATION

Communication in health care covers a wide field[3] including interpersonal skills, written skills for reports and, in today's world, professional social media skills. Interpersonal skills for effective communication encompasses many different elements. These include among many, active listening, use of individualized language, empathy, patient respect, hearing their concerns, understanding their beliefs, expectations and desired outcomes of management, providing information, encouraging questions and discussion to confirm understanding. Developing trust and rapport is the basis for a positive therapeutic relationship, ensuring the patient is an active participant in a genuine patient-clinician partnership. All elements of communication

are important and effective communication is central to the entire management period. In this section, comments are offered on practical aspects of some communication skills in the context of the initial assessment of patients with neck pain disorders.

Listening

Considerable information is required from a patient presenting with neck pain, or indeed any musculoskeletal disorder. Following the initial patient interview, the clinician wants to be assured that the patient has no "red flags". As well, information is required for the clinician to reason intelligently about pain mechanisms, possible underlying causes and pathophysiology, influences on functional activities, participation in work, recreational and daily activities, psychological or social moderators, influences of any health comorbidities and prognosis (see Chapter 8). Thus it is tempting to ask a series of questions supplemented by various questionnaires to "cover all bases". Although this may be an understandable approach for the novice clinician, it is one which risks missing important information and one that does not assure an optimal patient-clinician relationship.[4]

Information that is required can be better gained by inviting and encouraging the patient to tell the story of their neck pain disorder. The clinician should listen without distraction, responding to any concerns that the patient raises and requesting clarification when required.[5] The benefits of listening cannot be overestimated in relation to the quality of information gained.

Listening to how the patient describes their symptoms, how the disorder is affecting their function and participation and how the patient is dealing with the neck disorder will provide information not only on the biological components of the neck pain disorder but it provides insight into any concerns or anxieties that the patient has as well as any helpful or unhelpful beliefs or expectations. Being responsive to the patient with a comment or question, displays to them that the clinician has a genuine understanding of the condition from the patient's perspective. This is a skill that develops with experience,[5] but one to which all clinicians should aspire. Displaying empathy increases trust, assures the patient they are being understood and begins to validate the patient's complaint.

In the physical examination, the clinician can provide an appropriate commentary on what they are testing, for what reason, explaining the outcomes as relevant at that stage of the examination and respond to any questions the patient may have. Providing the patient with information will help them to understand and contribute to initial decisions about their care.

Language

Language should be individualized to the patient. In the initial examination, it begins by keying into terminology that the patient is using to describe their condition and using that terminology. For example, if the patient describes the symptom of light headedness with the word *fuzziness*, the clinician should adopt the term "fuzziness" when asking the patient for a response in any assessment of this symptom. Likewise, if pain is described as an ache, the term "ache" should be used. If the patient refers to their anxiety as "apprehension", this is the term that should be used from that point. Using the language of the patient contributes to assuring them of the clinician's understanding of their condition.

It is important to have consistent language or terminology between health care providers. Patients find it disturbing to receive differences of opinion about their neck pain disorder from different health care providers.[6] Thus even though a clinician might disagree with a previous diagnosis, it is better for the patient if the current clinician acknowledges that diagnosis rather than be dismissive or make derogatory statements about it. Unless the previous diagnosis is harmfully incorrect, the artful clinician can weave it into the explanation that they wish to provide about the patient's disorder to limit perceptions of differences of opinion.

Language is very important in explaining the patient's disorder. The "disadvantage" of having a neck disorder is that usually there is nothing readily visible to validate it. The "advantage" of having an extremity disorder is that it can often be seen (swelling, bruising, muscle wasting, painful to weight bear). Use of a simple analogy as an ankle sprain or overuse injury is often a good start to providing a basic explanation of what might be underlying a patient's neck pain. Alarmist explanations must be avoided, for example, "the x-rays show advanced degenerative changes at all levels, your neck is a real mess!" Such explanations sadly transfer a negative expectation of outcome to the patient, which may adversely shape their future attitudes and coping skills. When explaining the nature of the neck pain disorder to the patient, clinicians should avoid the use of professional jargon. As an example, telling a patient that their "C2 is rotated" and is the reason for their pain, is at best unhelpful and at worst mitigates against a good outcome. Patients often focus on the "rotated C2" and once the seed is planted by this explanation, they cannot get better until they are convinced it is "un-rotated". This is difficult if C2 was not rotated in the first instance, or the rotation is merely an epiphenomenon of head position.[7] This type of language can often lead to clinician induced, patient maladaptive beliefs!

Communication through touch

The power of touch is well recognized and there is continuing research investigating its physiological and therapeutic effects.[8,9] Touch is also a powerful nonverbal communication tool and can contribute substantially towards building a positive therapeutic relationship. Patients want to be assured that the clinician understands their neck pain and believes them.[10] Nothing can be more validating for the patient than when the clinician, without requesting patient feedback, can identify the painful cervical segment(s) during a skilled manual examination. This is very assuring to patients and they can gain considerable confidence in the clinician through this physical contact. Furthermore, patients can judge a clinician's mastery through such touch. As any educator could attest, patients can differentiate the lack of confidence in a novice compared with an expert's manual examination. The better the clinician's manual skills, the more confident the patient will become in the clinician.

Education

Systematic reviews have found that education as a stand-alone treatment is not efficacious for relieving neck pain,[11] whether the education is about advice to stay active, or advice on stress-coping skills, workplace ergonomics or self-care strategies. This is hardly surprising and is an unrealistic expectation of any monotherapy. Education has other outcomes. Ensuring patients have sufficient information and understanding of their neck pain disorder is critical if the patient is to contribute informed decisions about their own care, have positive expectations of management, see clear reasons to adhere to exercise programs as well as make any changes to lifestyle, i.e., have greater self-efficacy. Education forms part of a multimodal management approach for a patient with a neck pain disorder.

Information required is varied and patient specific. Patients' health literacy and learning styles need to be explored for effective education. The learning experience for the patient and their engagement in treatment and self-management is often a reflection of the communication and teaching skills of the clinician. Because the effectiveness of these skills has a powerful influence on patient uptake, it is salient for clinicians to reflect frequently, on their own skills and abilities as an educator.

Education on the neck pain disorder

Providing information and helping patients understand their neck pain condition is a vital first step in the education process and several topics are covered.

(1) The patient needs an understanding and validation of their neck pain disorder. Validation comes when the clinician acknowledges the patient's symptoms and the impact on their lives and offers a provisional pathoanatomical mechanism possibly using an analogy, such as a sprained ankle, an overuse injury or a flare up of an osteoarthritic knee. The clinical can provide a clear physical diagnosis based on the examination findings and explanation should encourage positive expectations of outcomes. It is important that conventional anatomical and medical terms are used and mystical, jargonish explanations are avoided.

(2) Pain education is an important aspect in the acute, subacute as well as persistent pain states.[12] Education should reflect the multidimensionality of pain incorporating sensory, emotional, cognitive and behavioural components. The educational content is best tailored to the patient's presentation. Information is provided on the sensory components or pain mechanisms in both the peripheral system and central nervous system (CNS). Where relevant, augmented CNS processing or central sensitization can be discussed, again avoiding alarmist terminology. Explanations of how emotions can influence the experience of pain through both CNS and hormonal processes can underpin treatment strategies to decrease stress or anxiety as relevant to the patient. Explanations of endogenous ascending and descending pain inhibitory mechanisms can likewise underpin discussions on management strategies. There is increasing interest in education in pain neurosciences and it makes a very important contribution to patient care. Pain education is relevant across all stages of musculoskeletal disorders although most research to date into its effectiveness is in chronic pain where it is proving helpful.[13] Similar to any intervention, some patients are more responsive than others.[14] Pain education's role in preventing the transition of acute to persistent back pain is currently being investigated.[15]

(3) The course of neck pain, prognosis and patient's expectations of recovery should be discussed. This may seem to be an eclectic group of topics but it is important to understand patient expectations of recovery to best contextualize explanations of the course of neck pain and prognosis. Patients may define their expectations of recovery in many different terms,[16,17] for example, complete pain relief versus relief until symptoms are manageable. Recovery may mean a return

to normal everyday activities or it may mean being able to undertake basic activities without hesitation. Expectations will also be guided by personal beliefs and past experiences.

The epidemiology of neck pain, regardless of aetiology, indicates that its course is typically of recurrences with variable degrees of recovery between episodes.[18–21] This relatively pessimistic message can be expressed in a positive and motivating way to support the need for self-management and maintenance programs in efforts to prevent or lessen recurrences.

Discussing "how long to get better" can be more challenging. Walton and colleagues[22] conducted a preliminary longitudinal study of patients presenting for treatment of mechanical neck pain and found that a mean linear trajectory for the population actually represented three different trajectories over a 1-month period. The majority (66%) had gradual improvement, some improved rapidly (20%) and some regressed (14%). People with more recent onset (< 6 months), and higher levels of pain were likely to improve more rapidly. Leaver et al.[23] made similar observations in patient cohort with an acute episode of neck pain. Those who reported recovery did so in a median of 6.4 weeks (75% recovered in 4 weeks). Thus it is difficult to estimate how long it will take for symptoms to ease for an individual, although the shorter duration of pain is a positive sign for a more rapid recovery.

There is some knowledge of prognostic indicators for recovery from a whiplash injury with which there can be strong confidence, but few for mechanical neck pain.[24,25] Risk factors for a poor prognosis after a whiplash injury include high pain intensity and high disability ratings at the initial presentation (strong confidence) and the presence of abnormal cold thresholds, posttraumatic stress symptoms and catastrophization (moderate confidence). Discussing outcomes with patients with poor prognostic indicators can be difficult. Not all patients presenting with initially high pain levels fail to recover. Informing a person that they will not recover would not be viewed well in a third-party insurance environment. However not informing a person of the poor prognosis could be another case of clinician-induced "catastrophic thoughts" as the patient worries that they are not getting better as the clinician advised

them that they should. These are areas of professional communication and care that need to be discussed and resolved. At present, it is probably reasonable to inform the patient that there are some symptoms of concern to alert them, but not automatically align them with a poor prognosis.

Education in anatomy and biomechanics

Education in basic cervical anatomy and biomechanics is not an intervention for neck pain. However, when considering self-management strategies and neck care, patients benefit from some anatomical and biomechanical knowledge of the cervical spine and shoulder girdle on which to problem solve so that they can self-manage effectively. It is important that patients understand the relationship between the loads induced by functional activities and pain so that they have the capability to develop appropriate strategies for their daily functional activities and develop an understanding of the value of undertaking exercise to improve physical support of their neck.

Education and use of behavioural strategies

Cognitive behaviour therapy (CBT) is a type of psychotherapy delivered by psychologists, which aims to help a person identify and challenge unhelpful thoughts and to learn practical self-help strategies to help improve quality of life. CBT has many forms. On current evidence, the benefits of CBT for neck pain disorders is marginal at best when its effectiveness is evaluated with pain as the primary outcome, although it can assist patients with chronic neck pain overcome fear of movement.[26] This marginal effect of CBT may not be a reflection of the potential benefit of CBT, but again may reflect the potential limitations of monotherapies, the lack of recognition of the heterogeneity of neck pain disorders and disregard of patient preferences. For example, Keefe et al.[27] advise that the patients most suitable for Pain Coping Skills training are those who accept that their pain is likely to persist and who are open to learn new skills for pain management. A CBT graded activity program may be suitable for some patients with persistent neck pain but may not be suitable for those patients with whiplash-associated disorders who display repetition-induced summation of activity-related pain.[28,29] Likewise a clinical trial is underway to test the efficacy of a CBT stress inoculation training program but for only those patients who exhibit early stress responses following an acute whiplash injury.[30]

CBT is a treatment method offered by trained health psychologists. This does not necessarily preclude physiotherapists or others from delivering a full CBT program, but it does take considerable training to meet psychologists' competency levels.[31,32] Nevertheless, physiotherapists do and should use psychologically informed practices.[33] Listening to the patient, acknowledging their pain, discussing and often normalizing a patient's anxieties and fears is central to a good patient/clinician relationship. In addition, physiotherapists have the skills to incorporate several of the CBT "lessons" into their management. These include (as relevant to the patient) progressive muscle relaxation, activity-rest cycling, pleasant activity scheduling and, importantly, problem solving.[34] An equally important lesson is helping the patient to recognize the signs of a potential relapse and providing them with strategies to abort or manage an acute episode of neck pain.

Self-Management

Self-management is a vital component of management, especially considering the recurrent nature of neck pain and in some cases, the persistence of neck pain. Patients ideally become involved in their own management from the beginning and the clinician may have to work to change patient behaviours. Their participation in treatment and compliance with home management programs is the foundation upon which to build an effective self-management program for use into the future. Patient compliance is essential to the success of any home or self-management program, and the skills and clinical attributes of the clinician influence this compliance.

From a content viewpoint, the patient requires knowledge and skills to manage their work practices and activities of daily living in ways that will not adversely overload the neck and cause unnecessary strain and pain. These will be very patient specific but may include best methods for working at a computer or other devices, best methods for driving, lifting and carrying, sleeping positions and pillows and gym and exercise, as examples. From a process point of view, some information will be delivered didactically, for example, data indicating that compared with a neutral head posture, using a device in a neck flexion position will increase the mechanical demand on extensor muscles by 3 to 5 times (and increase the resulting load on the cervical spine).[35] However, there is deeper learning when, after the patient identifies which are the aggravating activities or postures, they are helped to problem solve and find solutions or ways to perform the activity in a way that will not adversely load the neck and cause pain.

Self-management also includes an exercise component, which in the first instance will focus on rehabilitation strategies to ensure as optimal function as possible. Positive patient traits for self-management and exercise include greater self-efficacy for exercise and positive exercise outcome expectations.[36] A program usually consists of a manageable regime of exercises to help ease pain, restore movement and rehabilitate the neuromuscular and sensorimotor systems. The program should be patient specific and constantly modified and progressed throughout the management period. At all times, patients must have ready access to a description of the program. From a process viewpoint, determine the patient preference for receipt of this information. For example, one patient might be very happy to access exercise descriptions and demonstrations through an App downloaded onto a phone or tablet, another patient may prefer a hard copy of exercises.

Self-management should also include a simple and "do-able" maintenance program that a patient can continue after discharge from treatment to redress the recurrent nature of neck pain disorders. As well, the patient should have treatment strategies to implement if they recognize signs of a potential relapse and return of neck pain. Education should also address issue of general activity and fitness within the total management plan of patient care. The nature of these self-management strategies will be explored throughout the chapters on management.

REFERENCES

1. Ferreira P, Ferreira M, Maher C, et al. The therapeutic alliance between clinicians and patients predicts outcome in chronic back pain. Phys Ther 2013;93:470–8.
2. Scott W, Milioto M, Trost Z, et al. The relationship between perceived injustice and the working alliance: a

cross-sectional study of patients with persistent pain attending multidisciplinary rehabilitation. Disabil Rehabil 2016;38: 2365–73.

3. Higgs J, Ajjawi R, McAllister L, et al. Communicating in the health sciences. 3rd ed. Melbourne, Australia: Oxford University Press; 2012.

4. Potter M, Gordon S, Hamer P. The physiotherapy experience in private practice: the patients' perspective. Aus J Physiother 2003;49:195–202.

5. Opsommer E, Schoeb V. Tell me about your troubles': description of patient-physiotherapist interaction during initial encounters. Physiother Res Int 2014;19:205–21.

6. van Randeraad-van der Zee CH, Beurskens A, Swinkels R, et al. The burden of neck pain: its meaning for persons with neck pain and healthcare providers, explored by concept mapping. Qual Life Res 2016;25:1219–25.

7. Guenkel S, Scheyerer M, Osterhoff G, et al. It is the lateral head tilt, not head rotation, causing an asymmetry of the odontoid-lateral mass interspace. Eur J Trauma Emerg Surg 2016;42: 749–54.

8. Peled-Avron L, Goldstein P, Yellinek S, et al. Empathy during consoling touch is modulated by mu-rhythm: an EEG study. Neuropsychologia 2018, in press.

9. Zangrando F, Piccinini G, Tagliolini C, et al. The efficacy of a preparatory phase of a touch-based approach in treating chronic low back pain: a randomized controlled trial. J Pain Res 2017;10:941–9.

10. MacDermid J, Walton D, Miller J, et al. What is the experience of receiving health care for neck pain? Open Orthop J 2013;7(Suppl. 4: M5):428–39.

11. Gross A, Forget M, George KS, et al. Patient education for neck pain. Cochrane Database Syst Rev 2012;(3):CD005106.

12. Moseley G, Butler D. Fifteen years of explaining pain: the past, present, and future. J Pain 2015;16:807–13.

13. Louw A, Diener I, Butler D, et al. The effect of neuroscience education on pain, disability, anxiety, and stress in chronic musculoskeletal pain. Arch Phys Med Rehabil 2011;92: 2041–56.

14. Malfliet A, Oosterwijck JV, Meeus M, et al. Kinesiophobia and maladaptive coping strategies prevent improvements in pain catastrophizing following pain neuroscience education in fibromyalgia/chronic fatigue syndrome: an explorative study. Physiother Theory Prac 2017;33:6653–60.

15. Traeger A, Moseley G, Hübscher M, et al. Pain education to prevent chronic low back pain: a study protocol for a randomised controlled trial. BMJ Open 2014;4:e005505.

16. Carroll L, Jones D, Ozegovic D, et al. How well are you recovering? The association between a simple question about recovery and patient reports of pain intensity and pain disability in whiplash-associated disorders. Disabil Rehabil 2012;34:45–52.

17. Walton D, Macdermid J, Taylor T, et al. What does 'recovery' mean to people with neck pain? Results of a descriptive thematic analysis. Open Orthop J 2013;7:420–7.

18. Carroll L, Hogg-Johnson S, van der Velde G, et al. Course and prognostic factors for neck pain in the general population. Results of the bone and joint decade 2000-2010 task force on neck pain and its associated disorders. Spine 2008;33: S75–82.

19. Carroll L, Holm L, Hogg-Johnson S, et al. Course and prognostic factors for neck pain in whiplash-associated disorders (WAD). Spine 2008;33:S83–92.

20. Carroll LJ, Hogg-Johnson S, Cote P, et al. Course and prognostic factors for neck pain in workers - Results of the bone and joint decade 2000-2010 task force on neck pain and its associated disorders. Spine 2008;33:S93–100.

21. Hogg-Johnson S, van der Velde G, Carroll LJ, et al. The burden and determinants of neck pain in the general population - Results of the bone and joint decade 2000-2010 task force on neck pain and its associated disorders. Spine 2008;33: S39–51.

22. Walton D, Eilon-Avigdor Y, Wonderham M, et al. Exploring the clinical course of neck pain in physical therapy: a longitudinal study. Arch Phys Med Rehabil 2014;95:303–8.

23. Leaver A, Maher C, McAuley J, et al. People seeking treatment for a new episode of neck pain typically have rapid improvement in symptoms: an observational study. J Physiother 2013;59: 31–7.

24. Sterling M, Hendrik J, Kenardy J, et al. Assessment and validation of a prognostic model for poor functional recovery 12 months following whiplash injury: a multicentre inception cohort study. Pain 2012;153:1727–34.

25. Walton D, Carroll L, Kasch H, et al. An overview of systematic reviews on prognostic factors in neck pain: results from the International Collaboration on Neck Pain (ICON) Project. Open Orthop J 2013;7(Suppl. 4: M9):494–505.

26. Monticone M, Ambrosini E, Cedraschi C, et al. Cognitive-behavioral treatment for subacute and chronic neck pain: a Cochrane Review. Spine 2015;40:1495–504.

27. Keefe F, Beaupre P, Gil K, et al. Group therapy for patients with chronic pain. In: Turk D, Gatchel R, editors. Psychological approaches to pain management; a Practitioner's Handbook. 2nd ed. New York: Guilford Press; 2002. p. 234–54.

28. Mankovsky-Arnold T, Wideman T, Larivière C, et al. Measures of spontaneous and movement-evoked pain are associated with disability in patients with whiplash injuries. J Pain 2014;15: 967–75.

29. Mankovsky-Arnold T, Wideman T, Thibault P, et al. Sensitivity to movement-evoked pain and multi-site pain are associated with work-disability following whiplash injury: a cross-sectional study. J Occup Rehabil 2017;29:413–21.

30. Ritchie C, Kenardy J, Smeets R, et al. StressModEx–Physiotherapist-led stress inoculation training integrated with exercise for acute whiplash injury: study protocol for a randomised controlled trial. J Physiother 2015;61:157.

31. Bryant C, Lewis P, Bennell K, et al. Can physical therapists deliver a pain coping skills program? An examination of training processes and outcomes. Phys Ther 2014;94:1443–54.

32. Nielsen M, Keefe F, Bennell K, et al. Physical therapist-delivered cognitive-behavioral therapy: a qualitative study of physical therapists' perceptions and experiences. Phys Ther 2014;94: 197–209.

33. Main C, George S. Psychologically informed practice for management of low back pain: future directions in practice and research. Phys Ther 2011;91:820–4.

34. Keefe F, Kashikar-Zuck S, Opiteck J, et al. Pain in arthritis and musculoskeletal disorders: the role of coping skills training and exercise interventions. J Orthop Sports Phys Ther 1996;24: 279–90.

35. Vasavada A, Nevins D, Monda S, et al. Gravitational demand on the neck musculature during tablet computer use. Ergonomics 2015;58:990–1004.

36. Quicke J, Foster N, Ogollah R, et al. The relationship between attitudes, beliefs and physical activity in older adults with knee pain: secondary analysis of a randomised controlled trial. Arthritis Care Res 2017;69:1192–200.

14 MANAGEMENT OF JOINT AND MOVEMENT DYSFUNCTION

Painful cervical joint and movement dysfunction is managed in various ways depending on the underlying causes and contributors to the dysfunction. Information is sought throughout the patient interview and the physical examination to understand the relative contributions of external factors, for instance postures, poor muscle control and intrinsic factors such as articular changes, to the presenting joint and movement dysfunction. This information can direct initial management. Fig. 14.1 presents an example of clinical reasoning for a patient presenting with limited and painful cervical movement with associated cervical joint signs. It illustrates how the relative contributions of manipulative therapy, active mobilizing exercise and neuromuscular training may be apportioned in initial patient management on the basis of the examination findings. Nevertheless, regardless of their proportional contribution, the roles of manipulative therapy and neuromuscular training are synergistic.

This chapter discusses manipulative (or manual) therapy and exercise. The exercises in this context focus on active or assisted movement at a segmental or regional level to improve range and quality of movement. The patient must be an active participant. Any improvement gained in range and quality of motion in a treatment session must be supplemented by a home program of specific exercise because the immediate effects of manipulative therapy management, if not reinforced, will reduce.[1]

MANIPULATIVE THERAPY

Manipulative therapy (mobilization and manipulation) makes an important contribution to the management of patients with neck pain disorders, which are associated with painful segmental dysfunction. The evidence from systematic reviews indicates that manipulative therapy (manipulation and mobilization) is effective in reducing neck pain as a single modality[2,3] or as part of a multimodal program.[4] Furthermore evidence is emerging of its cost effectiveness when compared with exercise alone, advice or general practitioner care.[5–8] Manipulative therapy has shown benefit for acute, subacute and persistent or chronic neck pain disorders, for various age groups, including older patient groups with long-standing or chronic neck pain.[6,9] Yet manipulative therapy is not a panacea. It is not best practice when it is used as a sole treatment. Rather it is best positioned as part of a multimodal management approach. As with any intervention whether pharmacological, physical or psychological, patient suitability for and responsiveness to manipulative therapy will vary and the intervention should be abandoned if it is not producing the desired outcomes after a reasonable trial of treatment.

Benefits of manipulative therapy

The benefits of manipulative therapy are in relief of symptoms, be the symptoms of neck pain, neck-related arm pain, neck-related headache or dizziness.[2,9–12] Studies have indicated that manipulative therapy elicits

189

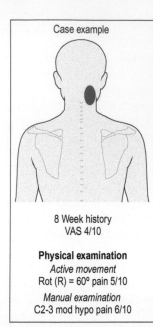

Case example

8 Week history
VAS 4/10

Physical examination
Active movement
Rot (R) = 60° pain 5/10

Manual examination
C2-3 mod hypo pain 6/10

Initial reasoning
Outcome of retest of scapular correction on ROM
retest manual examination after scapular muscle test

• ROM increases, Pain reduces to 1/10;   C2-3 no hypo; pain reduces to 1/10
  Reasoning: posture and muscle control major contributors to pain state
  Treatment priority (i) Muscle training and reeducation (80%)
                    (ii) MT for residual joint pain; active segmental exercise (20%)

• ROM slight increase, Pain reduces to 3/10;   C2-3 mod hypo; pain reduces to 3/10
  Reasoning: joint dysfunction, posture/muscle control equal contributors to pain state
  Treatment priority (i) Muscle training and reeducation (50%)
                    (ii) MT for joint pain; active segmental exercise (50%)

• ROM no change, Pain no change 5/10;   C2-3 mod hypo; pain no change 6/10
  Reasoning: joint dysfunction major contributor to pain state
  Treatment priority (i) MT for joint pain; active segmental exercise (70%)
                    (ii) Muscle training and reeducation (30%)

Additional features
• Hypomobility cervicothoracic region
• Fearful of movement
• Central sensitization present
• Reduced movement velocity, smoothness

Implication for management
Add MT and segmental/regional active exercise to C/Th region
Practice rotation in 4 point kneeling or within confined ranges
MT and exercise indicated but must not provoke pain
Practice increasing speed between fixed points in range

Fig. 14.1 ■ Example of clinical reasoning to inform on proportionate roles of manipulative therapy and muscle training in initial interventions. *C/Th*, cervicothoracic, *MT*, manipulative therapy, *ROM*, range of motion.

hypoalgesia both locally and remote to the neck and induces excitation of the sympathetic nervous system suggestive of systemic pain modulation effects.[13] Studies conducted on spinal and peripheral joints suggest the effects of manipulative therapy may be attributed to peripheral, spinal and supraspinal mechanisms.[13] For example, at the peripheral level, spinal manipulative therapy has been shown to significantly downregulate or reduce the production of inflammation-associated chemokines[14,15] which may be elevated in people with low-back and neck pain,[15,16] a change not observed following sham manipulation.[15] Similarly, manipulative therapy can promote changes in β-endorphin, anandamide, N-palmitoylethanolamide and serotonin levels.[17] Spinal mechanisms may include decreased activation of the dorsal horn of the spinal cord,[18] and changes in spinal reflex excitability[19,20] including a reduction of the H-reflex[21] and an increase in nociceptive flexion reflex threshold.[22] Finally, supraspinal responses with manipulative therapy shown at this time include decreased activation of areas in the brain associated with pain including the anterior cingulate (bilateral), frontal cortex (bilateral) and sensory motor cortex (contralateral).[18]

Manipulative therapy increases pressure pain thresholds both locally[23–25] and at remote distal sites,[23,26] but in contrast, thermal sensitivity seems to be unaffected.[22,24,25,27] Manipulative therapy also affects an immediate excitatory response in the sympathetic nervous system[24,26,28] as demonstrated by, for example, significant increases in skin conduction, breathing rate and heart rate.[24,28] Other mechanisms contributing to symptom relief could include the effects of placebo and patient expectations.[29,30] The physiological and therapeutic effects of hands on treatment also contribute to patient assurance and, indirectly, pain relief.

There is less certainty about the mechanical mechanisms of effect of manipulative therapy procedures.[27] For example, the technique of central posteroanterior (PA) glides, as its nomenclature suggests, should theoretically induce segmental translation at the target segment. In a magnetic resonance imaging study, cervical segmental motion was measured when a PA mobilization was performed centrally on C5 at a grade III technique (clinical definition—large amplitude of movement moving to the end of available range).[31] Not surprisingly with this large amplitude technique (over a segmental translation excursion of 1–1.5 mm), it was found that the mobilization induced extension in the levels above C5 and flexion in the levels below. In an earlier study of a grade IV PA technique, negligible to no intervertebral translation was observed.[32] In a similar vein, a cadaveric analysis of a localized high velocity, low amplitude C1–2 rotary thrust revealed that the displacement induced during the technique was unintentional, unpredictable and not reproducible.[33] Thus to base explanations of mechanism on a movement directional basis is not relevant for some techniques.

Several studies have investigated the effect of mobilization on tissue stiffness in the cervical spine (i.e., the resistance to deformation induced by the manual force or in clinical terms, the through range resistance and end feel). Stiffness tested segmentally in vivo is increased in patients with neck pain disorders, although there is no direct relationship between degree of stiffness and reported pain and disability.[34] The latter is understandable because stiffness is quite variable between individuals depending on collagen make up, age and gender. Cervical mobilization can reduce spinal stiffness and pain, although one study determined that this was not measurable until the short-term follow-up (4 days later) and was not related to any increase in range of movement.[35] In contrast, a study of unilateral PAs applied over the zygapophysial joints demonstrated an immediate, posttreatment reduction in segmental stiffness and an increase in range of movement.[36] Notably, the change was only determined when treatment was applied locally to the symptomatic and hypomobile segment, suggesting the need for localized application of treatment.

There is increasing clarity about potential neurophysiological mechanisms underpinning the symptomatic relief that can be afforded with manipulative therapy. However, more research is needed to better understand the importance of mechanical factors. This is both in relation to mechanisms of effect and also guidance for selection of manipulative therapy techniques.

What manipulative therapy cannot achieve

Manipulative therapy can modulate and help relieve symptoms such as pain, dizziness or light headedness or unsteadiness. Yet rehabilitation is also concerned with addressing impaired functions in the neuromuscular and sensorimotor systems to assist the return of normal safe function and in efforts to prevent recurrent episodes of neck pain. Thus the important question is whether manipulative therapy can address the impaired function as well as symptoms.

The immediate effect of cervical PA mobilization on muscle activity has been assessed by measuring sternocleidomastoid or longus colli muscle activity in the craniocervical flexion test (CCFT). There is evidence both for and against an immediate posttreatment change in muscle activity.[24,37,38] The change in muscle activity might relate to reduced pain following the PA technique. However, there is evidence from a randomized controlled trial that this immediate change is not sustained. No improvement in performance of the CCFT occurred in the short, medium or long term, despite the relief of neck pain and headache afforded by manipulative therapy.[10]

Dizziness and unsteadiness are not uncommon symptoms of cervical musculoskeletal disorders. They are associated with impairments in proprioception and balance. Manipulative therapy can efficiently alleviate these symptoms.[39] However this relief of symptoms was not accompanied by any substantive changes in measures of joint position sense in the short or long term. As found in other studies, neither techniques of mobilization or manipulation have been able to change balance sway measures.[12,40,41]

Thus manipulative therapy can successfully relieve symptoms, but symptom relief does not guarantee any improvement in impairments in neuromuscular and sensorimotor systems. Pain relief from manipulative therapy is the example used here, but it applies to pain relief by any modality and even pain relief over time.[42] This reinforces the need for multimodal management in a rehabilitation program for patients with neck pain disorders because aims are not just to address the episode of neck pain but to lessen future recurrent episodes.

Patients suitable for manipulative therapy

A systematic review of clinical trials, in which the intervention tested was cervical manipulative therapy, studied the inclusion criteria to reveal those patients who were deemed suitable for this therapy. The data from 30 trials revealed inclusion criteria of the broad categories of mechanical or idiopathic neck pain, cervical spondylitis, whiplash-associated disorders (WAD) and cervicogenic headache. The "manipulable lesion", if defined, was usually described as a positive response to a clinical test identifying abnormal segmental movement.[43] It is certainly not the ideal criteria especially when clinical tests based on identifying abnormal segmental movement are of themselves not highly reliable.[43,44]

Nevertheless, despite limitations, the basic framework to identify patients potentially suitable for manipulative therapy management remains: those with neck pain associated with impaired neck movement (usually painful), which is associated with symptomatic segmental joint dysfunction; and for whom there are no conditions or patient features which contraindicate the use of this therapy. Definitions are modified depending on the manipulative therapy approach followed, for example, detection of abnormal segmental motion and reproduction of pain during manual examination,[45] versus the reduction of pain and improvement of segmental/regional movement during manual examination.[46] Thus at this time, indications for manipulative therapy are in many ways, a definition essentially of exclusion of those unsuitable.

Another way to identify patients suitable for manipulative therapy is to recognize patients who are likely responders to manipulative therapy based on their clinical presentation. In this respect, most attention has been paid to developing classification schemes/subgrouping patients or developing clinical prediction rules.[44] Although of some assistance, these methods too have inherent limitations (see Chapter 1). An alternate method is to identify which clinical features indicate that patients are likely non-responders to manipulative therapy.[47] Discussion here has focussed on manipulative therapy, but the same challenge is still present for selecting patients who are suitable and will respond to most approaches or modalities used to treat neck pain.

Clinical reasoning throughout the entire clinical examination will inform selection of management strategies including manipulative therapy. The basic framework of impaired neck movement and associated symptomatic segmental joint dysfunction might be the appropriate guide. These indications for suitability for manipulative therapy treatment would be strengthened with evidence that relief of pain afforded by manipulative therapy is associated with resolution of the clinical signs that were used to detect the manipulable lesion.[43] This process of assessment and reassessment of the change in clinical signs in response to the intervention is used in clinical practice to guide the continuation or abandonment of the technique or approach. Suitable measures can and need to be included in clinical trials to provide the evidence of the validity of this guide.

Contraindications and cautions to manipulative therapy

Much attention has rightly been afforded to safety in practice. Texts have been devoted to nominating and clinically identifying serious spinal pathologies[48,49] as well as identifying conditions that might masquerade as spinal conditions[50] and would contraindicate the use of spinal manipulative therapy and indeed other physical therapies. The reader is referred to these sources for a comprehensive coverage of these conditions and their recognition. In the cervical spine, greatest concerns are vascular disorders (cervical arterial dissection, vertebrobasilar insufficiency, anticoagulant therapy) (see Chapter 10); any state which might reduce the integrity of cervical structures, such as acute trauma, metastases; inflammatory arthritides; traumatic or degenerative instability; connective tissue disease; congenital anomalies (Down syndrome); osteoporosis; infection and advanced degenerative disease with lateral and/or spinal canal stenosis with or without neurological signs.[51]

Fortunately, catastrophic adverse events associated with cervical manipulative therapy such as stroke or even death are rare. However, accurate estimates are not available as the quality of the literature on which estimates are based is still quite poor and all cases are not recorded in the literature. Best estimates vary widely from 1 in 20,000 to 1 in 250,000,000 manipulations.[52] To enhance accuracy, clinical trials that follow Consolidated Standards of Reporting Trials (CONSORT) guidelines now are required to report adverse events.[53] This might allow better analysis of practitioner, patient and technique characteristics associated with serious adverse events.[54] In perspective, a systematic review of adverse events with manipulative therapy (for either neck pain or low-back pain) confirmed that the risk of major adverse events was very low.[55] Nevertheless about one-half of the patients experienced minor to moderate adverse events, (often posttreatment pain) which lasted for a few to 72 hours. Of note, the incidence was similar for manipulative therapy and exercise. All clinicians should aim to eliminate these minor adverse events from practice, and this should be achievable with better understanding of the patient's pain state and skilled manual handling and exercise prescription.

Which manipulative therapy approach?

Manipulative therapy within physiotherapy incorporates several different approaches, which although not radically different, do have some unique philosophies and practices.[45,46,56–59] Each has an examination approach which underpins technique selection. This means that a patient's neck disorder or joint dysfunction could be treated with different techniques based on the clinicians' background training. Nevertheless, the evidence indicates that, when tested head to head, symptomatic outcomes are essentially the same between different manipulative therapy approaches.[2,39,60,61] Similarly, there is no consistent evidence that manipulation has superior outcomes to mobilization.[2,60,62–64] This encourages thought on mechanisms of effect, and the commonalities rather than differences between techniques. The commonalties would be neurophysiological effects and probably the changes the techniques afford in tissue stiffness. This then raises the question of the nature of tissue stiffness or altered tissue compliance underlying the segmental hypomobility. It could be reasoned that it is probably, in large part, muscle activity in response to a symptomatic joint when different techniques/movement directions all cause a similar change in tissue stiffness, and the change is achieved quite rapidly.

Selection and application of technique

The decision to use manipulative therapy and the selection of a particular technique is the culmination of clinical reasoning throughout the patient interview and physical examination. The process in different approaches varies slightly but is common, consideration is usually given to the nature and intensity of pain, functionally impaired movement or posture, the direction(s) of impaired and painful cervical motion and the local segmental test results.[45,46,56–59] The selection of a technique will usually relate to the pain response and direction of movement loss, noting that there are always different options (Figs 14.2A–C to 14.3A–C). The clinician must always test the response to the technique and, if it is not achieving the desired effect within a treatment, an alternate technique should be tried. Changes within a session can predict changes in subsequent treatments.[1] Nevertheless changes in impairments do not necessarily relate to changes in activity limitations,[65] which again emphasizes the need for multimodal treatment.

There has been discussion of whether it is necessary to be precise in treating the most dysfunctional cervical level.[44] A few studies have addressed this issue using a one-session, pre-post design in both the cervical and lumbar regions with some diverse outcomes.[36,66,67] Such pre-post single application studies have major limitations, but a systematic review found evidence to favour specific mobilization of the dysfunction cervical segment for pain relief.[68] Further research is required to evaluate whether treating the most symptomatic level produces superior treatment effects. Stronger questions and designs are necessary, for example, investigating effects

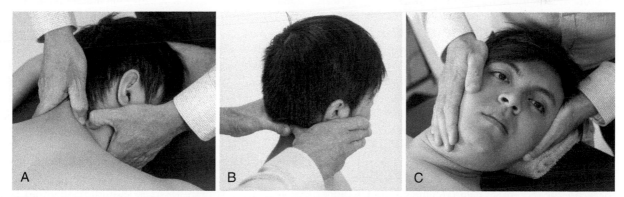

Fig. 14.2 ■ Techniques which can address a restriction in (R) C1–2 segmental motion. (A) Unilateral posteroanterior glide on C2 with the head and C1 positioned in slight (R) rotation. (B) A sustained natural apophysial glide on C1 with active (L) cervical rotation. (C) (R) lateral flexion mobilization of C0–1. (L) C1–2 rotation can be limited if there are restrictions in contralateral lateral flexion.

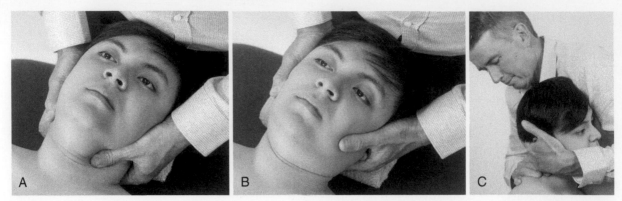

Fig. 14.3 ■ Techniques which can address a restriction in C3–4 lateral flexion. (A) An anteroposterior glide of C3 on C4 with a medial bias. The pad of the thumb is placed on the anterior surface of the transverse process of C3 and the thumb position is supported by the fingers gripping the lamina posteriorly. The grip around the segment remains constant and the movement is produced at the elbows. The thumb is the transmitter not the producer of the movement/force. If the movement is produced through thumb pressure, the technique will be painful. (B) A lateral flexion technique. The hands cradle the head and the index or middle finger is placed on the lamina of C3. The movement is a combination of a lateral flexion and medial glide to move the facet into lateral flexion. (C) Lateral flexion is performed in sitting. The spinous process and lamina of C4 is stabilised by a pincer grip of the (R) hand. The thenar eminence of the (L) hand grips C3 and the lateral flexion movement is produced by an arm/shoulder girdle movement.

of treating the most symptomatic cervical segment versus a random segment after three or four treatment sessions over, for instance, a 2-week period. Certainly, intuitively, treating the most symptomatic segment is logical clinical practice.

Nevertheless, upper thoracic spine mobilization and manipulation may also relieve neck pain.[69,70] However various trials have shown that although treatment of the upper thoracic region can relieve neck pain, this remote treatment is not as effective as local cervical treatment.[71–73] There are strong indications for including treatment to the upper thoracic region of patients with neck pain disorders because of the interdependent nature of cervical and upper thoracic motion and the need for upper thoracic movement to allow full head excursion. It is reasonable that both areas receive attention as required in management as is currently occurring.[62,63]

Various manipulative therapy approaches offer recommendations for the dosage of techniques, but it is an area that is not well researched. Various approaches have guides relevant to their approach, such as the grade of technique that might be used,[45] the position in range it might be performed[58] or the appropriate force to improve the impaired movement without causing pain.[46] Many factors influence "dosage" or how much mobiliza-

tion or manipulation is delivered. These include the nature and severity of the patient's pain, the acuteness of the condition, the irritability of the condition and patient preferences.

Preliminary research is providing some initial guidelines. For example, a study of the delivery of one to five sets of PA mobilizations, albeit on the lumbar spine of healthy individuals, found that at least 4 sets of 60 seconds mobilizations were required to elicit the best hypoalgesic response.[74] Another study investigated the effects of high (90 N mean peak force) versus low (30 N mean peak force) mobilization forces when delivering a PA mobilization to the most symptomatic segment of patients with chronic neck pain.[35] Better effects (reduced segmental stiffness and pain) were found with the higher force mobilization. However, these effects were not determined immediately posttreatment but at the follow-up up to 4 days later. Immediately posttreatment, pain levels were increased in the high force group, which may not be an optimal outcome. Dosage is a priority area for further research.

Application of techniques should at all times be comfortable for the patient (Fig. 14.4). Preferably, all treatment should cause nil or minimal pain. This is especially true when pain levels are high and/or when

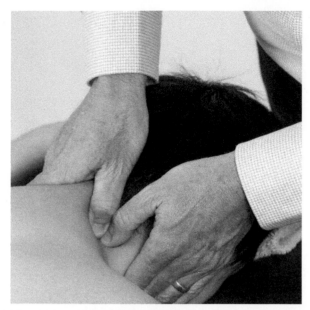

Fig. 14.4 ■ Unilateral posteroanterior (PA) glides C3-4. Unilateral PA glides should be performed painlessly and this can be achieved if the hands grip the side of C3 to support the position of the thumbs on the lamina to perform a unilateral PA. The movement is generated by the elbows/forearm and the thumbs are the transmission point, not the generator of force.

central sensitization is present as occurs in patients with cervicogenic headache, cervical radiculopathy and in some cases of whiplash.[75–77] Treatments that aggravate pain in these patients are counterproductive. Nevertheless, the presence of central sensitization does not mitigate against the use of manipulative therapy. It was thought that patients with WAD who displayed central sensitization would not respond as well to manipulative therapy,[78] but subsequent studies have not shown that this is the case.[79,80]

Treatment of the cervical spine for pain in adjacent areas

There has been much study into potential neurophysiological and biomechanical links between the cervical spine and disorders of the craniomandibular complex and upper limb.[81–85] Clinical trials have evaluated the effect of treating the neck for a craniomandibular or an upper-limb pain syndrome or conversely treating the craniomandibular disorder to ease neck pain.[28,82,84–87] Outcomes have been variable. In clinical practice,

patients can present with apparent "signs" in both the cervical spine and temporomandibular joint (TMJ). Clinicians need to undertake a disciplined assessment/reassessment process to determine the primary source of pain and dysfunction. Treatment of one region (e.g., the neck) might result in an immediate change in pain and range of motion in the TMJ. However, the critical issue is whether the treatment effect is maintained at the second treatment session. A basic guide is that at least 50% of any change gained in TMJ pain and motion in the previous treatment must be maintained to justify repeated treatments or a focus on the neck. Often the initial gains are from pain modulation, not true changes in the local dysfunction. Persisting with treatment that does not result in lasting changes is poor practice.

ACTIVE EXERCISE

Active exercise is a vital component of the management of joint and movement dysfunction. In this context, active exercise is used to regain active range of motion and to train movement velocity as indicated.

Range of motion

Active exercise is used to gently load the tissues during the healing process following acute trauma such as a whiplash or sporting injury. Active movement is used in idiopathic neck pain with movement and segmental dysfunction, to mobilize neck hypomobility at both segmental and regional levels. Active range of movement exercises as a sole treatment for neck pain is not optimal[88] but active exercises are an important part of a multimodal program.

In an acute phase of a neck disorder, patients may find it painful to perform range-of-motion exercises in the sitting position. Exercises are often easier to perform and less painful when head load and gravity are reduced. This is achieved by positioning the patient in four-point kneeling, prone on elbows or forward inclined sitting position as tolerated.

Active exercise should be prescribed to complement and supplement the manipulative therapy treatment to address the local segmental hypomobility. Fig. 14.5A–C illustrates examples of segmentally biased exercises. Early radiological studies demonstrated that an active regional movement does not mean that all segments are contributing.[89] Thus the segmental bias

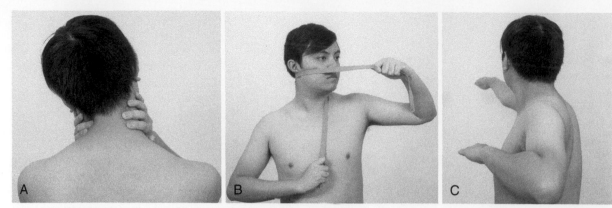

Fig. 14.5 ■ Segmentally biased active movement. (A) Lateral flexion C3–4. The patient places their index or middle finger on C4 and focusses lateral flexion at the C3–4 level. (B) A mobilization with movement technique to encourage C1–2 rotation. (C) The "archery exercise' ". This exercise compliments the passive mobilization of the cervicothoracic region with the lateral glide + active rotation technique (see Fig. 9.5). The patient keeps their eyes fixed on an imaginary target and draws the string back on an imaginary bow. They focus on producing and feeling the movement in the upper thoracic region. The action is performed on alternating sides.

to the regional exercise aims to ensure that the segments of interest are contributing to the motion. The segmental exercises are best taught and practised in conjunction with the manipulative therapy component of management. This helps the patient to understand and "feel" the movement that the treatment is trying to achieve. Patients replicate it with the active exercise. Teaching the active exercise at this time in treatment involves the patient immediately in management and does not divorce the active segmental mobilising exercise from the manipulative therapy treatment. Patients immediately understand the relevance of the exercise which might help compliance. This opportunity can be lost when teaching active exercise is relegated to the end of treatment and to a home program only.

Exercises for training movement velocity and accuracy

Recent research has investigated the use of both a customized neck virtual reality system and a laser and target for feedback during cervical kinematic training for impairments in range, velocity and accuracy of motion.[90,91] The applications are highly suitable for use in a home program of exercises. Training for range of motion, movement velocity and accuracy includes exercises such as quick active head movements, fine head movement control and stability in several movement directions (Fig. 14.6A and B). In the clinical

trial, patients had non-acute, persistent neck pain and performed exercises at home for 20 minutes, 4 times per week. Both forms of training (virtual reality and the laser and target system) improved patients cervical kinematics as well as their neck pain and disability in both the short and intermediate terms.[90,91] Because training with both the virtual reality and the laser and target system produced similar outcomes, the choice of training mode could depend on availability. Perhaps a more important consideration is the patient's preference, and in this technological age, a virtual reality device might be more appealing to some. Obliging with the patient's preference may facilitate exercise compliance.

SELF-MANAGEMENT

A home exercise program is a very necessary component of the management program. The small dosage of movement delivered and practised within a treatment session is insufficient. Dosage of either active segmentally biased exercise or exercises to address movement velocity will depend on the acuteness of the condition but low repetitions (e.g., 5–10 repetitions) performed several times during the day (e.g., 3–5 times) is a reasonable approach to commence the self-management program. Exercises will be progressed in nature and repetitions in line with the patient's and treatment progression.

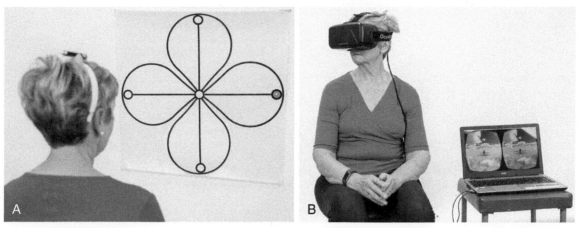

Fig. 14.6 ■ Exercises to train movement velocity, accuracy and range. (A) Kinematic training with a head mounted laser directed towards lines on a poster. Tasks include: moving as far as possible in all directions, moving quickly from the centre point to the circles placed in different directions and then stabilizing the laser before quickly returning to the centre and tracing the vertical and horizontal lines and then the curved pattern lines as accurately as possible with the laser using head motion. These exercises can be commenced in sitting and progressed to comfortable standing or more challenging stance conditions. (B) Kinematic home training using the virtual reality head mounted display, and customized software. Here, head motion controls a virtual airplane. Range of movement is challenged by gradually increasing the range of movement required to hit targets in flexion, extension, rotation left and right. Velocity of head motion is encouraged by motivating the participant to move quickly towards the target in random directions before it disappears. Finally, the player is directed to keep the head of the virtual pilot on a moving target up, down, right and left as accurately as they can.

The patient should be encouraged to think about how they can incorporate the exercise into their daily routines. The clinician needs to follow this up with the patient to demonstrate the importance of self-management to treatment outcome. Equally important is to determine how patients would like the exercises presented to them for home practice. Some patients, for instance, may prefer a hard copy description of the exercises, others may prefer a video of themselves performing the exercise to refer to at home.

Patient involvement with the development of the exercise program, which will evolve with the addition of other strategies into the self-management program, is a positive step towards compliance.

CONCLUSION

The treatment of painful cervical joint and movement dysfunction is an important element of the multimodal management program for patients with neck pain disorders. Manipulative therapy has effective and beneficial analgesic effects. Active movement exercises both segmentally directed and regional are vital and

necessary compliments to manipulative therapy to address the joint and movement dysfunction. All aspects of movement dysfunction need to be considered including the quality and range of movement, poor movement sense and velocity. Effective exercises need to be devised for the patient to practise efficiently and successfully.

REFERENCES

1. Tuttle N. Do changes within a manual therapy treatment session predict between-session changes for patients with cervical spine pain? Aust J Physiother 2005;51:43–8.
2. Gross A, Langevin P, Burnie S, et al. Manipulation and mobilisation for neck pain contrasted against an inactive control or another active treatment (Review). Cochrane Database Syst Rev 2015;(9):doi:10.1002/14651858.CD004249.
3. Wong J, Shearer H, Mior S, et al. Are manual therapies, passive physical modalities, or acupuncture effective for the management of patients with whiplash-associated disorders or neck pain and associated disorders? An update of the Bone and Joint Decade Task Force on Neck Pain and Its Associated Disorders by the OPTIMa collaboration. Spine J 2016;16:1598–630.
4. Sutton D, Côté P, Wong J, et al. Is multimodal care effective for the management of patients with whiplash-associated disorders or neck pain and associated disorders? A systematic review by the Ontario Protocol for Traffic Injury Management (OPTIMa) Collaboration. Spine J 2016;16:1541–65.

5. Korthals-de Bos IB, Hoving JlL, Tulder MW, et al. Cost effectiveness of physiotherapy, manual therapy, and general practitioner care for neck pain: economic evaluation alongside a randomised controlled trial. BMJ 2003;326:911.

6. Leininger B, McDonough C, Evans R, et al. Cost-effectiveness of spinal manipulative therapy, supervised exercise, and home exercise for older adults with chronic neck pain. Spine J 2016;16:1292–304.

7. Michaleff Z, Lin C, Maher C, et al. Spinal manipulation epidemiology: systematic review of cost effectiveness studies. J Electromyogr Kinesiol 2012;22:655–62.

8. Tsertsvadze A, Clar C, Court R, et al. Cost-effectiveness of manual therapy for the management of musculoskeletal conditions: a systematic review and narrative synthesis of evidence from randomized controlled trials. J Manipulative Physiol Ther 2014;37:343–62.

9. Uthaikhup S, Assapun J, Watcharasaksilp K, et al. Effectiveness of physiotherapy for seniors with recurrent headaches associated with neck pain and dysfunction: a randomized controlled trial. Spine J 2017;17:46–55.

10. Jull G, Trott P, Potter H, et al. A randomized controlled trial of exercise and manipulative therapy for cervicogenic headache. Spine 2002;27:1835–43.

11. Nee RJ, Vicenzino B, Jull GA, et al. Baseline characteristics of patients with nerve-related neck and arm pain predict the likely response to neural tissue management. J Orthop Sports Phys Ther 2013;43:379–91.

12. Reid S, Callister R, Snodgrass S, et al. Manual therapy for cervicogenic dizziness: long-term outcomes of a randomised trial. Man Ther 2015;20:148–56.

13. Bialosky JE, Bishop MD, Price D, et al. The mechanisms of manual therapy in the treatment of musculoskeletal pain: a comprehensive model. Man Ther 2009;14:531–8.

14. Teodorczyk-Injeyan J, Injeyan H, Ruegg R. Spinal manipulative therapy reduces inflammatory cytokines but not substance P production in normal subjects. J Manipulative Physiol Ther 2006;29:14–21.

15. Teodorczyk-Injeyan J, McGregor M, Triano J, et al. Elevated production of nociceptive CC-chemokines and sE-selectin in patients with low back pain and the effects of spinal manipulation: a non-randomized clinical trial. Clin J Pain 2018;34:68–75.

16. Teodorczyk-Injeyan J, Triano J, McGregor M, et al. Elevated production of inflammatory mediators including nociceptive chemokines in patients with neck pain: a cross-sectional evaluation. J Manipulative Physiol Ther 2011;34:498–505.

17. Degenhardt B, Darmani N, Johnson J, et al. Role of osteopathic manipulative treatment in altering pain biomarkers: a pilot study. J Am Osteopath Assoc 2007;107:387–400.

18. Malisza K, Stroman P, Turner A, et al. Functional MRI of the rat lumbar spinal cord involving painful stimulation and the effect of peripheral joint mobilization. J Magn Reson Imaging 2003;18:152–9.

19. Dishman J, Bulbulian R. Spinal reflex attenuation associated with spinal manipulation. Spine 2000;25:2519–24.

20. Dishman J, Burke J. Spinal reflex excitability changes after cervical and lumbar spinal manipulation: a comparative study. Spine J 2003;3:204–12.

21. Bulbulian R, Burke J, Dishman J. Spinal reflex excitability changes after lumbar spine passive flexion mobilization. J Manipulative Physiol Ther 2002;25:526–32.

22. Sterling M, Pedler A, Chan C, et al. Cervical lateral glide increases nociceptive flexion reflex threshold but not pressure or thermal pain thresholds in chronic whiplash associated disorders: a pilot randomised controlled trial. Man Ther 2010;15:149–53.

23. Coronado R, Gay C, Bialosky J, et al. Changes in pain sensitivity following spinal manipulation: a systematic review and meta-analysis. J Electromyogr Kinesiol 2012;22:752–67.

24. Sterling M, Jull G, Wright A. Cervical mobilisation: concurrent effects on pain, motor function and sympathetic nervous system activity. Man Ther 2001;6:72–81.

25. Vicenzino B, Collins D, Benson H, et al. An investigation of the interrelationship between manipulative therapy-induced hypoalgesia and sympathoexcitation. J Manipulative Physiol Ther 1998;21:448–53.

26. Vicenzino B, Collins D, Wright A. The initial effects of a cervical spine manipulative physiotherapy treatment on the pain and dysfunction of lateral epicondylalgia. Pain 1996;68:69–74.

27. Lascurain-Aguirreben I, Newham D, Critchley D. Mechanism of action of spinal mobilizations: a systematic review. Spine 2016;41:159–72.

28. Touche RL, París-Alemany A, Mannheimer J, et al. Does mobilization of the upper cervical spine affect pain sensitivity and autonomic nervous system function in patients with cervicocraniofacial pain? A randomized-controlled trial. Clin J Pain 2013;29:205–15.

29. Bialosky J, Bishop M, Penza C. Placebo mechanisms of manual therapy: a sheep in wolf's clothing? J Orthop Sports Phys Ther 2017;47:301–4.

30. Bishop M, Mintken P, Bialosky J, et al. Patient expectations of benefit from interventions for neck pain and resulting influence on outcomes. J Orthop Sports Phys Ther 2013;43:457–65.

31. Lee R, McGregor A, Bull A, et al. Dynamic response of the cervical spine to posteroanterior mobilisation. Clin Biomech (Bristol, Avon) 2005;20:228–31.

32. McGregor A, Wragg P, Gedroyc W. Can interventional MRI provide an insight into the mechanics of a posterior-anterior mobilisation? Clin Biomech 2001;16:926–9.

33. Buzzatti L, Provyn S, Roy PV, et al. Atlanto-axial facet displacement during rotational high-velocity low-amplitude thrust: an in vitro 3D kinematic analysis. Man Ther 2015;20:783–9.

34. Ingram L, Snodgrass S, Rivett D. Comparison of cervical spine stiffness in individuals with chronic non-specific neck pain and asymptomatic individuals. J Orthop Sports Phys Ther 2015; 45:162–9.

35. Snodgrass S, Rivett D, Sterling M, et al. Dose optimization for spinal treatment effectiveness: a randomized controlled trial investigating the effects of high and low mobilization forces in patients with neck pain. J Orthop Sports Phys Ther 2014;44: 141–52.

36. Tuttle N, Barrett R, Laakso L. Relation between changes in posteroanterior stiffness and active range of movement of the cervical spine following manual therapy treatment. Spine 2008;33:E673–9.

37. Jesus-Moraleida F, Ferreira P, Pereira L, et al. Ultrasonographic analysis of the neck flexor muscles in patients with chronic neck pain and changes after cervical spine mobilization. J Manipulative Physiol Ther 2011;34:514–24.

38. Lluch E, Schomacher J, Gizzi L, et al. Immediate effects of active craniocervical flexion exercise versus passive mobilisation of the upper cervical spine on pain and performance on the craniocervical flexion test. Man Ther 2014;19:25–31.

39. Reid S, Rivett R, Katekar M, et al. Comparison of mulligan sustained natural apophyseal glides and Maitland mobilizations for treatment of cervicogenic dizziness: a randomized controlled trial. Phys Ther 2014;94:466–76.

40. Fisher A, Bacon C, Mannion V. The effect of cervical spine manipulation on postural sway in patients with non-specific neck pain. J Manipulative Physiol Ther 2015;38:65–73.

41. Reid S, Callister R, Katekar M, et al. Effects of cervical spine manual therapy on range of motion, head repositioning, and balance in participants with cervicogenic dizziness: a randomized controlled trial. Arch Phys Med Rehabil 2014;95:1603–12.

42. Lee H, Nicholson LL, Adams RD. Cervical range of motion associations with subclinical neck pain. Spine 2004;29:33–40.

43. Smith J, Bolton P. What are the clinical criteria justifying spinal manipulative therapy for neck pain?- A systematic review of randomized controlled trials. Pain Med 2013;14:460–8.

44. Bialosky J, Simon C, Bishop M, et al. Basis for spinal manipulative therapy: a physical therapist perspective. J Electromyogr Kinesiol 2012;22:643–7.

45. Hengeveld E, Banks K. Maitland's vertebral manipulation: management of neuromusculoskeletal disorders. 8th ed. UK: Churchill Livingstone, Elsevier; 2013.

46. Hing W, Hall T, Rivett D, et al. The mulligan concept of manual therapy. Sydney: Churchill Livingstone, Elsevier; 2015.

47. Jull G, Stanton W. Predictors of responsiveness to physiotherapy treatment of cervicogenic headache. Cephalalgia 2005;25:101–8.

48. Greenhalgh S, Selfe J. Red Flags. Guide to identifying serious pathology of the spine. UK: Churchill Livingstone, Elsevier; 2006.

49. Greenhalgh S, Selfe J. Red Flags II. A Guide to solving serious pathology of the spine. UK: Churchill Livingstone, Elsevier; 2010.

50. Greenhalgh S, Selfe J. Masqueraders. In: Jull G, Moore A, Falla D, et al, editors. Grieve's modern musculoskeletal physiotherapy. 4th ed. UK: Elsevier; 2015. p. 343–7.

51. Puentedura E, March J, Anders J, et al. Safety of cervical spine manipulation: are adverse events preventable and are manipulations being performed appropriately? A review of 134 case reports. J Man Manip Ther 2012;20:66–74.

52. Nielsen S, Tarp S, Christensen R, et al. The risk associated with spinal manipulation: an overview of reviews. Syst Rev 2017;6:64.

53. Chaibi A, Benth J, Tuchin P, et al. Adverse events in a chiropractic spinal manipulative therapy single-blinded, placebo, randomized controlled trial for migraineurs. Musculoskelet Sci Pract 2017;29:66–71.

54. Kranenburg H, Schmitt M, Puentedura E, et al. Adverse events associated with the use of cervical spine manipulation or mobilization and patient characteristics: a systematic review. Musculoskelet Sci Pract 2017;28:32–8.

55. Carnes D, Mars T, Mullinger B, et al. Adverse events and manual therapy: a systematic review. Man Ther 2010;15:355–63.

56. Edwards BC. Manual of combined movements. 2nd ed. Edinburgh: Churchill Livingstone; 1999.

57. Kaltenborn F, Evjenth O, Kaltenborn TB, et al. Manual mobilization of the joints: the spine, vol. 2. 4th ed. Oslo: Norli. 2003.

58. McCarthy C. Combined movement theory. UK: Churchill Livingstone, Elsevier; 2010.

59. Mulligan B. Manual therapy 'NAGS', 'SNAGS', 'MWMS'. 5th ed. Wellington: Plane View Press; 1995.

60. Lopez-Lopez A, Perez JA, Gutierez JG, et al. Mobilization versus manipulations versus sustain apophyseal natural glide techniques and interaction with psychological factors for patients with chronic neck pain: randomized controlled trial. Eur J Phys Rehabil Med 2015;51:121–32.

61. Pérez H, Perez J, Martinez AG, et al. Is one better than another? A randomized clinical trial of manual therapy for patients with chronic neck pain. Man Ther 2014;19:215–28.

62. Dunning J, Butts R, Mourad F, et al. Upper cervical and upper thoracic manipulation versus mobilization and exercise in patients with cervicogenic headache: a multi-center randomized clinical trial. BMC Musculoskelet Disord 2016;17:64.

63. Griswold D, Learman K, O'Halloran B, et al. A preliminary study comparing the use of cervical/upper thoracic mobilization and manipulation for individuals with mechanical neck pain. J Man Manip Ther 2015;23:75–83.

64. Leaver A, Maher C, Herbert R, et al. A randomized controlled trial comparing manipulation with mobilization for recent onset neck pain. Arch Phys Med Rehabil 2010;91:1313–18.

65. Tuttle N, Laasko L, Barrett R. Change in impairments in the first two treatments predicts outcome in impairments, but not in activity limitations, in subacute neck pain: an observational study. Aust J Physiother 2006;52:281–5.

66. Aquino R, Caires P, Furtado F, et al. Applying joint mobilization at different cervical vertebral levels does not influence immediate pain reduction in patients with chronic neck pain: a randomized clinical trial. J Man Manip Ther 2009;17:95–100.

67. Chiradejnant A, Maher C, Latimer J, et al. Efficacy of "therapist-selected" versus "randomly selected" mobilisation techniques for the treatment of low back pain: a randomised controlled trial. Aust J Physiother 2003;49:233–41.

68. Slaven E, Goode A, Coronado R, et al. The relative effectiveness of segment specific level and non-specific level spinal joint mobilization on pain and range of motion: results of a systematic review and meta-analysis. J Man Manip Ther 2013;21:7–17.

69. Cleland J, Childs J, McRae M, et al. Immediate effects of thoracic manipulation in patients with neck pain: a randomized clinical trial. Man Ther 2005;10:127–35.

70. González-Iglesias J, Fernández-de-las-Peñas C, Cleland J, et al. Thoracic spine manipulation for the management of patients with neck pain: a randomized clinical trial. J Orthop Sports Phys Ther 2009;39:20–7.

71. Cleland J, Childs J, Fritz J, et al. Development of a clinical prediction rule for guiding treatment of a subgroup of patients with neck pain: use of thoracic spine manipulation, exercise, and patient education. Phys Ther 2007;87:9–23.

72. Puentedura E, Cleland J, Landers M, et al. Development of a clinical prediction rule to identify patients with neck pain likely to benefit from thrust joint manipulation to the cervical spine. J Orthop Sports Phys Ther 2012;42:577–92.

73. Puentedura E, Landers M, Cleland J, et al. Thoracic spine thrust manipulation versus cervical spine thrust manipulation in patients with acute neck pain: a randomized clinical trial. J Orthop Sports Phys Ther 2011;41:208–20.

74. Pentelka L, Hebron C, Shapleski R, et al. The effect of increasing sets (within one treatment session) and different set durations (between treatment sessions) of lumbar spine posteroanterior mobilisations on pressure pain thresholds. Man Ther 2012;17: 526–30.

75. Chien A, Eliav E, Sterling M. Whiplash (grade II) and cervical radiculopathy share a similar sensory presentation: an investigation using quantitative sensory testing. Clin J Pain 2008;24:595–603.

76. Chua N, Suijlekom HV, Vissers K, et al. Differences in sensory processing between chronic cervical zygapophysial joint pain patients with and without cervicogenic headache. Cephalalgia 2011;31:953–63.

77. Sterling M, Jull G, Vicenzino B, et al. Sensory hypersensitivity occurs soon after whiplash injury and is associated with poor recovery. Pain 2003;104:509–17.

78. Jull G, Sterling M, Kenardy J, et al. Does the presence of sensory hypersensitivity influence outcomes of physical rehabilitation for chronic whiplash? - a preliminary RCT. Pain 2007;129:28–34.

79. Castaldo M, Catena A, Chiarotto A, et al. Do subjects with whiplash-associated disorders respond differently in the short-term to manual therapy and exercise than those with mechanical neck pain? Pain Med 2017;18:791–803.

80. Michaleff Z, Maher C, Lin C, et al. Comprehensive physiotherapy exercise programme or advice for chronic whiplash (PROMISE): a pragmatic randomised controlled trial. Lancet 2014;384: 133–41.

81. Coombes B, Bisset L, Vicenzino B. Cervical dysfunction is evident in individuals with LE without obvious neck pain and may reflect central sensitization mechanisms. Further study of the nature of the relationship between cervical dysfunction and LE is required. J Manipulative Physiol Ther 2014;37:79–86.

82. Fernández-de-Las-Peñas C, Cleland J, Palacios-Ceña M, et al. The effectiveness of manual therapy versus surgery on self-reported function, cervical range of motion, and pinch grip force in carpal tunnel syndrome: a randomized clinical trial. J Orthop Sports Phys Ther 2017;47:151–61.

83. Grondin F, Hall T, Laurentjoye M, et al. Upper cervical range of motion is impaired in patients with temporomandibular disorders. Cranio 2015;33:91–9.

84. Mintken P, Cleland J, Carpenter K, et al. Some factors predict successful short-term outcomes in individuals with shoulder pain receiving cervicothoracic manipulation: a single-arm trial. Phys Ther 2010;90:26–42.

85. Piekartz H, Pudelko A, Danzeisen M, et al. Do subjects with acute/subacute temporomandibular disorder have associated cervical impairments: a cross-sectional study. Man Ther 2016;26:208–15.

86. Grondin F, Hall T. Changes in cervical movement impairment and pain following orofacial treatment in patients with chronic arthralgic temporomandibular disorder with pain: a prospective case series. Physiother Theory Pract 2017;33:52–61.

87. Piekartz H, Lüdtke K. Effect of treatment of temporomandibular disorders (TMD) in patients with cervicogenic headache: a single-blind, randomized controlled study. Cranio 2011;29:43–56.

88. O'Leary S, Jull G, Kim M, et al. Training mode-dependent changes in motor performance in neck pain. Arch Phys Med Rehabil 2012;93:1225–33.

89. Dvorak J, Froehlich D, Penning L, et al. Functional radiographic diagnosis of the cervical spine: flexion/extension. Spine 1988;13:748–55.

90. Bahat HS, Takasaki H, Chen X, et al. Cervical kinematic training with and without interactive VR training for chronic neck pain - a randomized clinical trial. Man Ther 2015;20:68–78.

91. Sarig-Bahat H, Croft K, Carter C, et al. Remote kinematic training for patients with chronic neck pain- a randomised controlled trial. Eur Spine J 2018;27:1309–23.

15 MANAGEMENT OF NEUROMUSCULAR DYSFUNCTION

■ ■

Exercise in the broader context is being discovered to have many and diverse benefits for physical and mental health. One of its valuable benefits in the musculoskeletal context is its hypoalgesic effect. This effect has been measured immediately after various exercise modes including aerobic,[1,2] dynamic resistance[3] and isometric exercise.[4,5] The mechanism is considered to involve a systemic analgesic process[6] with activation of central inhibitory pathways[7] as well as peripheral mechanisms.[8] However, specific research into immediate hypoalgesic effects following local neck or general exercise in people with neck pain is as yet quite sparse.[9–11] Nevertheless, in accord with patient centeredness and their desire for pain relief, current clinical trials and systematic reviews of interventions for neck pain all evaluate the effectiveness of exercise on the criterion of its pain relieving effect.[12–14] Evaluation is based on patient-centred outcomes of self-reported pain intensity and/or perceived disability immediately following the intervention and at intermediate and longer terms following intervention.

The benefits of exercise on pain are important but exercise that is also specially prescribed to address the neuromuscular dysfunction, a known feature of musculoskeletal disorders, is a key component of rehabilitation. It seems that with the emphasis on pain outcomes, there has been a recent loss of focus on exercise prescription for "rehabilitation". For instance, participant inclusion criteria in clinical trials usually do not include measures of muscle function that link to the intervention (e.g., presence of a muscle strength deficit for a strengthening program intervention). There

appears no major interest in whether or not exercise has addressed the neuromuscular deficits associated with neck pain (see Chapter 5) because measures of impairment are rarely included as primary (and often not even as secondary) outcomes. Exercise for pain relief is a very different construct to exercise for rehabilitating the neuromuscular system and neuromuscular impairments. We argue here for a reemphasis on the benefits of exercise for restoration of neuromuscular function in addition to its pain-relieving benefits.

An acute episode of neck pain usually resolves in a timely manner with appropriate management, although it can be incomplete.[15,16] The message that must be repeatedly emphasized is that for the majority of people neck pain is a recurrent or persistent disorder.[15,17] Together with low-back pain, neck pain accounts for more years lived with a disability than any other chronic disease.[18] The true personal and immense fiscal cost of neck pain is not in a single episode, but in the cost of repeated episodes, i.e., the repeated healthcare costs, the potential costs of harm from repeated use of medications such as nonsteroidal antiinflammatory drugs (NSAIDs), the personal cost of loss of quality of life as well as costs of lost work productivity. Managing an episode of pain is important but a pressing aim is to decrease recurrence rate. There are multiple features from biological, social and psychological perspectives that potentially contribute to the recurrent or persistent nature of neck pain. There will never be a perfect correlation between physical impairments and pain levels or states. Nevertheless, impaired neuromuscular function does not necessarily automatically resolve when pain

201

resolves, which cannot be good for neck health.[19–21] Although not the sole solution, rehabilitation of neuromuscular and sensorimotor impairments stands to make a positive contribution to both recovery and decreasing recurrence rate.

Exercise can relieve pain, but when a reduction in pain is the primary outcome, it does not appear to matter what exercise is prescribed, at least for those with chronic pain. Both low-load and high-load exercises can similarly reduce chronic neck pain.[19,22] Nevertheless, it does matter what exercises are prescribed if the aim is to restore the impaired elements of neuromuscular function. The evidence clearly indicates that changes in motor behaviour are best addressed through a low-load motor relearning approach in the first instance. Yet this exercise mode is clearly inadequate and inappropriate when the aim is to increase muscle strength and higher-level endurance where exercise against load is required.[23–27]

The exercise protocol presented in this chapter is informed by research into the changes in neuromuscular function that are induced by neck pain and injury, as well as research which has informed the need for specificity of exercise to address each impaired function (see Chapter 5). Muscle facilitation and training in the clinical setting is always accompanied by a home program of exercises, which will change as the patient progresses through the program. We will recommend certain exercises, but this is not to suggest that they are the only exercises that can be used or necessarily the best exercise for a certain patient. The final choice of an exercise is at the clinician's discretion. What is necessary is that the effect of any exercise is constantly monitored with a measure to ensure that the desired effect on the related impairment is being achieved.

EXERCISE ADHERENCE

It does not matter how research informed and effective an exercise program is, it will not be successful unless the patient complies with and adheres to the recommended program. There is a growing body of research examining adherence because it is relevant for successful management across a whole spectrum of health interventions.

Communication with a patient-centred style is valuable and can provide a motivational basis to help the patient engage in appropriate self-management behaviours.[28,29] The clinician and patient need to work together to identify motivators or enablers as well as barriers to exercise.[30,31] A prime motivator for exercise is a decrease in neck pain. Every opportunity should be undertaken during examination and treatment to link a proposed exercise with pain relief, for example, how a change in spinal or scapular posture can change neck pain and range of motion, or how facilitation of scapular or neck flexor muscles can decrease palpable joint pain (see Chapters 9 and 14). Patients are growing more cognizant of the need for evidence-based treatments. Thus it is relevant to both demonstrate and discuss with them the evidence for the nature of neuromuscular impairments that can be associated with neck pain, the fact that these impaired functions do not automatically and consistently improve when the pain resolves and the need for good muscle function towards preventing any recurring episodes of neck pain.

Other enablers can be as simple as adopting an established routine for exercise, identifying and supplying equipment and intensive monitoring.[31] A first criterion is that a program is straight forward and manageable in current "time-limited" contemporary lifestyles. Initially during the low-load movement control phase of training, we advocate a routine of formal training for no longer than 5 to 10 minutes, twice per day (before starting the day and after work or before retiring for the night). The formal exercises are supplemented by functional exercises (e.g., correcting posture), which can be conducted repeatedly during the day, without interrupting the patient's daily activities, to gain the necessary dosage of muscle activation or movement skill to achieve the desired change. Small equipment such as sports tape to facilitate cervical segmental exercise (see Chapter 14), a laser and targets for position and movement sense training (see Chapter 16) and the pressure biofeedback device for assessing and progressing deep cervical flexor training are all very simple pieces of equipment which enable exercise and most importantly, provide feedback on performance. It is vital to monitor progress, provide feedback on performance and advance the exercise program to maintain a patient's interest and adherence.

Any potential barriers to exercise need to be identified. Studies have recognized barriers, such as pain with exercise and lack of motivation.[30,31] It is counterproductive for exercises to cause pain, especially in the motor-relearning phase. It has been shown experimentally that nociceptive input modulates cortical neuroplasticity associated with novel motor training and may impair the ability to learn a motor task.[32] Motivation to exercise can be promoted with links to the pain relieving effects of exercise. In addition, motivation is enhanced with intensive monitoring of both the exercise and the gains made by the patient.[31] Measures of muscle impairment and changes in performance can be constantly monitored both to motivate adherence and to progress the exercise program. Effective long-term adherence is essential for good self-management.

THE HOME PROGRAM

A home program of exercises is a key element of rehabilitation and self-management programs. The patient must actively contribute to its development to facilitate adherence. Box 15.1 lists some pointers to consider when developing the home exercise program. Adherence to the home exercise program is necessary for successful training and it should be given due time for reassessment and development in each treatment session.

NEUROMUSCULAR TRAINING

Neuromuscular training consists of a program of exercise that usually commences with a low-load exercise and posture training program and progressively adds movement complexity and load to train:

- the activation and endurance capacity of the deep cervical postural muscles (flexors and extensors) and axioscapular muscles.
- coordination between the deep and superficial layers of the neck muscles and axioscapular muscles in movement and postural tasks of increasing difficulty.
- muscle control within functional and work activities.
- muscle endurance at different contraction intensities.
- muscle strength tailored to the functional demands of the patient.

Principles of motor relearning (segmentation, simplification, augmented feedback) are followed especially in

---

BOX 15.1
POINTERS FOR HOME EXERCISE PROGRAM DEVELOPMENT

The program must be patient specific and tailored to the patient's needs and not a generic handout of exercises.

Establish patients' preferences for recording the home program. For example, some may prefer to receive written descriptions and illustrations of the exercises. Other patients may prefer the clinician to video them performing the exercises on their phones or tablets for home reference. Others may prefer a combination of methods. Establish and act on patients' preferences.

Assist the patient to identify suitable times for exercise that fit their lifestyle and work—times for formal exercise and intermittent exercise during the day.

Ensure exercises are relevant and contained to a minimum. Balance the program, too many exercises may be too time consuming, which might deter adherence, too few exercises may be insufficient to be effective.

Ensure there is variety in exercises to capture and maintain interest.

Provide clear instruction on exercise dosage.

Establish progressive goals for training muscle groups and related outcome measures on which to regularly monitor improvement.

Demonstrate the importance of the home exercise program by prioritizing its review, rather than leaving it to the end of the treatment session. The latter can give the patient the impression that it is of low priority in management.

Do not presume that the exercises are being performed correctly. Review exercises in each treatment session to ensure that performance is correct. Correction is required more often than not.

Ensure that as exercises are added in the progressive program, exercises that have been superseded are removed.

When the program has progressed to strength training, it may be appropriate to train strength on 3 days per week, refresh activation and patterning exercises on the alternate 3 days, and have 1 day a week without formal exercises.

---

the early to intermediate phases of the program.[33] Precision in exercise is emphasized, and exercises are performed in a pain free manner and in the initial phases, short of fatigue. Attention is given to use of correct movement patterns and to the need for multiple repetitions in skill learning.

From the outset, it is important to ensure that improvements in muscle control from specific training are translated to the patient's specific functional or work activity to address any provocative activity. It is ideal to observe the patient in their own work environment, but when this is not possible, it is advantageous to mock-up or replicate their pain provoking work, sporting or daily activity. Training control and muscle coordination directly in the functional task is often necessary because it cannot be assumed that there will always be an automatic translation from formal training to the function.[34] It is also important to review any gym or fitness program in which the patient is participating. The patient must be given all encouragement to continue these programs, but exercises should be reviewed to ensure that they are "neck safe" and "neck friendly".

The precise training program for an individual patient is guided by and responsive to the nature and extent of neuromuscular dysfunction documented in the physical examination (see Chapter 9). In this chapter, a full training program is presented but all exercises may not be necessary for all patients, and patients will progress through the program at different rates. Precise exercise selection and progression, as indicated, is based on the findings of the initial examination, continual monitoring of the patient's progress as well as knowledge concerning the patient's functional demands and lifestyle. Exercises for posture and the neck flexor, extensor and axioscapular muscles are integrated from the first treatment as needed and continued as the patient achieves progressive goals. Posture training is described first because it is an integral functional exercise for training all muscle groups.

POSTURE TRAINING

Poor working postures or drifting into poor working postures has been implicated in neck pain disorders of several occupations.[24,35,36] Specific training of posture is indicated when the patient interview and physical examination reveal that poor postural behaviours contribute to the individual's neck disorder. Correcting to the upright neutral posture reduces passive, often end-range load on cervical structures, which can be pain relieving in itself. "Postural correction" as an exercise is nevertheless prescribed for most patients because it is a key functional exercise to repeatedly activate spinal postural muscles and axioscapular muscles during the day as is required in the motor learning process.[37] Assuming an upright posture will activate the deep cervical flexors,[37] and further activation can be achieved by adding a "neck lengthening" strategy to the postural correction strategy.[38] Repeated practice of the postural correction alone will improve performance on the craniocervical flexion test,[39] confirming it as an important exercise strategy.

Postural training commences in the first treatment. As mentioned, it is an important component of cervical and axioscapular muscle training because it provides the opportunity for the multiple repetitions required in the motor learning process. It is a functional exercise that can be included in a patient's working day. Postural correction is also beneficial as a preventative or pain-relieving strategy during the working day. These aspects are discussed with the patient so that they understand the importance of the exercise in their rehabilitation.

Spinal posture

Postural training is specific to the activity identified as problematic, and this is commonly the sitting posture. The spinal regions are interdependent, and all regions are given attention. Patients may sit in a good neutral lumbopelvic posture but often they sit in an unacceptable extended or most commonly, a flexed lumbar posture. In this latter circumstance, correction to a neutral lumbar lordosis is initiated from the lumbopelvic region that facilitates lumbar multifidus activity.[37,40] The thorax should move upwards and forwards to position the shoulders over the hips. Thoracolumbar extension is undesirable because it emphasizes activity in the thoracolumbar extensors rather than the lumbar extensors.[41] There are many ways to facilitate postural correction. One simple way, which patients quickly learn, is to roll the pelvis to an upright position to form a normal lumbar lordosis with faciliatory pressure on the L5 spinous process (Fig. 15.1). The patient is taught self-facilitation by placing their own thumb on the L5 spinous process. They can use this strategy until they gain an awareness of the position. The thoracic and cervical postures often correct automatically with correction of the lumbopelvic position. If not, the patient is encouraged to subtlety lift or depress the sternum to correct any residual thoracic kyphosis or thoracic extension, respectively. On occasions, patients have

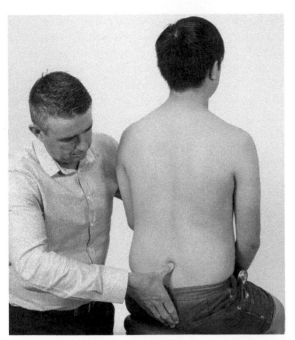

Fig. 15.1 ■ Facilitation of a neutral posture with a pressure stimulus on spinous process of L5.

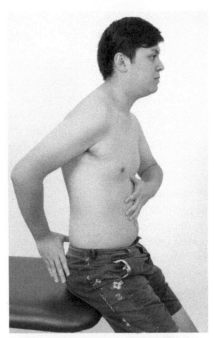

Fig. 15.2 ■ The patient preflexes the thoracolumbar region by placing the thumb on the sternum and the little finger in the naval and drawing them together. Lumbopelvic motion is practised in this position and once the patient learns the movement, it is practised without the thoracolumbar restraint.

difficulty dissociating lumbopelvic movement from thoracolumbar extension. In these cases, lumbopelvic movement may be more easily performed when the patient sits on the edge of a raised treatment bed. Visual feedback from a photo on the patient's mobile phone or a set of mirrors may be helpful for patients who feel that the position is quite foreign.

If the patient sits with an extended spinal posture, they first learn to relax into flexion. The extended posture frequently includes extension from the lumbar to the thoracolumbar, low thoracic regions. It is often necessary to first train proprioceptive awareness of lumbopelvic movement, dissociated from thoracolumbar extension. For patients with a very fixed pattern of extension, it may be necessary to practice lumbopelvic movement with the thoracolumbar region set in a preflexed position in either a high-seated position (Fig. 15.2) or in side lying. Once awareness is gained, the patient trains posture with an unrestrained thoracolumbar region.

Scapular posture

Scapular posture is trained as indicated and directed by the response to scapular correction in the physical examination. Active correction of scapular posture facilitates appropriate muscle activity.[42,43] Training usually commences in the first treatment session once the patient has mastered correction of spinal posture with little effort and concentration. When patients find correction of spinal posture takes much concentration, adding a second task of scapular correction may be too challenging. In concentrating on the scapulae, they lose the spinal position. In these cases, teaching scapular correction is undertaken in the second session or subsequent sessions. When scapular posture is protective of neural tissue (an elevated shoulder posture), treatment of neural tissue takes priority in management because correction may be provocative.

As with spinal posture, instructions/methods for correcting an aberrant scapular posture are many and the clinician should use the one that the patient finds easiest to implement. The clinician may try to repeatedly manually position the patient's scapula into a neutral position to give the patient the sense of the corrected position so that they can develop cognitive strategies to self-correct scapular posture. When patients find it difficult to determine their own strategies, the clinician may provide them with one. One we find very patient friendly is for them to visualize the correction from cues on the front of their chest. The manual correction of scapular posture undertaken in the physical examination (see Fig. 9.2C) informs the clinician on the movements required to correct scapular posture. Patients are asked to imagine strips of elastic attached to the front of their chests. If the scapula is in downward rotation and protraction, the elastic strip runs at 45 degrees from mid sternum to the tip of the shoulder. The instruction to the patient is to lift up the tips of the shoulders and spread the tips of the shoulders out to stretch the elastic. If the scapulae are protracted, the elastic band runs across the chest horizontal to the floor. If the scapulae are in anterior tilt, then the elastic bands run vertically (like a set of braces). Scapular positions often contain elements of one or two directions. The clinician modifies the angles of the imaginary elastic bands to suit the individual patient and observes, from behind, how well the instructions correct scapular position. Some further modification of the angles of the band/instructions may be required, but if the patient can achieve a reasonable position, that is acceptable. Further refinement can be made in subsequent sessions if required, but it is easy to frustrate the patient with too detailed a correction, which can deter compliance. On occasions, taping may be used to facilitate the correct posture.

Head and neck posture

The third element of posture correction is instructing the patient to gently lengthen the back of their neck. This will automatically correct neck and head posture and no other instruction is required. No mention is made of chin position. This is an important component of the correction as it enhances activity of the deep cervical flexors and is an important functional exercise for these muscles.[38]

Dosage for posture training: The patient is encouraged to gently hold the corrected posture for 10 seconds and to practice the exercise, ideally, 3 to 4 times an hour. The exercise is incorporated into activities in sitting, standing or walking. Appropriate muscle activity can be augmented, (e.g., pressing the hands on the thighs or the elbows on the arms of an office chair enhances

the contraction of serratus anterior and the lower trapezius).[44] The postural correction exercise is a vital part of self-management. Although we advocate that the exercise is performed 3 to 4 times per hour, patients in our study on posture correction complied twice per hour for, on average, 8 hours per day. With this dosage, they achieved a positive muscle training effect in the deep cervical flexors in 2 weeks.[39] The patient needs to consider how to remember to undertake regular postural correction. Some elect to have a sound reminder on their mobile phones or a pop up on their computer at work. The clinician can send a strong message to the patient of the importance of posture correction to neck health at the second treatment session, by prioritizing enquiry of the reminders the patient has adopted for the posture exercise before asking any other questions about their neck condition. Posture correction is a key exercise in both management and maintenance programs.

TRAINING THE ACTIVATION AND ENDURANCE OF THE DEEP CERVICAL AND AXIOSCAPULAR MUSCLES

Cervical flexor training

Initial training is directed towards the deep cervical flexors, the longus capitis and longus colli to improve the muscles' activation and endurance capacity. Impairment in the deep cervical flexors performance is characteristic of neck pain disorders (see Chapter 5) and training commences in the first treatment session. There is one contraindication to the training regime, i.e., when the upper cervical flexion neural provocation test is positive (provokes neck pain or headache) (see Chapter 9). In these cases, training begins with self-resisted isometric contractions against the fist positioned under the chin with a 10% effort. Other circumstances such as high levels of pain or suspected cervical instability are not contraindications. In relation to pain, deep cervical flexor training is a low-load exercise performed in supine crook lying and is rarely pain provocative. When ligamentous instability is suspected, training muscle control is indicated as a key component of management.

The outcome measure to assess the effects of training is the craniocervical flexion test (CCFT). The aim is for the patients to be able to perform 10, 10-second isometric holds on the pressure level of 30 mmHg.

Training the craniocervical movement pattern

Findings in the physical examination will inform the initial approach to deep cervical flexor training. If the patient was unable to perform appropriate craniocervical flexion and used a retraction action or other substitution strategy (see Chapter 9), then training begins by facilitating the correct pattern of motion. Attention is given to endurance, only when the correct movement/muscle action is mastered. The movement of craniocervical flexion is taught in supine crook lying with the craniocervical region positioned in a neutral position (folded towels may be placed under the head if necessary, to achieve the neutral position as done in the formal test). The simple instruction of "feel the back of your head slide up the bed to nod your chin" facilitates the correct sagittal rotation action and the patient receives feedback from the surface of the bed. A focus on the sliding sensation negates a tendency to retract the chin. Movement is performed slowly, with control. As large a range as possible from craniocervical extension to craniocervical flexion is used because this makes it easier for the patient to feel and understand the correct movement. Training the movement is augmented with eye movement to facilitate the craniocervical flexors (eyes looking down) and craniocervical extensors (eyes up and back). The patient can palpate the sternocleidomastoid and they practice through a full excursion of motion without feeling sternocleidomastoid activity (Fig. 15.3). Practicing the movement, 10 repetitions, 2 to 3 times per day for a few days in a home program is usually sufficient to learn the pattern and be able to progress to training deep cervical flexor endurance.

Training the endurance of the deep cervical flexors

Training the low-level endurance of the longus capitis and colli commences when the patient can perform the craniocervical flexion movement correctly. The pressure biofeedback unit (Stabilizer, Chattanooga, USA) is used to teach the exercise and to provide feedback on performance. It is very difficult without this feedback for the clinician or patient to know if the deep cervical flexor contraction is being maintained. Training is commenced at the pressure level, determined in the physical examination that the patient was able to achieve with a good movement pattern and hold steady without dominant use of the superficial flexor muscles. This is often at test levels 22 or 24 mmHg. Again, the movement is facilitated by the feel of the back of the head sliding up the bed, and the patient slowly nods to the target pressure level. They then hold the position using the feedback from the dial to confirm performance. Failure is signalled when the needle on the dial drops below the target pressure, or the patient has to constantly reposition to the target pressure. The clinician monitors the head movement to ensure a correct movement pattern.

The feedback assists the patient to learn the low-load, endurance exercise but they typically train at home without the feedback. The reason is that many patients while focussing on the dial, do not concentrate on performing the correct action and the pressure is kept steady with an incorrect strategy. To prepare to train at home without feedback, the patient practices first with the feedback and concentrates on the feeling to maintain the position. They repeat the exercise with the feedback and then turn the dial away and attempt to hold the position without feedback. Here, it is vital for the patient to be actively looking down which is a facilitatory strategy for the deep cervical flexors (Fig. 15.4A and B). The dial is turned back, and the patient checks their success or not. Once they can hold the position, the patient then trains to locate the target without feedback, checking accuracy with the feedback. The aim of the practice is that the patient can target the training pressure and hold it steady without feedback for 10 seconds. Most patients will learn the exercise with 5 to 10 minutes of unsupervised practice. However,

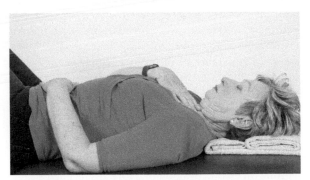

Fig. 15.3 ■ The patient trains the craniocervical flexion movement pattern through the full excursion of the flexion, extension movement. They facilitate the flexors with eyes looking down and monitor that the sternocleidomastoid and scalene muscles remain relaxed.

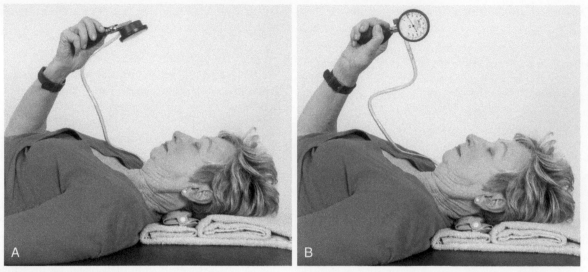

Fig. 15.4 ■ Towards effective craniocervical flexor muscle endurance training at home, (A) the patient practices first with the feedback, then (B) practices without feedback by turning the dial away and then turns the dial back to check their performance with the feedback.

this can be challenging for a patient with poor neck proprioception and in that case, careful training with the feedback may be necessary in the first instance. In home training, they aim to replicate the feel of the contraction. It is helpful to include descriptors of what the patient felt to achieve the task in the instructions for home exercise.

Dosage: Home practice is encouraged at least twice daily, with a pattern of practice being, for example, before arising in the morning and when retiring at night. The aim is for patients to practice 10 repetitions of 10-second holds of the craniocervical flexion exercise. On some occasions, training is commenced with a lesser dosage when the patient fatigues or cannot retain a good pattern of craniocervical flexion for the 10 repetitions. On return for follow-up treatment, the patient's performance in the CCFT is retested. If improvement is present, they then train with the assistance of the feedback to target the next pressure level. This process continues until the patient can achieve 10 × 10-second holds at the 30 mmHg level without effort. Most patients are capable of achieving this goal.[19] Of interest, a biproduct of this training is improvement in joint position sense,[45] which probably results from the relocation practice inherent in the training protocol. The time taken to reach the 30 mmHg target is variable but is

usually achieved in 4 to 6 weeks.[19] It depends on many variables including levels of pain and degree of presenting impairment.[46,47] Patients with very poor baseline movement and muscle activation often require longer whereas others without complexities achieve the goal in a shorter time. During this formal training period, other exercises are added to train the deep cervical flexors (see later sections) at levels commensurate with their capacity.

Formal testing of the deep cervical flexors as well as monitoring and progressing training with the pressure biofeedback unit promotes accuracy in performance and prescription. Equally as important, the objective feedback is a powerful motivator for the patient and assists in adherence to the exercise program.

Cervical extensor training

The initial training protocol for the suboccipital and neck extensor muscles replicates the movements and tests used in the physical examination. The exercises can be performed in the four-point kneeling position, a prone on elbows position or a forward reclined sitting position as suitable for the individual patient. Care is taken with patient positioning in relation to spinal and scapular postures. Ensure that the hips are positioned above the knees and the lumbar lordosis, thoracic kyphosis and cervical lordosis are in neutral. Muscles, such as serratus anterior and lower trapezius, may need to be facilitated so that the patient holds a neutral position of the scapulae. All cervical extensor muscles work to hold the weight of the head against gravity, but each exercise is designed to target muscle groups.

Craniocervical extensors

The exercise targets rectus capitis major and minor in a craniocervical extension and flexion (head nodding) exercise while maintaining the cervical spine in its neutral position. This action is usually instantly learnt by the patient as the familiar action of saying yes. These muscles have key proprioceptive functions as well as controlling movement of the upper cervical joints.

Craniocervical rotators

The exercise targets the obliquus capitis superior and inferior muscles while the cervical spine is maintained in the neutral position. Best instructions are to gently shake the head as if saying no. The range should be less than 40 degrees to each side to focus on C1–2 rotation. Manual facilitation is provided for those patients identified in the physical examination to have difficulty in localizing C1–2 rotation (Fig. 15.5). A facilitatory strategy for home use is to have the patient fix their gaze on a spot between their hands and rotate their head as if saying 'no' while maintaining their fixed gaze. This technique is not suitable for patients who have impaired gaze stability (see Chapter 16). An alternate cue is for the patient to imagine drawing a straight line between the hands with their nose.

Deep cervical extensors

The exercise targets the deep cervical extensors, the semispinalis cervicis and multifidus by mechanically disadvantaging the more powerful torque producing extensors of the head and neck (e.g., splenius and semispinalis capitis) by keeping the craniocervical region in a neutral position during the extension movement.[48] Even at this early stage of the exercise, the deeper extensor muscles work in coactivation with the deep cervical flexor muscles that control the craniocervical neutral position. The exercise is performed as per the test. A pen is placed between the wrists (four-point kneeling) or between the elbows (prone on elbows or inclined sitting) and the patient curls their neck down

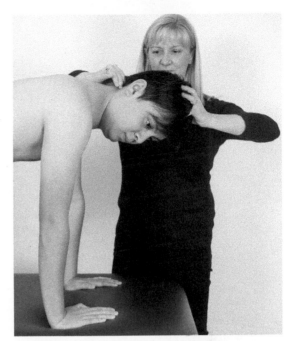

Fig. 15.5 ■ C1–2 rotation can be facilitated by stabilizing C2 and guiding the "spin" of the head to target activity of the obliquus capitis superior and inferior.

to look at their knees/chest and then curls their neck back as far as possible but keeping their gaze fixed on the pen. If patients are having difficulty performing the correct movement, the clinician can guide the movement in the learning process by facilitating the movement through C2 and encouraging a craniocervical neutral position with a hand on the head (Fig. 15.6). In addition, a more segment-specific contraction of the deep extensors, relative to the splenius capitis is gained with localized resistance over the vertebral arch (Fig. 15.7).[49,50]

Dosage: Exercises to train all three muscle groups are performed to the patient's capability because correct movement and muscle use are key considerations. For example, if the patient can only perform cervical extension from the flexed position back to the neutral position, this range is practiced initially. With training, the range will improve, and the patient concentrates on the quality of the movement until they can achieve the normal excursion of approximately 20 to 30 degrees while maintaining the craniocervical region in neutral. Training of C1–2 rotation may begin with excursions of 10 degrees to each side. The aim is for local movement

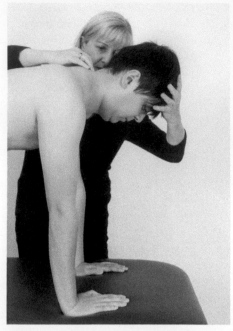

Fig. 15.6 ■ Facilitation of cervical extension. The clinician grips C2 and controls a craniocervical neutral position with the hand on the head. The clinician can pattern the movement with the patient in an assisted active movement.

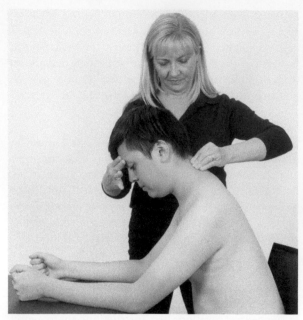

Fig. 15.7 ■ Manual resistance applied over the lamina of the cephalad vertebra (e.g., C4) can enhance the activation of the deep neck extensors (semispinalis cervicis) relative to the superficial extensors (splenius capitis) at the caudal level (i.e., C5).

of C1–2 and facilitation of the obliquus capitis superior and inferior. Range will increase with practice as patients gain more proprioceptive awareness of the movement.

Craniocervical and cervical extensor muscle training is added to the home exercise program. Initial dosage for training may be three sets of five repetitions of each of craniocervical extension, rotation and cervical extension, with a rest between each set. This can be progressed by improving range of movement within the exercises and adding repetitions until the patient can comfortably perform three sets of 10 repetitions through full excursions of movement.

Scapular muscle training

The capacity of the axioscapular muscles (particularly the three parts of trapezius and serratus anterior) is trained to sustain correct postural alignment. Specific scapular postural correction strategies, as well as exercise to improve scapular motion control in specific directions, are trained progressively as required by the individual patient. Many different exercises can be used,[51] and some examples are provided.

When weakness and fatigability of the upper trapezius[52] has been found in the physical examination, often in association with a downwardly rotated scapular posture, initial emphasis is placed on the specific action of upper trapezius. The patient is taught to upwardly rotate their scapula by visualizing the upward movement of the distal end of the clavicle, i.e., a controlled shrugging (Fig. 15.8). This action also relaxes the levator scapulae which downwardly rotates the scapula. The exercise is performed in sitting or standing and the clinician may manually facilitate the upward rotation initially. The exercise is initially performed without load and then progressed as able, against resistance with hand weights. In some patients, better activation of the upper trapezius may be achieved by performing the shrug exercise with the arms abducted to at least 30 degrees (Fig. 15.9).[53]

Dosage: Upper trapezius is trained, as an example, by performing three sets of 10 repetitions of scapular

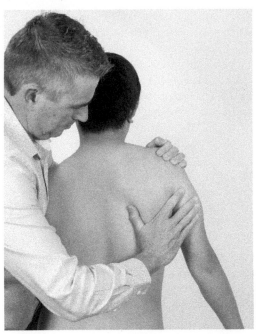

Fig. 15.8 ■ Facilitation of upper trapezius. The patient upwardly rotates their scapula by visualizing the upward movement of the distal end of the clavicle to ensure a correct action.

upward rotation with the emphasis placed on scapular control. The exercise is progressed with increasing arm load. Again, the dosage and progressions will depend on the patient's ability to perform the exercise with precision.

For a particular focus on lower trapezius, training may be commenced in side lying with the arm elevated to approximately 140 degrees. This position deters use of latissimus dorsi and pre-sets the scapula in some upward rotation. The exercise is easy to perform at home using pillows to support arm weight. The cues for the patient are to lengthen their arm by drawing the scapula upward and forward in line with their arm and actively hold and concentrate on the forward action (upper trapezius and serratus anterior). The patient then shortens their arm by drawing the scapula across and down their chest wall and again holds the position (lower trapezius) (Fig. 15.10). The clinician can manually facilitate the scapular movement to enhance learning. The angle of the arm can be varied to better target the middle portion of the trapezius when required.

Dosage: In the home program, the patient practices, for example, 10 × 10-second holds in this formal exercise.

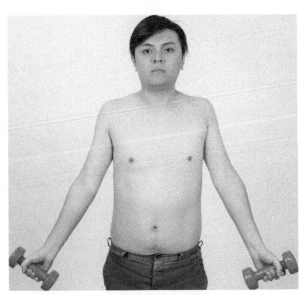

Fig. 15.9 ■ The upward rotation shrug exercise for upper trapezius. The arms are abducted to approximately 30 degrees to pre-position the scapula in upward rotation before commencing the exercise against load.

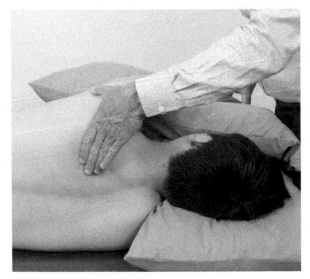

Fig. 15.10 ■ The patient trains the endurance of the scapular muscles in side lying. The arm is positioned in approximately 140 degrees and supported on pillows. Serratus anterior is facilitated by an arm lengthening manoeuvre to draw the scapula forwards and upwards. Lower trapezius is facilitated by shortening the arm by drawing the scapula across and downwards on the chest wall.

This muscle training is reinforced with frequent activation of the scapular supporting muscles in the posture training exercise which is undertaken frequently during the day.

TRAINING MUSCLE CONTROL AND COORDINATION IN MOVEMENT AND POSTURAL TASKS

The training program is progressed as the targets for training the activation and endurance capacity of the deep cervical flexors, extensor and axioscapular muscles are met.

Training the cervical flexor and extensor muscles

Training coactivation

The deep cervical flexor and extensor muscles are described as a deep muscle sleeve which supports the cervical segments.[54] Functionally, these muscles coactivate during neck movements.[55] Once the activation of the deep flexor and extensor muscles has been trained, this functional coactivation is trained with self-resisted alternating isometric exercises. The exercise is performed sitting, with the posture corrected and the back of the neck 'lengthened' to prefacilitate the deep cervical flexors. Gentle resistance is applied by the palm of the patient's hands in an axial rotation direction, alternately to the left and right. The muscles are facilitated by the patient looking toward their hand before resistance being applied. Resistance should match about a 10% effort so that the focus remains on the deeper muscles. Holds for a few seconds can be performed, and this is a portable exercise that the patient can practice at convenient times during the day.

Training control and coordination between deep and superficial neck flexors

Cervical extension in the upright position is a common functional movement requiring both eccentric and concentric control and coordination between deep and superficial neck flexors. It is a movement commonly reported functionally as provocative of symptoms. Coordinated control and sufficient strength and endurance of the deep and superficial flexors are required to sustain the extension position in various functional tasks.

Control of the movement into extension is trained in the first instance within the capacity of particularly, the deep cervical flexors. The movement is initiated by craniocervical extension with the patient looking to the ceiling behind the head. The return to neutral is initiated by craniocervical flexion. The patient only extends to a range that is pain free and that they can control. The key feature of the exercise is the eccentric and concentric work of the deep cervical flexors in coordination with the sternocleidomastoid and anterior scalene muscles. Both clinician and patient should monitor the smooth movement into extension and the ability to return to neutral initiating with craniocervical flexion. A deficit in either component indicates that the deep cervical flexors are loaded beyond their capacity. Extension is practised in a range that the deep cervical flexors can control. The range to which the head is moved into extension is gradually increased as control is improved and any pain permits.

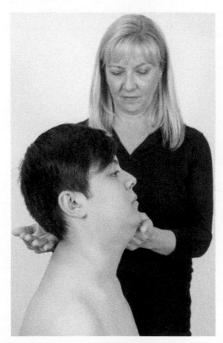

Fig. 15.11 ■ Training the endurance of the craniocervical and cervical flexors against the load of gravity and head weight is interposed with training control in the movement pattern of extension. Control of chin position is monitored. If the chin extends, it signals that the load has exceeded the capacity of the deep cervical flexors.

The second stage of the exercise adds isometric holds in positions through range, which begins the strength and endurance training of the cervical flexor synergy. The patient extends the head and neck to a predetermined position in range that is able to be controlled and is pain free. The clinician supports the head in this position and the patient relaxes. The holding contraction is initiated by looking down together with a slight craniocervical flexion action. Controlling this position, the patient then initiates a head lift, just taking the weight of the head off the clinician's hand (Fig. 15.11). For home practice, the support of the clinician's hand is replaced by that of the patient.

Dosage: In the second stage of training, the aim is to hold the position for up to 5 seconds before curling the neck back up to the neutral upright position. In practice, building up to five repetitions of 5 second holds is often a sufficient dose for most patients, although others may require higher dosages depending on functional requirements. The exercise is progressed by progressively increasing the range of extension in which the exercise is performed.

Training scapular control with arm movement and light load

As soon as the patient masters correction of scapular posture, training is progressed to challenge this control with arm movement and then load. Such exercises are very relevant for patients reporting aggravating activities such as keyboard or mouse use, bench top light processing work, similar household activities or lifting and carrying. Arm activities require a stable base of support. Emphasis is placed on maintaining a correct scapular position while performing either open or closed chain upper limb exercises at a load that the patient can control. Training may commence with free arm movements (e.g., shoulder flexion, abduction [to approximately 40–60 degrees] and internal/external rotation) and then against resistive straps such as Theraband (Pro-Med Products Inc) or light-hand weights in line with the patient's functional needs. Once this is achieved, the axioscapular muscles' control can be challenged with the addition of more rapid arm movement. In addition, closed chain exercises can be performed in sitting with a corrected scapular position using hand resistance against the thigh or the edge of the desk to particularly facilitate serratus anterior in patients with scapular winging.

Scapular control often needs to be trained through full arm elevation with the focus on the timing and quality of scapular movement.[51] Patients with both idiopathic neck pain and whiplash-associated disorders may have delayed onset of serratus anterior during arm elevation and reduced duration of serratus muscle activity in arm elevation and lowering.[56] Correcting spinal posture first has been shown to enhance the effect on serratus anterior activity compared with exercising with a forward head posture.[57]

Training often needs to be progressed for serratus anterior and the tripartite trapezius muscle for patients where winging of the scapula is an issue. The push up and push up plus exercises are efficient exercises for this purpose.[44,58] Training can be commenced by performing the push up against the wall, and once there is good control under these lighter load conditions, the starting position can be progressed to a four-point kneeling position. The patient concentrates on pushing through the arms to raise the chest rather than use the common substitution strategy of thoracic flexion. Training can be made efficient, by combining this exercise with training for the neck extensor muscles.

TRAINING MUSCLE ENDURANCE AND STRENGTH

As patients gain muscle control and coordination, the deficits in neck flexor and extensor strength and endurance are addressed by progressive resistance training. Progression to higher-load exercise is important to address the cervical muscle atrophy that may present in patients with idiopathic neck pain or whiplash[59] to promote hypertrophy.[60] Muscle endurance is trained at low-contraction, moderate-contraction and higher-contraction intensities[61] and deficits in strength are trained to meet the patient's functional demands.

Neck flexors

Progression to higher load strength and endurance training incorporates the action of both the deep and superficial flexors. The focus remains on performing controlled movement. In all exercises, craniocervical flexion is monitored to ensure that the load is within the capacity of the deep cervical flexors. A drift of the chin into extension indicates their capacity has been exceeded and load should be reduced.

The neck flexors can be progressively challenged with antigravity head lifts by gradually increasing the effect of gravity. Exercises can begin as head lifts off the wall from a sitting position with the back supported at an angle such that the patient can perform the exercise painlessly (Fig. 15.12). The exercise is initiated by looking down, followed by craniocervical flexion and the chin position is controlled throughout the exercise. Exercise dosage initially is usually 5-second holds × 5 repetitions, increasing to 10 repetitions or greater. The exercise is progressed by increasing the effect of gravity by progressively moving the chair away from the wall to the extent of approximately 25 cm from the wall. After this point, the exercise progresses to head lifts in supine from two to three pillows using the same technique as followed in the wall exercises and building up to 10 repetitions of 5-second holds. For many patients, progression to head lifts from one pillow is sufficient. These exercises are readily translated to a home program. Some patients will require further training to meet the strength demands of their sport or occupation, and in these circumstances, resistance can be increased with the use of pulleys and weights. Alternately, a variety of equipment can be used to assist strength training including pulleys, weights and dynamometers.[62–64]

Neck extensors

Exercise for the cervical extensors is progressed to isotonic strength training. Training is conducted with the two patterns of extension, (1) with the craniocervical region in neutral to emphasize the deeper cervical extensors and (2) allowing the movement to proceed with craniocervical extension, which will permit a full contribution from the superficial extensors.

Exercises can be performed in prone lying,[65] four-point kneeling, sitting or standing using weights, Theratube or a pulley system to provide resistance (Fig. 15.13).[62,64] Exercises are tailored to the patient's functional demands. For example, if the patient's neck pain is related to poor extensor endurance in flexion, the

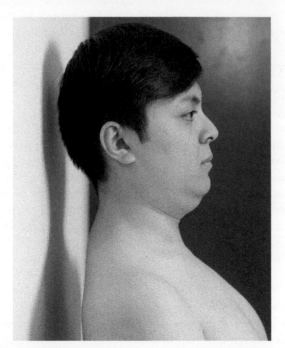

Fig. 15.12 ■ Cervical flexor endurance and strength training begins with head lifts from the wall. The patient performs the familiar action of sliding the back of the head up the wall to preflex the craniocervical spine, and holding that position, just takes the weight of the head off the wall. Concentration is on keeping the chin flexed position.

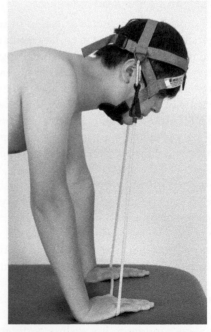

Fig. 15.13 ■ Neck extensor strength training. Many forms of resistance can be used including weights, Theratube or a pulley system attached to a head harness.

exercises can be undertaken in the functional ranges of concern as well as the upright posture. The emphasis is on endurance, and dosage is advanced proportionally more by time rather than load. Nevertheless, for most patients, exercise should also incorporate strength parameters (higher load and less repetitions) to address known strength deficits and muscle atrophy.[59] Maintaining a neutral craniocervical position when performing any extension exercise in prone will continue to bias the deep cervical extensors.[48] Likewise, it has been shown that when resisting an isometric flexion force in sitting with the head in a neutral posture, a vertical resistance or a pulley angle declined 15 degrees from the horizontal, results in higher activity in the deep extensors relative to the superficial flexors.[64] As with the neck flexors, extensor training must be designed to meet the strength demands of the patient's sport or occupation.

Dosage: Progressive resistance exercise for the neck follows guidelines for facilitating changes in muscle endurance, strength and hypertrophy.[66,67] When progressing flexor and extensor strength and endurance training, attention is given to the relative exercise load of these muscle groups. In healthy individuals, the cervical extensors are approximately 1.75 times stronger than the cervical flexors.[68] The extensors have at least twice the capacity for endurance compared with the flexor muscles under the same relative load (sustained contractions at 50% of maximal strength).[69] These factors should be considered in exercise prescription. As an example, endurance exercises for the extensors may need to be sustained for longer or more repetitions performed compared with endurance training for the flexors, particularly in the later stages of the exercise program.

Training scapular muscle endurance and strength

Training scapular muscle strength, endurance and patterns of movement are indicated when the examination reveals that poor scapular posture and muscle control are contributing to the neck pain disorder. This often occurs when patients report activities with their arms as ones provoking their neck pain (e.g., lifting, carrying).[70–72] The axioscapular muscles can be challenged with progressive resistance from pulleys, Theraband[62] or hand weights or by progressing exercises such as the push up plus on unstable surfaces.[73]

DOSAGE AND INTERVENTION TIMELINES

There are several issues which influence the design and duration of an exercise program making it difficult to answer the frequent question: "How long must I do the exercises for?" For instance, there is wide variation in deep cervical flexor activation capacity between patients.[46,47] It is most probable that patients with very poor activation will require a longer time for rehabilitation of deep cervical flexor function than those presenting with fair activation. Furthermore, a certain dose of exercise may address one impairment but not another. Our study of patients with mechanical neck pain revealed that after training the deep cervical flexors for a designated 6 weeks, performance in the CCFT improved to reflect a normal pattern of behaviour between the deep and superficial flexors.[26] However this training dosage failed to fully resolve the delay in onset of the deep cervical flexors in response to a rapid arm movement. Unpublished pilot data suggests that it might be possible to resolve the delay, but it could take up to 12 to 16 weeks of training. Time for strength training is variable, and time for change can range from 6 up to 20 weeks depending on the age of the patient, the intensity of training and goals. Thus giving definitive training time periods for individual patients is difficult, although approximate periods could be estimated.

Throughout the intervention period, the patient and clinician work towards effective self-management. There are often economic pressures to curb the number of sessions with the clinician and therefore costs of treatment. As indicated, time is needed to complete the exercise program and patients will undertake many of the exercises within a self-management exercise program, especially once symptoms have eased. Nevertheless, patients should be checked (e.g., once per month) to progress exercise and to maintain motivation, which is enhanced when the program is monitored.[31] Evidence from a meta-analysis investigating exercise adherence supports this practice with evidence that booster sessions with a physiotherapist assisted people, albeit with hip/knee osteoarthritis, to better adhere to exercise.[74] Follow-up does not always have to be in person. The advent of telepractice provides an alternate, convenient and inexpensive way to support adherence.[75,76] Many people have access to devices and programs that permit free video calls. Effectiveness of self-management is enhanced when patients have access to, and regular, support.

MAINTENANCE PROGRAM

Neck pain is a recurrent disorder[17] and recovery from an acute episode is frequently incomplete.[15,16] It is pertinent to think about the potential effect of subclinical pathology and the effect of arthrogenous muscle inhibition on muscle function following the rehabilitation period.[20,77–79] Our study of the effects of different training modes on various measures of craniocervical flexor performance illustrate the reason for concern.[63] The 10-week follow-up of a motor relearning program showed "normalized" performance in the CCFT. Yet by the 6 month follow-up, the performance had deteriorated, i.e., sternocleidomastoid activity was increasing again in the CCFT indicating a decline in function of the deep cervical flexors[80] (Fig. 15.14). An interesting observation was that the gains in craniocervical flexor strength and endurance with an endurance training program (training at 20% and 50% of maximum voluntary capacity) were maintained at the 6-month follow-up.[63] This is one study, but it does illustrate the vulnerability of the neuromuscular system in neck pain disorders and, particularly, the postural supporting muscles.

The need for a maintenance program is clearly supported by factors as the recurrent nature of neck pain, the presence of subclinical pathology, the effect of arthrogenous muscle inhibition and the quite rapid deterioration of muscle performance following cessation of training. The maintenance program is a long-term commitment. Only a very small percentage of people are likely to commit in the long term, to a 30-minute program of neck exercises 3 or 4 times a week. Thus a maintenance program must be realistic and contain exercises with a high possibility of adherence. They should be easy to do, convenient and not disruptive to work or lifestyle. The aim is for the patient to develop "preventative habits" for their neck akin to other personal hygiene habits, the best example being the lifetime preventative habit of cleaning the teeth.

At present, there is no research informed maintenance program for the neck, and if patients search the internet for exercises, they commonly encounter advice for range of movement exercises. However, these exercises alone do little to improve muscle function.[63] The following suggestion for developing a long-term preventative habit to maintain muscle function has no evidence base although it does have a research-informed rationale. The key exercises are the postural correction exercise and a mobilising exercise. The evidence to support

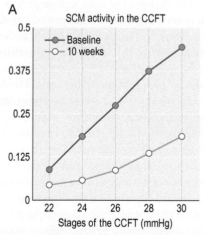
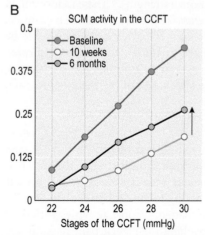

Fig. 15.14 ■ Sternocleidomastoid (SCM) activity at each stage of the craniocervical flexion test (A) Following a 10-week motor learning program, SCM activity decreased significantly in all stages of the test indicating improved performance in the deep cervical flexors after training.[80] (B) Follow-up at 6 months (*dotted line*) indicated a regression in muscle performance as in evidence with the increased SCM activity across the craniocervical flexion test stages. (Modified from O'Leary S, Jull G, Kim M, et al. Training mode-dependent changes in motor performance in neck pain. Arch Phys Med Rehabil 2012;93:1225–1233.)

the suggestion of a postural correction exercise is as follows.

- Assuming an upright neutral lumbopelvic position facilitates lumbar multifidus and the deep cervical flexors (longus capitis and colli).[24]
- Elongating the back of the neck facilitates longus colli,[38] and there is evidence that correction of spinal and neck posture will effectively exercise the deep cervical flexors.[39]
- Correcting scapular posture facilitates the scapular supporting muscles.[42,43] The active correction can decrease any neck tenderness via reciprocal relaxation of muscles as levator scapulae and the neck extensors.[9]
- When the exercise is performed sitting in an office chair with arms, further facilitation of serratus anterior and lower trapezius is gained by gently pushing down on the arms of the chair through the forearms.[44]

Thus the postural correction exercise can help maintain the activation and low-load endurance capacity of the deep neck and scapular postural supporting muscles. It brings the spine into a neutral position, which will take end-range loading strains off the joints. Based on our trial, sufficient exercise dosage could be holding posture correction for 10 seconds twice per hour for at least 8 hours of a day.[39]

The mobilizing exercise for the maintenance regime is the archery exercise (see Fig. 14.4C). This exercise promotes a rotation mobilization thoughout the functional cervical spine C0–1 to upper/mid thoracic region. It is an easy and portable exercise that can be performed at any convenient time of the day.

Future research is needed to judge whether the combination of regular performance of the postural correction and the rotation mobility exercise are an effective maintenance program and can lessen the frequency, intensity and duration of episodes of neck pain. However, there is some confidence in the rationale for this simple "neck-health" program.

Relapse prevention

The chance that patients will have another episode of neck pain is relatively high based on current evidence. Thus good advice to the patient is to self-check their ability to perform key exercises. This could be a monthly routine, and if loss of performance is found, the patient should have exercises to recommence to help prevent another episode of pain. Another key part of the development of the self-management program is a discussion with the patient on what measures they can take if their neck becomes painful or they feel that another episode of neck pain is pending. The relapse prevention program should be based on the key features of the individual's neck pain and how they have responded to various interventions. For example, advice may be to recommence a self-sustained natural apophysial glide (SNAG) or mobilization with movement for the painful joint.[81] Home applied heat or ice or, if necessary, simple analgesics may also be useful to help settle pain, rather than the patient resorting to NSAIDs with their inherent side effects. The muscles will react to the pain and a list of the appropriate exercise strategies to ensure adequate muscle control are an important component of a relapse prevention program. Patients may need to return to low-load exercises if in pain and then progress to their former exercise status. The strategy developed should be patient specific with the patient feeling confident in their ability to implement the self-management program. They can be advised to contact their health care practitioner if they are unable to successfully self-manage.

CONCLUSION

Research has provided evidence that neuromuscular adaptations are a common and expected reaction to neck pain and injury. Changes occur in motor output, muscle behaviour and muscle properties. The evidence also points to the need for assessment-driven targeted exercises for people with neck pain if neuromuscular function is to be improved. Relief of pain does not guarantee that the many aspects of neuromuscular function will return to their preinjury status. Neck pain is frequently characterized by recurrent episodes over many years. Training the neuromuscular system is vital to not only restore muscle function in respect of the current episode of pain but as a protection against future episodes of pain. In this respect, maintenance programs are an important element of self-management.

REFERENCES

1. Gurevich M, Kohn P, Davis C. Exercise-induced analgesia and the role of reactivity in pain sensitivity. J Sports Sci 1994;12:549–59.

2. Hoffman M, Shepanski M, Ruble S, et al. Intensity and duration threshold for aerobic exercise-induced analgesia to pressure pain. Arch Phys Med Rehabil 2004;85:1183–7.

3. Koltyn K, Arbogast R. Perception of pain after resistance exercise. Br J Sports Med 1998;32:20–4.

4. Koltyn K, Trine M, Stegner A, et al. Effect of isometric exercise on pain perception and blood pressure in men and women. Med Sci Sports Exerc 2001;33:282–90.

5. Kosek E, Ekholm J. Modulation of pressure pain thresholds during and following isometric contraction. Pain 1995;61:481–6.

6. Hoffman M, Shepanski M, Mackenzie S, et al. Experimentally induced pain perception is acutely reduced by aerobic exercise in people with chronic low back pain. J Rehabil Res Dev 2005;42:183–90.

7. Lima L, Abner T, Sluka K. Does exercise increase or decrease pain? Central mechanisms underlying these two phenomena. J Physiol 2017;595:4141–50.

8. Cooper M, Kluding P, Wright D. Emerging relationships between exercise, sensory nerves and neuropathic pain. Front Neurosci 2016;10:372.

9. Lluch E, Arguisuelas M, Quesada OC, et al. Immediate effects of active versus passive scapular correction on pain and pressure pain threshold in patients with chronic neck pain. J Manipulative Physiol Ther 2014;37:660–6.

10. Lluch E, Schomacher J, Gizzi L, et al. Immediate effects of active craniocervical flexion exercise versus passive mobilisation of the upper cervical spine on pain and performance on the craniocervical flexion test. Man Ther 2014;19:25–31.

11. O'Leary S, Falla D, Hodges PW, et al. Specific therapeutic exercise of the neck induces immediate local hypoalgesia. J Pain 2007;8:832–9.

12. Bertozzi L, Gardenghi I, Turoni F, et al. Effect of therapeutic exercise on pain and disability in the management of chronic non-specific neck pain: systematic review and meta-analysis of randomized trials. Phys Ther 2013;93:1026–36.

13. Fredin K, Lorås H. Manual therapy, exercise therapy or combined treatment in the management of adult neck pain - A systematic review and meta-analysis. Musculoskelet Sci Pract 2017;31:62–71.

14. Gross A, Paquin J, Dupont G, et al. Exercises for mechanical neck disorders: A Cochrane review update. Man Ther 2016;24:25–45.

15. Hush J, Lin C, Michaleff Z, et al. Prognosis of acute idiopathic neck pain is poor: a systematic review and meta-analysis. Arch Phys Med Rehabil 2011;92:824–9.

16. Leaver A, Maher C, McAuley J, et al. People seeking treatment for a new episode of neck pain typically have rapid improvement in symptoms: an observational study. J Physiother 2013;59:31–7.

17. Haldeman S, Carroll L, Cassidy J. Findings from the Bone and Joint Decade 2000 to 2010 task force on neck pain and its associated disorders. J Occup Environ Med 2010;52:424–7.

18. Collaborators GDaIIaP. Global, regional, and national incidence, prevalence, and years lived with disability for 310 diseases and injuries, 1990-2015: a systematic analysis for the Global Burden of Disease Study 2015. Lancet 2016;388:1545–602.

19. Jull G, Trott P, Potter H, et al. A randomized controlled trial of exercise and manipulative therapy for cervicogenic headache. Spine 2002;27:1835–43.

20. Lee H, Nicholson LL, Adams RD. Cervical range of motion associations with subclinical neck pain. Spine 2004;29:33–40.

21. Sterling M, Jull G, Vicenzino B, et al. Development of motor system dysfunction following whiplash injury. Pain 2003;103:65–73.

22. Ylinen J, Nikander R, Nykänen M, et al. Effect of neck exercises on cervicogenic headache: a randomised controlled trial. J Rehabil Med 2010;42:344–9.

23. Falla D, Jull G, Hodges P, et al. An endurance-strength training regime is effective in reducing myoelectric manifestations of cervical flexor muscle fatigue in females with chronic neck pain. Clin Neurophysiol 2006;117:828–37.

24. Falla D, Jull G, Russell T, et al. Effect of neck exercise on sitting posture in patients with chronic neck pain. Phys Ther 2007;87:408–17.

25. Falla D, Lindstrøm R, Rechter L, et al. Effectiveness of an 8-week exercise programme on pain and specificity of neck muscle activity in patients with chronic neck pain: a randomized controlled study. Eur J Pain 2013;17:1517–28.

26. Jull G, Falla D, Vicenzino B, et al. The effect of therapeutic exercise on activation of the deep cervical flexor muscles in people with chronic neck pain. Man Ther 2009;14:696–701.

27. O'Leary S, Jull G, Kim M, et al. Training mode dependent changes in motor performance in neck pain. Arch Phys Med Rehabil 2012;93:1225–33.

28. Lonsdale C, Hall A, Murray A, et al. Communication skills training for practitioners to increase patient adherence to home-based rehabilitation for chronic low back pain: results of a cluster randomized controlled trial. Arch Phys Med Rehabil 2017; 98:1732–43, e7.

29. Gross DP, Park J, Esmail S, et al. Motivational interviewing for workers with disabling musculoskeletal disorders: results of a cluster randomized control trial. J Occup Rehabil 2017;98:2355–63.

30. Gay C, Eschalier B, Levyckyj C, et al. Motivators for and barriers to physical activity in people with knee osteoarthritis: a qualitative study. Joint Bone Spine 2018;in press.

31. Sandford F, Sanders T, Lewis J. Exploring experiences, barriers, and enablers to home- and class-based exercise in rotator cuff tendinopathy: a qualitative study. J Hand Ther 2017;30:193–9.

32. Boudreau S, Romaniello A, Wang K, et al. The effects of intra-oral pain on motor cortex neuroplasticity associated with short-term novel tongue-protrusion training in humans. Pain 2007;132: 169–78.

33. Magill R. Motor learning: concepts and applications. 6th ed. USA: McGraw-Hill; 2001.

34. Falla D, Jull G, Hodges P. Training the cervical muscles with prescribed motor tasks does not change muscle activation during a functional activity. Man Ther 2008;13:507–12.

35. Ohlendorf D, Erbe C, Hauck I, et al. Kinematic analysis of work-related musculoskeletal loading of trunk among dentists in Germany. BMC Musculoskelet Disord 2016;17:427.

36. Szeto G, Straker L, Raine S. A field comparison of neck and shoulder postures in symptomatic and asymptomatic office workers. Applied Ergonom 2002;33:75–84.

37. Falla D, O'Leary S, Fagan A, et al. Recruitment of the deep cervical flexor muscles during a postural-correction exercise performed in sitting. Manual Ther 2007;12:139–43.

38. Fountain FP, Minear WL, Allison PD. Function of longus colli and longissimus cervicis muscles in man. Arch Phys Med Rehabil 1966;47:665–9.

39. Beer A, Treleaven J, Jull G. Can a functional postural exercise improve performance in the craniocervical flexion test? - A preliminary study. Man Ther 2012;17:219–24.

40. Claus A, Hides J, Moseley G, et al. Different ways to balance the spine: subtle changes in sagittal spinal curves affect regional muscle activity. Spine 2009;34:E208–14.

41. Caneiro J, O'Sullivan P, Burnett A, et al. The influence of different sitting postures on head/neck posture and muscle activity. Man Ther 2010;15:54–60.

42. Mottram S, Woledge R, Morrissey D. Motion analysis study of a scapular orientation exercise and subjects' ability to learn the exercise. Man Ther 2009;14:13–18.

43. Wegner S, Jull G, O'Leary S, et al. The effect of a scapular postural correction strategy on trapezius activity in patients with neck pain. Man Ther 2010;15:562–6.

44. Andersen C, Zebis M, Saervoll C, et al. Scapular muscle activity from selected strengthening exercises performed at low and high intensities. J Strength Cond Res 2012;26:2408–16.

45. Jull G, Falla D, Treleaven J, et al. Retraining cervical joint position sense: The effect of two exercise regimes. J Orthop Res 2007;25:404–12.

46. Falla D, O'Leary S, Farina D, et al. Association between intensity of pain and impairment in onset and activation of the deep cervical flexors in patients with persistent neck pain. Clin J Pain 2011;27:309–14.

47. Falla D, O'Leary S, Farina D, et al. The change in deep cervical flexor activity after training is associated with the degree of pain reduction in patients with chronic neck pain. Clin J Pain 2012;28:628–34.

48. Elliott J, O'Leary S, Cagnie B, et al. Muscle functional magnetic resonance imaging of cervical extensor muscles during different cervical extension exercises. Arch Phys Med Rehabil 2010; 91:1418–22.

49. Schomacher J, Erlenwein J, Dieterich A, et al. Can neck exercises enhance the activation of the semispinalis cervicis relative to the splenius capitis at specific spinal levels? Man Ther 2015;20: 694–702.

50. Schomacher J, Petzke F, Falla D. Localised resistance selectively activates the semispinalis cervicis muscle in patients with neck pain. Man Ther 2012;17:544–8.

51. Sahrmann SA. Diagnosis and treatment of movement impairment syndromes. St. Louis: Mosby; 2002.

52. Falla D, Farina D. Muscle fiber conduction velocity of the upper trapezius muscle during dynamic contraction of the upper limb in patients with chronic neck pain. Pain 2005;116:138–45.

53. Pizzari T, Wickham J, Balster S, et al. Modifying a shrug exercise can facilitate the upward rotator muscles of the scapula. Clin Biomech (Bristol, Avon) 2014;29:201–5.

54. Mayoux-Benhamou MA, Revel M, Vallee C. Selective electromyography of dorsal neck muscles in humans. Exp Brain Res 1997;113:353–60.

55. Conley MS, Meyer RA, Bloomberg JJ, et al. Non-invasive analysis of human neck muscle function. Spine 1995;20:2505–12.

56. Helgadottir H, Kristjansson E, Einarsson E, et al. Altered activity of the serratus anterior during unilateral arm elevation in patients with cervical disorders. J Electromyog Kinesiol 2011;21:947–53.

57. Weon J, Oh J, Cynn H, et al. Influence of forward head posture on scapular upward rotators during isometric shoulder flexion. J Bodyw Mov Ther 2010;14:367–74.

58. Horsak B, Kiener M, Pötzelsberger A, et al. Serratus anterior and trapezius muscle activity during knee push-up plus and knee-plus exercises performed on a stable, an unstable surface and during sling-suspension. Phys Ther Sport 2017;23:86–92.

59. Elliott J, Pedler A, Jull G, et al. Differential changes in muscle composition exist in traumatic and non-traumatic neck pain. Spine 2014;39:39–47.

60. O'Leary S, Jull G, vanWyk L, et al. Morphological changes in the cervical muscles of female patients with chronic whiplash can be modified with exercise - a pilot study. Muscle Nerve 2015;52:772–9.

61. O'Leary S, Jull G, Kim M, et al. Craniocervical flexor muscle impairment at maximal, moderate, and low loads is a feature of neck pain. Man Ther 2007;12:34–9.

62. Johnston V, O'Leary S, Comans T, et al. A workplace exercise versus health promotion intervention to prevent and reduce the economic and personal burden of non-specific neck pain in office personnel: protocol of a cluster-randomised controlled trial. J Physiother 2014;60:233.

63. O'Leary S, Jull G, Kim M, et al. Training mode-dependent changes in motor performance in neck pain. Arch Phys Med Rehabil 2012;93:1225–33.

64. Rivard J, Unsleber C, Schomacher J, et al. Activation of the semispinalis cervicis and splenius capitis with cervical pulley exercises. Musculoskelet Sci Pract 2017;30:56–63.

65. Lee H, Nicholson L, Adams R. Neck muscle endurance, self-report, and range of motion data from subjects with treated and untreated neck pain. J Manipulative Physiol Ther 2005;28:25–32.

66. Bird S, Tarpenning K, Marino F. Designing resistance training programmes to enhance muscular fitness. A review of the acute programme variables. Sports Med 2005;35:841–51.

67. Wernbom M, Augustsson J, Thomee R. The influence of frequency, intensity, volume and mode of strength training on whole muscle cross-sectional area in humans. Sports Med 2007;37:225–64.

68. van Wyk L, Jull G, Vicenzino B, et al. A comparison of craniocervical and cervicothoracic muscle strength in healthy individuals. J Appl Biomech 2010;26:400–6.

69. ÓLeary S, Fagermoen CL, Hasegawa H, et al. Differential strength and endurance parameters of the craniocervical and cervicothoracic extensors and flexors in healthy individuals - Technical Note. J Appl Biomech 2017;33:166–70.

70. McLean S, Moffett J, Sharp D, et al. An investigation to determine the association between neck pain and upper limb disability for patients with non-specific neck pain: a secondary analysis. Man Ther 2011;16:434–9.

71. Osborn W, Jull G. Patients with non-specific neck disorders commonly report upper limb disability. Man Ther 2013;18: 492–7.

72. See K, Treleaven J. Identifying upper limb disability in patients with persistent whiplash. Man Ther 2015;20:487–93.

73. Torres R, Pirauá A, Nacimento V, et al. Shoulder muscle activation levels during the push-up plus exercise on stable and unstable surfaces. J Sport Rehabil 2017;26:281–6.

74. Nicolson P, Bennell K, Dobson F, et al. Interventions to increase adherence to therapeutic exercise in older adults with low back pain and/or hip/knee osteoarthritis: a systematic review and meta-analysis. Br J Sports Med 2017;51:791–9.

75. Cottrell M, Hill A, O'Leary S, et al. Patients are willing to use telehealth for the multidisciplinary management of chronic musculoskeletal conditions: a cross-sectional survey. J Telemed Telecare 2018;in press.

76. Wall L, Ward E, Cartmill B, et al. Adherence to a prophylactic swallowing therapy program during (chemo) radiotherapy: impact of service-delivery model and patient factors. Dysphagia 2017;32:279–92.

77. Callaghan M, Parkes M, Hutchinson C, et al. Factors associated with arthrogenous muscle inhibition in patellofemoral osteoarthritis. Osteoarthritis Cartilage 2014;22:742–6.

78. Hurley M, Newham D. The influence of arthrogenous muscle inhibition on quadriceps rehabilitation of patients with early, unilateral osteoarthritic knees. Br J Rheumatol 1993;32:127–31.

79. Young A. Current issues in arthrogenous inhibition. Ann Rheum Dis 1993;52:829–34.

80. Jull G, Falla D. Does increased activity of the superficial neck flexor muscles during performance of the craniocervical flexion test reflect reduced activation of the deep flexor muscles in people with neck pain? Man Ther 2016;25:43–7.

81. Hing W, Hall T, Rivett D, et al. The mulligan concept of manual therapy. Sydney: Churchill Livingstone, Elsevier; 2015.

16 MANAGEMENT OF SENSORIMOTOR CONTROL DISTURBANCES

■ ■ ■ ■ ■ ■ ■ ■ ■ ■ ■ ■ ■ ■ ■ ■ ■ ■ ■

Management of disturbances in proprioception, eye movement control, coordination and postural stability have not been studied as extensively as the management of other cervical musculoskeletal impairments. However, evidence is growing for the efficacy of specific rehabilitation strategies to positively influence altered sensorimotor control and cervicogenic dizziness. Strategies include treatments directed locally to the neck muscles and joints as well as exercises to integrate the visual, vestibular and cervical sensorimotor control systems. The close connections between these systems and the adaptations that occur in the sensorimotor control system warrants problem orientated, tailored, multimodal management that addresses both the primary cervical musculoskeletal causes as well as any secondary adaptive sensorimotor control changes.

APPROACHES TO MANAGEMENT

Addressing the cervical musculoskeletal pain and dysfunction

Several different treatments for neck pain and cervical musculoskeletal dysfunction have improved dizziness and sensorimotor control. More specifically, dizziness has improved with the use of manual therapy for cervical joint dysfunction,[1–4] specific neck muscle training,[5] acupuncture,[1] and multimodal treatment (manual therapy, electrotherapy and muscle relaxation exercises).[6] Cervical joint position sense (JPS) has improved following manual therapy,[1–4] craniocervical flexion training,[7] and acupuncture.[1] Likewise balance has shown

some improvement following cervical extensor muscle endurance training[8] and acupuncture.[9]

Studies are beginning to provide evidence of long-term benefits for patients with chronic cervicogenic dizziness from treatments of cervical musculoskeletal dysfunction.[10,11] Malmstrom et al.[11] showed that multimodal cervical musculoskeletal treatment reduced neck pain and dizziness in the long term. Reid et al.[10–12] demonstrated the effectiveness of short periods of manipulative therapy to reduce dizziness (both sustained natural apophysial glides [Fig. 16.1] and posteroanterior glides) over four to six treatments. Both methods of manual therapy had immediate and sustained (up to 2 years) effects and reduced the intensity and frequency of chronic cervicogenic dizziness.

Treating cervical musculoskeletal pain and dysfunction will improve the symptoms of cervicogenic dizziness, but treatments must also be directed towards the sensorimotor impairments to enhance treatment outcomes. Reid et al.[3,10] found that although manual therapy improved dizziness, objective changes in sensorimotor control (joint position error and balance) in these patients were minimal. Similarly, specific neck muscle exercises improved dizziness in some patients with whiplash-associated disorders (WAD), but many others continued to report dizziness and still had signs of impaired sensorimotor function after the intervention.[5] Thus the aims of specific training are to improve not only the symptoms but also the sensorimotor impairments, to normalize the system with the aim of preventing recurrence and optimizing function.

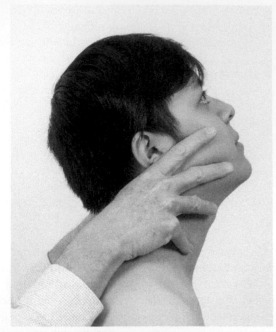

Fig. 16.1 ■ Sustained natural apophysial glides used in the management of cervicogenic dizziness when the patient reports dizziness on cervical extension.

Addressing the adaptive changes in the sensorimotor control system

Specific training to improve disturbances in sensorimotor control should address the adaptive changes in the sensorimotor control system that occur with altered cervical afferent input. Specific training of sensorimotor impairments has been investigated and there is evidence of wider effects of training. For instance, training gaze stability, eye-head coordination and head on trunk relocation can improve both sensorimotor impairments and patients' neck pain and disability without any treatment of local cervical musculoskeletal dysfunction.[13–16] Revel and colleagues,[13] with an 8-week training program consisting of gaze stability exercises, eye head coordination and head on trunk relocation practice, improved neck pain and disability as well as cervical joint position error (JPE). Similar outcomes were described by Jull et al.[7] and Humphreys et al.[14] for multimodal sensorimotor programmes. Balance has improved with a program of oculomotor rehabilitation.[16] In turn, balance training has improved JPE[17] and JPE training has improved cervical flexor neuromuscular control.[18,19]

Cervical movement sense/accuracy has been improved with cervical kinematic training using either a virtual reality environment or a laser on a target[20,21]. In other examples, Heikkila and Astrom[22] tested a multimodal approach (body awareness training, a behaviour therapy–based exercise approach and multiprofessional advice and education) and demonstrated improvements in JPE. Moreover, Hansson and colleagues[23] used a vestibular rehabilitation program for patients with chronic WAD and demonstrated improved balance and reduced dizziness. Vestibular rehabilitation programmes may also be useful for persons with concussion.[24,25] Of note, although vestibular training improved dizziness and balance, it did not improve neck pain or movement in a cohort of patients with chronic WAD.[26]

Despite these examples of cross-over effects of training, there is little direct correlation between the various sensorimotor measures, i.e., proprioception, eye movement control and balance.[27,28] This suggests that exercises used to treat eye movement control for instance, may not be the most effective for balance or JPS deficits. Thus even though there might be some cross over in training effects, the preferred approach is to prescribe exercises for each deficit found in the evaluation of cervical joint position and movement sense, oculomotor function, co-ordination and static and dynamic balance. The exercise program is individualized and responds to each specific deficit identified in the physical examination. We regard this as the best clinical approach.[29–31] A clinical trial is currently underway to confirm whether this specificity is always justified in sensorimotor programs.[32]

Combining cervical musculoskeletal and sensorimotor approaches

Patients with neck pain and symptoms of dizziness have impaired musculoskeletal and sensorimotor function. Not surprisingly, several studies have combined management of the cervical musculoskeletal and sensorimotor systems.[1,33,34] The success of combining cervical musculoskeletal and vestibular interventions was apparent in the management of young adults with persistent neck pain, dizziness and headaches following concussion. The combined treatment approach resulted in improved times to return to sport[35] and stimulated recommendations for its adoption for patients with neck trauma and concussion.[36–38]

A combined approach is supported for the management of patients with cervicogenic dizziness and visual disturbances. It is logical that attention is paid directly to any impaired proprioception, eye movement control, coordination or postural stability as well as to the source of the altered cervical somatosensory input (e.g., impaired muscle function, painful restricted joint motion). A multimodal program might include education, assurance to assist any anxiety, manipulative therapy and active exercise, specific muscle rehabilitation as well as a tailored program to train as indicated, cervical joint position and movement sense, oculomotor control, coordination and balance. The program recognizes the associations between the cervical somatosensory, vestibular and ocular systems and addresses all potential causes of altered cervical somatosensory input.

PRINCIPLES FOR TAILORED SENSORIMOTOR CONTROL EXERCISES

Sensorimotor changes occur early after the onset of neck pain[39–41] and thus exercises should be commenced as soon as possible. A progressive program is devised based on specific impairments identified in the examination. The level of difficulty of initial exercises will depend on the presenting symptoms, their degree of severity as well as the level of impairment. The program is progressed to the functional requirements of the patient.

The home program is vital as repetition is required to achieve improvements. Exercises for each impairment should be performed in short sessions (e.g., 30 seconds or 5–10 repetitions as fits the exercise), 2 to 5 times per day depending on severity and irritability of the patient's symptoms. Temporary reproduction of mild to moderate dizziness or visual disturbances is acceptable however exacerbation of nausea, neck pain or headache is not. If the latter occurs, the exercises can be modified by decreasing the number of repetitions, range of motion or altering the patient's position to a more supported one such as supine lying.

Starting levels for the exercises are adjusted to suit the individual patient, their presenting symptoms and the degree of impairment demonstrated in the physical examination. Subsequent progression of each exercise set is directed by constant reassessment of performance.

Exercises are progressed by altering the duration, repetitions, frequency and the degree of difficulty of the task. Degrees of difficulty can be increased by altering the speed and range of head movement, the amount of visual feedback (eyes open, restricted peripheral vision or eyes closed) and the visual focus point (single point compared with a word or group of words), background (plain, striped or checkered), position of the patient (supine, sitting, standing) and condition. Exercises can also be progressed by combining activities. For example, oculomotor tasks, cervical movement or position sense practice can be undertaken with a balance task, for example, while sitting on an unstable surface such as a therapy ball or standing with an unstable base of support (e.g., tandem or single leg stance).

All exercises should be performed at a speed, movement range and starting position that allows the patient to perform the task with precision and without exacerbating pain or headache. Larger ranges of motion at slower speeds will bias the cervical afferents and should be conducted first. Faster smaller ranges will challenge the vestibular system and can be used as a progression when indicated.

EXERCISES TO TRAIN SENSORIMOTOR CONTROL

A variety of exercise strategies are used to train the various aspects of sensorimotor control assessed to be impaired in the particular patient. Patients must be carefully instructed in the exercises. As indicated, short sessions of training are used, and the patient must be provided with a clear self-management program to be performed at home. Regular review is important to progress the exercise program. How quickly a patient progresses and how quickly symptoms resolve is a very individual characteristic.

Training cervical joint position sense

The test of relocation to the natural head posture used in assessment of cervical JPS converts to a training method. A target is printed on A4 size paper to the dimensions calculated by Roren et al.[42] and provides feedback to the patient on performance—the inner three circles reflect a good performance (0–3 degrees of error) the next circle a fair performance (3–4.5 degrees of error) and the outer circle and beyond an abnormal performance greater than 4.5 degrees of error is used (see Fig. 9.19). The patient sits 90 cm from the wall wearing a laser mounted on a headband. The target is placed on a wall so that the laser projects into the centre of the target. The patient practices the relocation task in directions assessed to be abnormal (> 4.5° relocation error). This may be any or all of flexion, extension, right and left rotation directions depending on the assessment findings. The patient concentrates on the starting position, closes their eyes and moves in the direction to be trained. They return to the neutral position as accurately as possible, then open their eyes to check their performance, using the feedback from the laser beam on the target. The patient readjusts their head back to the neutral position as required before practising the task again. Some patients find this task very difficult and, in those cases, patients can perform the movement initially with the eyes open to gain constant feedback from the laser. When ready, they again attempt the task with the eyes closed. The position sense task can be progressed by the patient attempting to find different points in range, for example, at 20° intervals throughout the available range of movement with their closed eyes, again checking and correcting performance with eyes open at each interval. Further progressions can include performing the tasks in standing and then with decreasing bases of support.

For most effective training of JPS, the patient is provided with a laser and a printed target for home use. Commercial head mounted lasers or simple inexpensive homemade head mounted lasers (plastic head band, key chain laser and self-adhesive cord clip to maintain the "on" button of the laser) and targets are given or loaned to the patient. The accurate feedback not only helps to enhance performance, but it provides the patient with a powerful incentive to perform the exercise and improve adherence.

Retraining cervical movement sense

Movement sense is trained using the head mounted laser to project on to targets consisting of patterns of various difficulty. Patients again sit 90 cm from the wall. They perform fine head movements to trace lines and patterns with the laser as accurately as possible concentrating on accuracy rather than speed. Again, the level chosen to start training will depend on the findings in the assessment of cervical movement sense. The easiest

level of training is tracing simple, short straight lines, progressing to larger ranges of movement and patterns. The task is further increased in difficulty with the patient tracing more complex patterns such as curves, zigzags and the alphabet presented on A4 size paper (Fig. 16.2). Again, for best practice, a laser and target are given to the patient to practise movement sense exercises at home.

Recently Sarig-Bahat et al.[20] assessed the use of a neck virtual reality system to train cervical movement sense/accuracy. In the virtual environment, the patient had to accurately follow a target moving at 10° per second in single movement planes. It was tested against a system to train cervical movement accuracy similar to that described earlier where the patient had to trace stationary lines in different movement directions (initially flexion, extension, rotation left and right) and then progressing to more complex patterned movements) on a larger target (70 cm × 70 cm) using a laser attached to a headband for feedback. Improvements were evident in both the short and intermediate terms with both the virtual reality system and the target and laser tasks.[20,21] Thus the choice of which application to use could be the availability of a device or the patient's

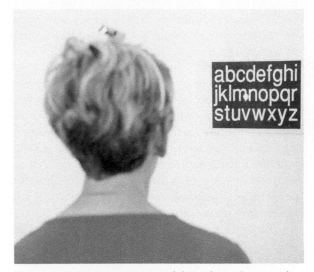

Fig. 16.2 ■ **Movement sense training. The patient practises to accurately trace a pattern with the laser mounted on the headband (see also Fig. 9.21). As the patient improves, the task can be progressed by having them trace more complex patterns. Tracing the alphabet as shown is a challenging task. The laser guides and provides feedback on performance.**

preferred method of training—an important feature to encourage adherence.

Smooth-pursuit eye-movement exercises

Training eye-movement control initially uses the same task as the smooth-pursuit neck torsion test. The starting position chosen is dependent on the assessment findings. The patient can commence the exercise with the head in the neutral position if this is impaired. However, the exercise can be commenced with the trunk prerotated, if assessment has shown poorer eye follow performance in the torsioned (compared with neutral) position of the neck. The patient follows a slow (20° per second) moving target with their eyes through visual angles of about 40° without moving their head. Different movement directions can be practised but horizontal movements are most often required. The moving target can be provided by the patient themselves which aids home practice. They hold the laser and project it onto a wall and move it in backward and forward, up and down directions as required (Fig. 16.3). Alternatively, the patient can throw a ball from one hand to the other while following the trajectory of the ball with the eyes. The instruction is to follow the moving object as accurately as possible with the eyes, while keeping the

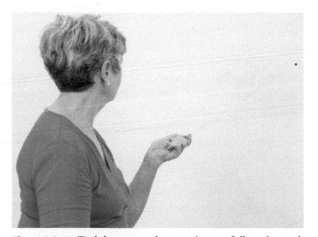

Fig. 16.3 ■ **Training smooth pursuit eye follow in neck torsion. The patient holds the laser and slowly moves their hand projecting the laser back and forwards on a wall to provide the visual feedback. The patient follows the laser with their eyes without moving their head. Training can be conducted with the neck in the neutral or in the more challenging torsioned position.**

head still. Again, it is advantageous for accuracy and compliance with practice, to provide the patient with a laser for home practice.

Gaze stability exercises

Exercises to train gaze stability are usually commenced in sitting but can be performed in supine lying if pain is exacerbated in the sitting position. In these circumstances, the clinician performs passive or assisted active head movements. The patient is to maintain focus on an object directly in the midline as the head is moved.

Most patients commence training in sitting. The patient keeps their eyes fixed on a point while performing slow controlled head and neck movements. Movement may be into rotation and/or flexion-extension as directed by assessment findings. The patient aims to perform "pure plane" movements. If the patient performs awkward or combined plane motions, the gaze stability exercise is practised in front of a mirror. A focus point is marked on the mirror and the reflections provide feedback to the patient on the quality of the head movement. The patient practises the task with slow movements initially, concentrating on accuracy and quality of head movement.

Exercise difficulty can be advanced by progressively increasing the range of movement to approximately 45° or by providing increased visual conflict, by changing the fixation point from a dot, to several words, to a busy background (stripes or a checkerboard pattern under the dot or group of words) (Fig. 16.4). These exercises are similar to gaze stability exercises in vestibular rehabilitation protocols.[43] The differences are that movements are performed slowly and through larger ranges of head motion to bias the cervical afferents. Exercises are usually practiced in smaller doses and thus are more easily tolerated by the patient. It is important that clear instruction is provided to the patient for home practice at every stage of progression.

Eye-head coordination exercises

The movement directions (vertical; horizontal) practised in the eye-head coordination exercises are guided by examination findings. The aim of the exercises is for the patient to perform dissociated head and eye movements. Training is undertaken in sitting and the patient is asked to look between two points. The two points can be created by the patient holding their fingers

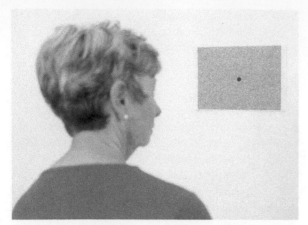

Fig. 16.4 ■ **Gaze stability. The patient trains gaze stability by keeping their eyes fixed on a point while performing slow controlled head and neck movements. An example of more advanced gaze stability training is depicted where a single focus point is placed on a busy background.**

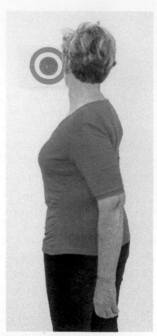

Fig. 16.5 ■ **Trunk head coordination. The patient tries to hold their head still while rotating their trunk to the left and right. The precision of the exercise is enhanced by the patient aiming to hold the laser light on a target. Alternatively, a mirror can be used to make this task easier.**

approximately 30° apart from the midline or two dots can be placed on a wall 30° apart. The patient focuses on the point in the midline, then moves the eyes first, without moving the head, to the point at 30°. Once there, eyes remain focused on the point while the patient brings the head in line with this target. They then return their eyes back to the midline without moving the head and next bring the head back to that point while maintaining their focus.

The exercise can be progressed in several ways. The patient can practise moving the head to one direction, while their eyes maintain focus on a target, which is moving to the opposite direction. The patient can perform progressively larger ranges of arm, head and trunk movement to challenge the control of eye movements. The focus point and background can be altered as was done for the gaze stability exercises. Finally, peripheral vision can be restricted by blackening out some swimming goggles to increase the difficulty level of this task. Of importance, the patient's performance must be continually evaluated and the program progressed accordingly. The home program must also be continually adjusted.

Trunk head coordination exercises

For training trunk head coordination, movement of the body is best performed by rotating from the hips

and torso on stable feet, rather than using thoracic rotation. The patient is asked to keep the head still while rotating the trunk, pelvis and hips to the left and/or right as directed by assessment findings. Initially, patients often require feedback on performance and this can be gained by looking into a mirror to ensure that the head is kept still while they move the trunk. The clinician can assist by keeping the head still while the patient moves the trunk, or alternatively, the patient maintains head stability while the clinician passively rotates the trunk.

Training trunk head coordination is progressed by increasing the range and speed of trunk motion. The exercise increases in difficulty by using the head-mounted laser beam projected onto a target (as per joint position and movement sense training). The patient must hold the laser point still, which more precisely keeps the head still while moving the trunk (Fig. 16.5). Use of the mirror and then the laser is easily incorporated in the home program.

Static balance training

Balance training and progressions follow relatively standard procedures. Starting positions and progressions are based on the assessed deficits and the patient's functional requirements respectively. Static balance is trained with eyes open and then closed, on a firm then soft surface (such as a piece of foam or a soft mat). Stance positions are progressed in difficulty starting in comfortable stance and advancing to narrow, tandem and single leg stance. The patient trains to maintain each increasingly difficult position for up to 30 seconds at a time without excessive movement or rigidity.

Balance training can be further challenged by adding head movement, oculomotor tasks and or coordination exercises to the balance task. Patients with neck pain disorders often need to be challenged by these higher-level exercises. It is important when developing the home program with the patient that they are conscious of performing the balance exercises in a safe environment, for example, in a corner with the safety of two walls or near a fixed bench or table.

Functional, dynamic balance training

Dynamic balance training is a functional progression. It is particularly indicated in patients who report functional difficulties such as feeling light headed or unsteady when walking or moving quickly and in whom this task is found to be impaired on examination. Training focuses on the skill of walking with head movement. It commences with the patient walking with a shoulder width base, slowly turning the head as far as possible to one side and then the other. Walking is also practised moving the head up and down through full range of head motion. The patient should not try to focus on a specific point. Rather the head and eyes should move together in the same direction. If the task is too difficult or provokes symptoms, the gaze can be stabilized to the midline initially. Training can be progressed to faster neck movements and also to tandem walking while performing neck movements (Fig. 16.6). Again, when developing the home program, an emphasis must be placed on safety. Performing these exercises in a hallway is safe practice.

Vestibular rehabilitation and vision therapy

Some patients may have concomitant vestibular and visual deficits. For example, when a person sustains

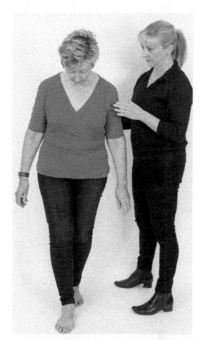

Fig. 16.6 ■ Walking with head turns. The patient is asked to walk in tandem walk, slowly moving the head through full range of flexion and extension.

trauma to the neck they also suffer a concussion or, vice versa, trauma to the head may involve the neck. In these cases, specific oculomotor and balance exercises are directed more specifically towards the vestibular and oculomotor systems. Treatment for Benign paroxysmal positional vertigo (BPPV) might also be provided when indicated. Vestibular rehabilitation aims to assist the individual to habituate, compensate or adapt to any explicit deficits or imbalance in the vestibular system. In general, when the patient has both neck pain and vestibular disorders, cervical sensorimotor and musculoskeletal deficits are best managed in the first instance to facilitate performance of exercises for the vestibular system that might involve fast head motion.[43] There is some overlap in the exercises used for cervical sensorimotor rehabilitation with those used for vestibular rehabilitation, especially exercises for balance and oculomotor control. These can be useful as a starting point in patients with concomitant sensorimotor and vestibular deficits. Visual disturbances can exacerbate cervical symptoms. When the visual system is of particular concern, it is often the first focus of management.

Treatment includes oculomotor exercises. Some patients may require multidisciplinary management with treatment also from a behavioural or neuro-optometrist or vision therapist who may prescribe prism glasses, lenses, filters or other devices to encourage specific eye movements to facilitate and maximize the effects of training.[44,45]

Psychological considerations

Just as pain and general distress can be related, so can symptoms of dizziness interact with psychological distress. In some individuals, dizziness may contribute to psychological distress, whereas in others, psychological distress can manifest as vertigo or dizziness. Anatomic and neurophysiological overlap between the vestibular system and the pathways implicated in emotional states might explain these close links.[46] Thus, the clinician should be aware that psychological factors may affect clinical presentations and therapeutic outcomes in some[47] but not others.[48] Likewise addressing the symptoms and signs of sensorimotor disturbances may help to decrease psychological distress.[49]

SELF-MANAGEMENT

Best management tailors treatment to address the impairments identified in the physical examination of the individual patient. As emphasized throughout this chapter, a home program of training must be developed with the patient, and it must be constantly modified as the patient progresses through their individualized rehabilitation program. Part of the development of the self-management program is a discussion with the patient on measures they can take if they feel that symptoms of light headedness or unsteadiness, for example, are returning so that any relapse is prevented or minimized.

Individual patients have different presentations and comorbidities with respect to their musculoskeletal and sensorimotor deficits of cervical, visual and/or vestibular origin. The nature and amount of rehabilitation that the patient requires to improve sensorimotor control may depend on the nature and magnitude of concomitant disturbances in the vestibular and/or visual systems and the extent to which cervical function may need to be optimized to compensate for any permanent changes in the visual or vestibular systems. This is particularly important in older patients who have age-related changes

to vision and the vestibular system and in persons with permanent vestibular impairment associated with vestibular pathology or trauma. In these circumstances, more extensive rehabilitation is often required. Patients with any permanent changes in the visual or vestibular systems should routinely be provided with strategies and remedial exercises for relapse management and prevention because they will require the cervical spine to be functioning at an optimal level to compensate for such deficits. This usually includes exercises to maintain and optimize both cervical musculoskeletal and sensorimotor function.

CONCLUSION

Evidence is growing for the need to target sensorimotor control disturbances in persons with neck pain disorders. Problem orientated, tailored, multimodal management that addresses both the primary cervical musculoskeletal causes as well as any secondary adaptive sensorimotor control changes is currently recommended. Tailored sensorimotor control exercises could include exercises aimed at addressing impairments in proprioception, head and eye movement control, coordination and postural stability. In some patients, additional management directed towards the vestibular and/or visual systems may be required and consideration of any psychological components when present, should be part of the approach.

REFERENCES

1. Heikkila H, Johansson M, Wenngren BI. Effects of acupuncture, cervical manipulation and NSAID therapy on dizziness and impaired head repositioning of suspected cervical origin: a pilot study. Man Ther 2000;5:151–7.
2. Palmgren PJ, Sandstrom PJ, Lundqvist FJ, et al. Improvement after chiropractic care in cervicocephalic kinesthetic sensibility and subjective pain intensity in patients with non-traumatic chronic neck pain. J Manipulative Physiol Ther 2006;29: 100–6.
3. Reid SA, Callister R, Katekar MG, et al. Effects of cervical spine manual therapy on range of motion, head repositioning, and balance in participants with cervicogenic dizziness: a randomized controlled trial. Arch Phys Med Rehabil 2014;95:1603–12.
4. Yang J, Lee B, Kim C. Changes in proprioception and pain in patients with neck pain after upper thoracic manipulation. J Phys Ther Sci 2015;27:795–8.
5. Treleaven J, Peterson G, Ludvigsson ML, et al. Balance, dizziness and proprioception in patients with chronic whiplash associated disorders complaining of dizziness: a prospective randomized

study comparing three exercise programs. Man Ther 2016;22: 122–30.

6. Bracher ES, Almeida CI, Almeida RR, et al. A combined approach for the treatment of cervical vertigo. J Manipulative Physiol Ther 2000;23:96–100.

7. Jull G, Falla D, Treleaven J, et al. Retraining cervical joint position sense: the effect of two exercise regimes. J Orthop Res 2007;25:404–12.

8. Stapley PJ, Beretta MV, Dalla Toffola E, et al. Neck muscle fatigue and postural control in patients with whiplash injury. Clin Neurophysiol 2006;47:610–22.

9. Fattori B, Borsari C, Vannucci G, et al. Acupuncture treatment for balance disorders following whiplash injury. Acupunct Electrother Res 1996;21:207–17.

10. Reid SA, Callister R, Snodgrass SJ, et al. Manual therapy for cervicogenic dizziness: long-term outcomes of a randomised trial. Man Ther 2015;20:148–56.

11. Malmstrom EM, Karlberg M, Melander A, et al. Cervicogenic dizziness - musculoskeletal findings before and after treatment and long-term outcome. Disabil Rehabil 2007;29:1193–205.

12. Reid SA, Rivett DA, Katekar MG, et al. Comparison of Mulligan sustained natural apophyseal glides and Maitland mobilizations for treatment of cervicogenic dizziness: a randomized controlled trial. Phys Ther 2014;94:466–76.

13. Revel M, Minguet M, Gergory P, et al. Changes in cervicocephalic kinesthesia after a proprioceptive rehabilitation program in patients with neck pain: a randomized controlled study. Arch Phys Med Rehabil 1994;75:895–9.

14. Humphreys B, Irgens P. The effect of a rehabilitation exercise program on head repositioning accuracy and reported levels of pain in chronic neck pain subjects. J Whiplash and Related Disorders 2002;1:99–112.

15. Treleaven J. A tailored sensorimotor approach for management of whiplash associated disorders. A single case study. Man Ther 2010;15:206–9.

16. Storaci R, Manelli A, Schiavone N, et al. Whiplash injury and oculomotor dysfunctions: clinical-posturographic correlations. Eur Spine J 2006;15:1811–16.

17. Beinert K, Taube W. The effect of balance training on cervical sensorimotor function and neck pain. J Mot Behav 2013;45: 271–8.

18. Izquierdo TG, Pecos-Martin D, Girbes EL, et al. Comparison of craniocervical flexion training versus cervical proprioception training in patients with chronic neck pain: a randomized controlled clinical trial. J Rehabil Med 2016;48:48–55.

19. Ernst M. Comparison of craniocervical flexion training versus cervical proprioception training in patients with chronic neck pain: a randomized controlled clinical trial. Physioscience 2016;12:167–76.

20. Sarig Bahat H, Croft K, Carter C, et al. Remote kinematic training for patients with chronic neck pain: a randomised controlled trial. Eur Spine J 2017;1–15.

21. Sarig Bahat H, Takasaki H, Chen X, et al. Cervical kinematic training with and without interactive virtual reality training for chronic neck pain - a randomized clinical trial. Man Ther 2015;20:68–78.

22. Heikkila H, Astrom PG. Cervicocephalic kinesthetic sensibility in patients with whiplash injury. Scand J Rehabil Med 1996;28:133–8.

23. Hansson EE, Mansson NO, Ringsberg KAM, et al. Dizziness among patients with whiplash-associated disorder: a randomized controlled trial. J Rehabil Med 2006;38:387–90.

24. Alsalaheen BA, Mucha A, Morris LO, et al. Vestibular rehabilitation for dizziness and balance disorders after concussion. J Neurol Phys Ther 2010;34:87–93.

25. Gurley JM, Hujsak BD, Kelly JL. Vestibular rehabilitation following mild traumatic brain injury. Neurorehabilitation 2013;32:519–28.

26. Hansson EE, Persson L, Malmstrom EM. Influence of vestibular rehabilitation on neck pain and cervical range of motion among patients with whiplash-associated disorder: a randomized controlled trial. J Rehabil Med 2013;45:906–10.

27. Treleaven J, Jull G, LowChoy N. The relationship of cervical joint position error to balance and eye movement disturbances in persistent whiplash. Man Ther 2006;11:99–106.

28. Swait G, Rushton AB, Miall C, et al. Evaluation of cervical proprioceptive function. Spine 2007;32:E692–701.

29. Jull G, Sterling M, Falla D, et al. Whiplash, headache and neck pain. London: Elsevier; 2008.

30. Treleaven J. Sensorimotor disturbances in neck disorders affecting postural stability, head and eye movement control. Man Ther 2008;13:2–11.

31. Treleaven J. Sensorimotor disturbances in neck disorders affecting postural stability, head and eye movement control - Part 2: Case studies. Man Ther 2008;13:266–75.

32. Uthaikhup S, Sremakaew M, Jull G, et al. Effects of local treatment with and without sensorimotor and balance exercise in individuals with neck pain: protocol for a randomized controlled trial. BMC Musculoskelet Disord 2018;19:48.

33. Oddsdottir G. Cervical induced balance disturbances after motor vehicle collisions: The efficacy of two successive physical treatment approaches. Reykjavik: University of Iceland; 2006.

34. Provinciali L, Baroni M, Illuminati L, et al. Multimodal treatment to prevent the late whiplash syndrome. Scand J Rehabil Med 1996;28:105–11.

35. Schneider KJ, Meeuwisse WH, Nettel-Aguirre A, et al. Cervicovestibular rehabilitation in sport-related concussion: a randomised controlled trial. Br J Sports Med 2014;48:1294–8.

36. Ellis MJ, Leddy JJ, Willer B. Physiological, vestibulo-ocular and cervicogenic post-concussion disorders: an evidence-based classification system with directions for treatment. Brain Inj 2015;29:238–48.

37. Marshall CM, Vernon H, Leddy JJ, et al. The role of the cervical spine in post-concussion syndrome. Phys Sportsmed 2015;43:274–84.

38. Broglio SP, Collins MW, Williams RM, et al. Current and emerging rehabilitation for concussion: a review of the evidence. Clin Sports Med 2015;34:213–31.

39. Sterling M, Jull G, Vicenzino B, et al. Development of motor system dysfunction following whiplash injury. Pain 2003;103: 65–73.

40. Sterling M, Jull G, Vicenzino B, et al. Characterization of acute whiplash-associated disorders. Spine 2004;29:182–8.

41. Jull G, Kenardy J, Hendrikz J, et al. Management of acute whiplash: a randomized controlled trial of multidisciplinary stratified treatments. Pain 2013;154:1798–806.

42. Roren A, Mayoux-Benhamou MA, Fayad F, et al. Comparison of visual and ultrasound based techniques to measure head repositioning in healthy and neck-pain subjects. Man Ther 2009;14:270–7.

43. Herdman S, Clendaniel RA. Vestibular rehabilitation. 4th ed. Philadelphia Davis Company; 2014.

44. Padula WV, Argyris S. Post trauma vision syndrome and visual midline shift syndrome. Neurorehabilitation 1996;6:165–71.

45. Padula WV, Capo-Aponte JE, Padula WV, et al. The consequence of spatial visual processing dysfunction caused by traumatic brain injury (TBI). Brain Inj 2017;31:589–600.

46. Kutay O, Akdal G, Keskinoglu P, et al. Vestibular migraine patients are more anxious than migraine patients without vestibular symptoms. J Neurol 2017;264:37–41.

47. MacDowell SG, Trommelen R, Bissell A, et al. The impact of symptoms of anxiety and depression on subjective and objective outcome measures in individuals with vestibular disorders. J Vestib Res 2018;27:295–303.

48. Obermann M, Bock E, Sabev N, et al. Long-term outcome of vertigo and dizziness associated disorders following treatment in specialized tertiary care: the dizziness and vertigo registry (diver) study. J Neurol 2015;262:2083–91.

49. Miyazaki H, Nomura Y, Mardassi A, et al. How minimally invasive vestibular neurotomy for incapacitating Ménière's disease improves dizziness and anxiety. Acta Otolaryngol 2017;137:707–11.

17

MANAGEMENT OF NERVE TISSUE

S ome neck pain disorders involve sensitized or compromised nerve tissue that require specific management approaches targeting nerve tissue. Correctly identifying involvement of nerve tissue is essential (see Chapters 4 and 9) because it may indicate the need for a change in management strategy. Significantly compromised nerve function in the presence of a severe cervical myelopathy or radiculopathy, signals a safety concern for the patient and may require immediate specialist medical consultation. For the most part, neck pain disorders involving nerve tissue do not involve immediate safety concerns for the patient and are effectively treated conservatively. Nerve related cervical conditions do, however, require a gentle approach because they may easily be aggravated by overzealous physical treatments. The status of nerve function may occasionally deteriorate and requires diligent monitoring over the duration of management. There is the potential for conditions presenting initially as only a sensitized nerve state, to progress to a state of compromised function (i.e., worsening nerve conduction) with potentially irreversible longer-term consequences for the patient if not identified early. Effective management of nerve-related neck pain disorders requires an understanding of the potential mechanisms underlying the condition (see Chapter 4), so that management approaches can be applied appropriately, and symptoms and signs signalling worsening of the condition can be identified and interpreted accurately. This chapter discusses the management strategies for nerve-related neck pain disorders, including neurophysiological

mechanisms proposed to underlie successful management approaches.

NEUROPHYSIOLOGICAL MECHANISMS UNDERPINNING NERVE TISSUE MANAGEMENT

Mechanisms of effect underlying nerve tissue management approaches are underpinned by neurophysiological processes to restore homeostasis in and around the affected nerve.[1]

Restoring homeostasis around the nerve

In the first instance, the neuropathy may be addressed by treating the musculoskeletal tissues determined in the examination to be directly causing the nerve irritation and/or compression. Treatments aim to resolve perineural inflammation resulting from injury or pathology of interfacing musculoskeletal structures (e.g., disc lesions).[2–4] Acute or chronic perineural inflammation along a nerve trunk is known to induce nerve pain, potentially nerve damage[5–11] as well as nerve mechanosensitivity.[12–15] Furthermore, degenerative or injured spinal or peripheral musculoskeletal interfaces may entrap or compress the nerve, potentially affecting nerve conduction and mechanosensitivity.[16–19] Restoring the normal status of these musculoskeletal tissues by resolving inflammation, as well as restoring normal movement (joint mobility) and physical support (neuromuscular function) will directly reduce nerve interface factors contributing to a neuropathy. In one experimental animal study[20] where inflammatory mediators were placed around the dorsal root ganglion of a rat, spinal mobilization resulted in faster resolution of dorsal root ganglion hyperexcitability and resultant hyperalgesia compared with no intervention. The authors hypothesized that potential mechanisms of effect of the spinal mobilization may have included improved blood supply and nutrition to the affected dorsal root ganglion with a faster resolution of inflammation and excitability.

Restoring homeostasis within the nerve

An aim of management is to return homeostasis within injured nerve tissue that may have been disturbed by injury and associated perineural oedema or nerve entrapment/compression. Disturbances in intraneural homeostasis may include reduced circulation to the nerve, intraneural ischaemia, neuroinflammation and intraneural oedema[21–25] that can result in nerve conduction loss and mechanosensitivity.[16–19] Neurodynamic treatment methods, usually in the form of manual therapy or exercise directed at the nerve tissue or nerve-musculoskeletal interfaces, aim to have positive mechanical and neurophysiological effects. Movement/mobilization of the nerve and its connective tissues results in intraneural pressure changes that are proposed to decrease excitability of dorsal horn cells by altering axoplasmic flow, improving intraneural circulation, and reducing intraneural oedema.[1,26] Mechanistic studies have supported the effect of neural mobilization modalities on dispersion and reduction of intraneural oedema.[27–29] Neurodynamic mobilization in animal studies has also shown that such mobilization may impact neuro-inflammatory responses (decreasing nerve growth factor concentration and glial cell activation) in the dorsal root ganglia and spinal cord that potentially influence mechanisms associated with the occurrence of more widespread pain in neuropathic pain states.[30,31]

Restoring tolerance to motion and resolving mechanosensitivity

Treatment may be directed towards restoring the capacity of nerves to tolerate motion, compression and stretch forces relative to their musculoskeletal interfacing structures during movement.[32–35] Studies have shown that affected nerves may have a reduced capacity for motion or mechanosensitivity to motion and/or compression.[13,14] This is detected in the examination as a positive response to neurodynamic tests and palpation (see Chapter 9).[33,36–39] Manual therapy techniques, such as the lateral glide mobilization, can improve the tolerance of nerve tissues to motion, and have been shown to reduce protective muscle responses during neurodynamic tests in mechanosensitive individuals.[40] Furthermore, neurodynamic techniques both in humans[41] and animals[42] have shown mechanisms (e.g., reduced temporal summation) suggestive of the activation of descending inhibitory systems. Although there is evidence that treatment may improve nerve tolerance to motion, there is little evidence currently that treatment can increase the excursion of nerve motion[1] known to be reduced in some compressive neuropathies such as carpal tunnel syndrome.[43–46]

MATCHING MANAGEMENT TO THE NATURE OF THE NERVE-RELATED CONDITION

Management approaches to nerve-related neck pain disorders vary depending on the patient's presentation and examination findings. In some presentations, involvement of nerve tissue may be a minor secondary component of the condition (i.e., mild mechanosensitivity) that resolves spontaneously as other more substantial musculoskeletal impairments are addressed. In other conditions, the nerve component may be more significant with more marked signs of nerve mechanosensitivity or changes in nerve conduction. Techniques aimed specifically at resolving these nerve tissue–related impairments are a priority. Where there is marked nerve mechanosensitivity, other examination findings (e.g., elevated scapular postures, marked active or passive movement restrictions) may be protective responses to mechanosensitive nerves. Attempts to improve scapular posture or perform exercise may aggravate the condition. Instead, attention is given immediately to resolving the underlying nerve mechanosensitivity. In summary, interpreting the level of nerve involvement and priority for specifically addressing nerve tissue within a management approach will depend on the findings from the patient examination, and may change over the duration of a management period as the patient's condition progresses.

When specific attention to nerve tissue is a priority, techniques chosen will depend on the stage of the condition and the nature of the nerve involvement. For example, in the acute stages of a condition, there may be an emphasis on reducing perineural and/or intra-neural inflammation. In subacute and chronic conditions, the focus may be more on restoring pain free mobility, the function of nerve tissue and the musculoskeletal interfaces. If it is suspected that a nerve is compressed or entrapped, treatment is focused on reducing compression to the nerve. Irrespective of approach, the potentially irritable nature of mechano-sensitive nerve tissue warrants that physical treatments be undertaken with care so as not to further provoke the patient's symptoms.[47,48]

A multimodal mechanistic approach to management of cervical nerve-related conditions is taken because mechanisms underlying conditions, such as cervical radiculopathy, may vary from individual to individual. Nerve tissue exposed to perineural inflammation and/or compression secondary to injury of a musculoskeletal structure, may present as a loss of nerve conduction,[49] as a mechanosensitive nerve painful to movement or pressure[13,14] or as a variable mix of both. Therefore there is no one set approach to managing conditions such as radiculopathy. The presentation of this disorder may vary significantly between patients, thus requiring a patient-centred management approach. Determining an appropriate course of management requires judicious initial examination and continual reassessment of treatment response.

Patient education and advice

Management is underpinned by comprehensive patient education and advice regarding the clinical presentation with collaborative discussion concerning management strategies. Informing patients of the involvement of nerve tissue within their disorder is important for safety reasons for certain nerve-related cervical conditions. Firstly, patients with compromised nerve conduction, such as cervical radiculopathy or myelopathy, should be informed of signs of deteriorating nerve function and the need to seek advice if deterioration is suspected. Secondly, nerve tissue has a propensity to be irritable. Patients who have been given exercises to address nerve mechanosensitivity need to be cautioned to commence and progress slowly and be analytical regarding their symptomatic response to a new exercise intervention. The concept of performing exercise for nerve mechanosensitivity is usually foreign to patients and careful explanation as to the rationale for their inclusion is necessary for optimal compliance.

Addressing contributing factors

There may be significant patient (e.g., postural) and environmental (e.g., ergonomic) factors that underlie nerve irritation in neck pain disorders.

Postural/movement–based strain to nerve

When considering nerve tissue mechanosensitivity, clinicians need to be cautious in addressing aberrant postures if they appear to be protective of nerve tissue. However, it is also possible for postures to be contributing to the nerve mechanosensitive state. Poor cervical and shoulder girdle muscle control can underlie persisting nerve-related disorders. Some cases of persistent cervicobrachial mechanosensitivity appear to be related to aberrant shoulder girdle function. In particular, a downwardly rotated and/or depressed scapula (a sensitizing component of neurodynamic tests of the brachial plexus) may induce continuous excessive strain to the brachial plexus. Patients with symptoms (pain and/or paraesthesia) in relaxed upright standing may experience immediate reduction in these symptoms when the clinician manually corrects this aberrant scapular posture. A link between scapular posture and nerve symptoms may be confirmed by taping the corrected scapular posture over a longer time period. Although these patients demonstrate positive signs of nerve mechanosensitivity, mobilizing techniques to address mechanosensitivity may have limited effect if the underlying postural and movement–based impairments of the scapula are not addressed first (see Chapter 15).

Adequate neuromuscular function of the cervico-thoracic region and shoulder girdle is essential in the long-term management and prevention of recurrence of nerve-related conditions including cervical radiculopathy and cervical myelopathy. If pain is severe in the early stages of management, gentle isometric exercises are commenced initially. Exercise to improve neuromuscular function can be progressed (see Chapter 15), as long as an exercise does not compromise integrity of the neural structures and nerve function.

Ergonomic factors and nerve strain

Consistent with the management approach to other cervical conditions, ergonomic and work-related modifications may need to be considered in cervical nerve-related conditions. This is particularly relevant for ergonomic factors affecting the upper limb such as overreaching associated with poor work station design. Nerve entrapments of the upper limb such as carpal tunnel syndrome, which may be associated with concurrent cervical disorders (i.e., double crush), often have ergonomic or work-related contributing factors that need to be addressed. For example, the prevalence of carpal tunnel syndrome is approximately 3.8% in the general population[50] and 21% in occupations involving repetitive hand tasks.[51] Similarly the ulnar nerve may become entrapped as it passes through the cubital tunnel of the elbow particularly in individuals in occupations that involve repetitive tasks such as manipulating tools.[52] Addressing these work-related contributing factors may include the modification of work equipment or work practices (e.g., technique modification, incorporation of work breaks).

Manual therapy

This section considers the application of manual therapy techniques for both nerve mechanosensitivity and nerve conduction deficits. For many patients, these features coexist in a variable mix. The choice of technique and progression will depend on the priority features of the condition, and the continued evaluation of the response to treatment.

Manual techniques directed at nerve mechanosensitivity

Manual therapy techniques targeting the nervous system are well described for managing neck pain disorders exhibiting positive signs of neuromechanosensitivity.[53,54] Techniques may either directly mobilize the relevant musculoskeletal interface (e.g., joint mobilization), or specifically mobilize nerve tissue. Techniques such as a cervical lateral glide mobilization (Fig. 17.1) target the restoration of pain-free relative motion of the cervical nerve-musculoskeletal interface.[53,54]

Signs of cervical nerve mechanosensitivity may resolve with manual therapy techniques targeted at improving painful or restricted cervical segmental motion without the need for specific nerve-based

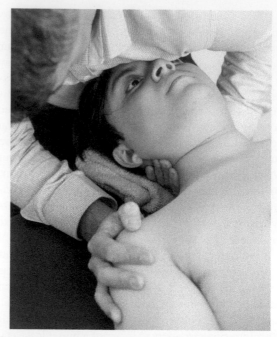

Fig. 17.1 ■ Cervical lateral glide. This technique is applied with the clinician's index finger gently wrapped around the posterolateral aspect of the uppermost vertebrae (i.e., C5 for a C5–6 technique) on the symptomatic side such that a lateral glide can be applied to C5 relative to C6. In this example, the clinician's force application produces a left lateral glide for a right sided neural mechanosensitivity issue. The clinician's right hand stabilizes the patient's right shoulder girdle. The patient's right arm can be positioned in neutral or in a progressively more advanced upper limb neurodynamic test position.

techniques. However, in many cases, a better effect is gained from manual therapy techniques directed to the nerve interface. The cervical lateral glide mobilization technique has been shown to immediately reduce protective muscle responses associated with neurodynamic tests[40] with positive effects on mobility and pain[55] in those who are mechanosensitive. In a clinical trial, Nee et al.[56] showed that management including education, manual therapy (lateral glide technique) and nerve mobilizing exercises provided immediate clinically relevant benefits beyond advice to remain active. Evidence from a systematic review and meta-analysis supports the use of cervical lateral glide techniques in people with nerve-related neck and arm pain. The technique had a positive effect on pain, with clinically meaningful effect sizes.[57] The lateral glide technique is often progressed by prepositioning the arm from the neutral position to a progressively more advanced upper limb neurodynamic test position, as well as incorporating active mobilization of the upper limb.

Dosage: Manual therapy techniques directly addressing nerve tissue mechanosensitivity are initially conservative (e.g., 1–2 sets of 30 second durations of mobilizations, at a grade short of symptom reproduction). They can be progressed with regard to increased sets, repetitions, and grade of mobilization. Once the risk of an adverse response to treatment has been negated, techniques may be progressed to symptom reproduction within the individual's tolerance. As indicated, the cervical lateral glide mobilization may be progressed by progressively increasing positions of the relevant positive upper limb neurodynamic test (e.g., median nerve biased test) or reported provoking functional upper limb position (e.g., arm overhead). Progression is guided by symptom response and symptom irritability.

Manual techniques for altered nerve conduction

For conditions such as cervical radiculopathy with changes in nerve conduction, traction may assist in alleviating symptoms associated with this nerve compression.[58] Traction generally has not shown efficacy in the management of non-specific neck pain disorders,[59–61] but in cervical radiculopathy, mechanical traction may provide additional clinical benefit to other therapeutic modalities such as exercise.[58] Nevertheless, evidence of the benefits of traction have been mixed.[62–64] If traction is to be trialled in a patient with cervical radiculopathy, the preference is to first apply manual traction (e.g., traction to C5/6 in the presence of C6 radiculopathy) to permit the appropriate adjustment of technique in

response to patient comfort for these potentially irritable nerve conditions.

Cervical radiculopathies may also respond well to manual techniques targeting restricted or painful cervical segmental motion, including cervical lateral glide techniques as described for neural mechanosensitivity. In the early stages of management, techniques that potentially compromise an already compressed or inflamed nerve (e.g., C5/6 right lateral flexion mobilization in the presence of right C6 nerve conduction deficits) may need to be avoided. Irrespective of the technique applied, there needs to be diligent monitoring of nerve conduction status to ensure techniques are having a positive impact, and importantly, not an adverse impact.

Dosage: Techniques addressing cervical radiculopathies should initially be conservative. Traction and other mobilization techniques should not reproduce symptoms and initially be applied in a trialled manner to assess the effect on symptoms. Traction can be progressed in duration and force and mobilization techniques by increased sets/repetitions, once the risk of an adverse response to treatment has been negated.

Self-mobilization with home exercise

Exercises to self-mobilize neural tissue for the management of nerve mechanosensitivity have long been advocated. Techniques broadly include those commonly referred to as *sliders* that combine movements which simultaneously shorten and lengthen the nerve bed at adjacent joints (Fig. 17.2A–C), respectively. The other techniques are referred to as *tensioners* that aim to mobilize a nerve by elongation of the nerve bed (Fig. 17.3A and B).[54,65,66] Mechanistic studies in the upper limb have shown that nerve sliding techniques may

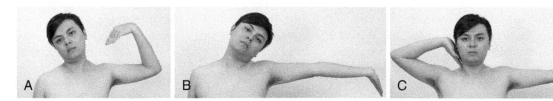

Fig. 17.2 ■ Nerve "slider" self-mobilization technique (median nerve bias). The neural tissue mobilization techniques combine movements which simultaneously shorten and lengthen the nerve bed at adjacent joints to create gentle excursion of nerve tissue relative to their interfaces. (A) The nerve bed is lengthened in the cervical spine and shortened at the wrist and elbow. (B) The nerve bed is lengthened at the wrist and elbow and shortened in the cervical spine. (C) the nerve bed can be moved in the cervical region by shortening and lengthening the nerve bed alternately in each upper limb.

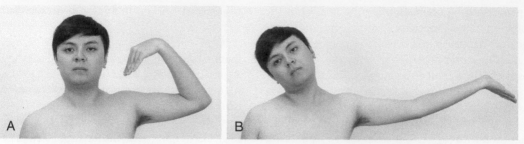

Fig. 17.3 ■ Nerve "tensioner" self-mobilization technique (median nerve bias). These neural tissue mobilisation techniques combine movements which move and then elongate the nerve bed from (A) the starting position to (B) end position of the exercise

result in greater nerve excursion compared with tensioning techniques[67] particularly between the two moving joints.[68] As such, sliding techniques for managing neural mechanosensitivity are generally recommended because they expose the nervous system to more mobilization and less strain.[35,68] However, the choice and progression of neural mobilizing exercises may differ depending on the initial presentation and stage of individual's recovery. For example, tensioning techniques may be appropriate in non-irritable presentations if sliding techniques are not proving effective, particularly if they best expose the nerve and musculoskeletal interface to the mechanical forces that they will need to tolerate for optimal return to function (e.g., fully outstretched positions such as reaching, tennis serve). The initial choice of exercise and exercise progressions are based on clinical reasoning processes.[69]

Exercise to address nerve mechanosensitivity may also involve exercises directed towards sensitive dura. Some presentations of headache and neck pain appear to be related to movement sensitivity of the dura as evident by pain with cervical (or craniocervical) flexion (see Chapter 9). Exercises may target dural tissue initially with slider type exercises using pain-free ranges of concurrent craniocervical flexion/ankle plantarflexion, alternated with concurrent craniocervical extension/ankle dorsiflexion. Exercises are progressed as able to a sitting position incorporating cervical flexion/knee flexion alternated with cervical extension/knee extension. When symptoms are severe or irritable, nerve mechanosensitivity may need to be addressed with manual therapy initially because these direct neural mobilizing exercises may be potentially aggravating.

Dosage: Exercises to mobilize nerve tissue should be commenced at a low dosage (e.g., 1 set of 10 or less repetitions per session, twice per day) and short of symptom reproduction. Exercises can be progressed with increased sets and repetitions once the absence of an adverse response has been ascertained.

Referral to medical physicians

Although most neuropathies can be managed conservatively, some may require medical attention or a multidisciplinary approach. In particular, neurological signs of absent or significantly altered reflexes or muscle strength may indicate severe compressive neuropathy (or myelopathy). Further investigation, such as magnetic resonance imaging, may be indicated to determine the presence of nerve or spinal cord compromise, with potential treatment options that may include surgery. Patients with severe or recalcitrant neuropathic pain usually require good pharmaceutical pain management by a medical practitioner. Such medications currently include tricyclic antidepressants, pregabalin, gabapentin and lidocaine patches.[70] However, even in these more severe cases where medication is required, there is a still a role for physiotherapy within a multidisciplinary approach. Physiotherapy is particularly important with regard to education on activity modification and the restoration of pain-free postural and movement function with the use of manual therapy techniques and progressive exercise as is appropriate to the patient's condition.

CONCLUSION

When neck pain disorders involve sensitized or compromised nerves, management approaches may need to specifically target nerve tissue. Correctly identifying the nature of nerve involvement will guide management.

Some presentations involving significantly compromised nerve function may signal safety concerns for the patient requiring medical consultation, however most neck pain disorders involving nerve tissue can be effectively treated conservatively. Effective management requires an understanding of the potential mechanisms underlying the condition so that interventions can be applied appropriately and the status of neural function can be judiciously monitored.

REFERENCES

1. Coppieters MW, Nee R. Neurodynamic management of the peripheral nervous system. Grieve's modern musculoskeletal physiotherapy. 4th ed. China: Elsevier; 2015.
2. Kang JD, Georgescu HI, McIntyre-Larkin L, et al. Herniated cervical intervertebral discs spontaneously produce matrix metalloproteinases, nitric oxide, interleukin-6, and prostaglandin E2. Spine 1995;20:2373–8.
3. Furusawa N, Baba H, Miyoshi N, et al. Herniation of cervical intervertebral disc: immunohistochemical examination and measurement of nitric oxide production. Spine 2001;26:1110–16.
4. Bogduk N. The anatomy and pathophysiology of neck pain. Phys Med Rehabil Clin N Am 2011;22:367–82, vii.
5. Benoliel R, Wilensky A, Tal M, et al. Application of a pro-inflammatory agent to the orbital portion of the rat infraorbital nerve induces changes indicative of ongoing trigeminal pain. Pain 2002;99:567–78.
6. Eliav E, Herzberg U, Ruda MA, et al. Neuropathic pain from an experimental neuritis of the rat sciatic nerve. Pain 1999;83:169–82.
7. Chacur M, Milligan ED, Gazda LS, et al. A new model of sciatic inflammatory neuritis (SIN): induction of unilateral and bilateral mechanical allodynia following acute unilateral peri-sciatic immune activation in rats. Pain 2001;94:231–44.
8. Gazda LS, Milligan ED, Hansen MK, et al. Sciatic inflammatory neuritis (SIN): behavioral allodynia is paralleled by peri-sciatic proinflammatory cytokine and superoxide production. J Peripher Nerv Syst 2001;6:111–29.
9. Eliav E, Gracely RH. Sensory changes in the territory of the lingual and inferior alveolar nerves following lower third molar extraction. Pain 1998;77:191–9.
10. Milligan ED, Maier SF, Watkins LR. Sciatic inflammatory neuropathy in the rat: surgical procedures, induction of inflammation, and behavioral testing. Methods Mol Med 2004;99:67–89.
11. Eliav E, Tal M, Benoliel R. Experimental malignancy in the rat induces early hypersensitivity indicative of neuritis. Pain 2004;110:727–37.
12. Eliav E, Benoliel R, Tal M. Inflammation with no axonal damage of the rat saphenous nerve trunk induces ectopic discharge and mechanosensitivity in myelinated axons. Neurosci Lett 2001;311:49–52.
13. Bove GM, Ransil BJ, Lin HC, et al. Inflammation induces ectopic mechanical sensitivity in axons of nociceptors innervating deep tissues. J Neurophysiol 2003;90:1949–55.
14. Dilley A, Lynn B, Pang SJ. Pressure and stretch mechanosensitivity of peripheral nerve fibres following local inflammation of the nerve trunk. Pain 2005;117:462–72.
15. Eliav E, Benoliel R, Herzberg U, et al. The role of IL-6 and IL-1beta in painful perineural inflammatory neuritis. Brain Behav Immun 2009;23:474–84.
16. Devor M. Sodium channels and mechanisms of neuropathic pain. J Pain 2006;7(1 Suppl. 1):S3–12.
17. Moalem G, Grafe P, Tracey DJ. Chemical mediators enhance the excitability of unmyelinated sensory axons in normal and injured peripheral nerve of the rat. Neuroscience 2005;134:1399–411.
18. Sorkin LS, Xiao WH, Wagner R, et al. Tumour necrosis factor-alpha induces ectopic activity in nociceptive primary afferent fibres. Neuroscience 1997;81:255–62.
19. Grossmann L, Gorodetskaya N, Baron R, et al. Enhancement of ectopic discharge in regenerating A- and C-fibers by inflammatory mediators. J Neurophysiol 2009;101:2762–74.
20. Song XJ, Gan Q, Cao JL, et al. Spinal manipulation reduces pain and hyperalgesia after lumbar intervertebral foramen inflammation in the rat. J Manipulative Physiol Ther 2006;29:5–13.
21. Rydevik B, Lundborg G, Bagge U. Effects of graded compression on intraneural blood blow. An in vivo study on rabbit tibial nerve. J Hand Surg Am 1981;6:3–12.
22. Rydevik B, Lundborg G. Permeability of intraneural microvessels and perineurium following acute, graded experimental nerve compression. Scand J Plast Reconstr Surg 1977;11:179–87.
23. Mueller M, Leonhard C, Wacker K, et al. Macrophage response to peripheral nerve injury: the quantitative contribution of resident and hematogenous macrophages. Lab Invest 2003;83:175–85.
24. Moalem G, Tracey DJ. Immune and inflammatory mechanisms in neuropathic pain. Brain Res Rev 2006;51:240–64.
25. Moalem G, Xu K, Yu L. T lymphocytes play a role in neuropathic pain following peripheral nerve injury in rats. Neuroscience 2004;129:767–77.
26. Basson A, Olivier B, Ellis R, et al. The effectiveness of neural mobilizations in the treatment of musculoskeletal conditions: a systematic review protocol. JBI Database System Rev Implement Rep 2015;13:65–75.
27. Schmid AB, Elliott JM, Strudwick MW, et al. Effect of splinting and exercise on intraneural edema of the median nerve in carpal tunnel syndrome–an MRI study to reveal therapeutic mechanisms. J Orthop Res 2012;30:1343–50.
28. Brown CL, Gilbert KK, Brismee JM, et al. The effects of neurodynamic mobilization on fluid dispersion within the tibial nerve at the ankle: an unembalmed cadaveric study. J Man Manip Ther 2011;19:26–34.
29. Gilbert KK, Smith MP, Sobczak S, et al. Effects of lower limb neurodynamic mobilization on intraneural fluid dispersion of the fourth lumbar nerve root: an unembalmed cadaveric investigation. J Man Manip Ther 2015;23:239–45.
30. Giardini AC, Dos Santos FM, da Silva JT, et al. Neural mobilization treatment decreases glial cells and brain-derived neurotrophic factor expression in the central nervous system in rats with neuropathic pain induced by CCI in rats. Pain Res Manag 2017;2017:7429761.

31. Santos FM, Silva JT, Giardini AC, et al. Neural mobilization reverses behavioral and cellular changes that characterize neuropathic pain in rats. Mol Pain 2012;8:57.

32. McLellan DL, Swash M. Longitudinal sliding of the median nerve during movements of the upper limb. J Neurol Neurosurg Psychiatry 1976;39:566–70.

33. Coppieters MW, Alshami AM, Babri AS, et al. Strain and excursion of the sciatic, tibial, and plantar nerves during a modified straight leg raising test. J Orthop Res 2006;24:1883–9.

34. Gelberman RH, Hergenroeder PT, Hargens AR, et al. The carpal tunnel syndrome. A study of carpal canal pressures. J Bone Joint Surg Am 1981;63:380–3.

35. Coppieters MW, Butler DS. Do 'sliders' slide and 'tensioners' tension? An analysis of neurodynamic techniques and considerations regarding their application. Man Ther 2008;13:213–21.

36. Byl C, Puttlitz C, Byl N, et al. Strain in the median and ulnar nerves during upper-extremity positioning. J Hand Surg Am 2002;27:1032–40.

37. Dilley A, Lynn B, Greening J, et al. Quantitative in vivo studies of median nerve sliding in response to wrist, elbow, shoulder and neck movements. Clin Biomech (Bristol, Avon) 2003;18: 899–907.

38. Wilgis EF, Murphy R. The significance of longitudinal excursion in peripheral nerves. Hand Clin 1986;2:761–6.

39. Wright TW, Glowczewskie F Jr, Cowin D, et al. Radial nerve excursion and strain at the elbow and wrist associated with upper-extremity motion. J Hand Surg Am 2005;30:990–6.

40. Coppieters MW, Stappaerts KH, Wouters LL, et al. Aberrant protective force generation during neural provocation testing and the effect of treatment in patients with neurogenic cervicobrachial pain. J Manipulative Physiol Ther 2003;26: 99–106.

41. Bialosky JE, Bishop MD, Price DD, et al. A randomized sham-controlled trial of a neurodynamic technique in the treatment of carpal tunnel syndrome. J Orthop Sports Phys Ther 2009;39:709–23.

42. Santos FM, Grecco LH, Pereira MG, et al. The neural mobilization technique modulates the expression of endogenous opioids in the periaqueductal gray and improves muscle strength and mobility in rats with neuropathic pain. Behav Brain Funct 2014;10: 19.

43. Hough AD, Moore AP, Jones MP. Reduced longitudinal excursion of the median nerve in carpal tunnel syndrome. Arch Phys Med Rehabil 2007;88:569–76.

44. Korstanje JW, Scheltens-De Boer M, Blok JH, et al. Ultrasonographic assessment of longitudinal median nerve and hand flexor tendon dynamics in carpal tunnel syndrome. Muscle Nerve 2012;45:721–9.

45. Allmann KH, Horch R, Uhl M, et al. MR imaging of the carpal tunnel. Eur J Radiol 1997;25:141–5.

46. Erel E, Dilley A, Greening J, et al. Longitudinal sliding of the median nerve in patients with carpal tunnel syndrome. J Hand Surg [Br] 2003;28:439–43.

47. Elvey R. Physical evaluation of the peripheral nervous system in disorders of pain and dysfunction. J Hand Ther 1997;10: 122–9.

48. Sterling M, Treleaven J, Jull G. Responses to a clinical test of mechanical provocation of nerve tissue in whiplash associated disorders. Man Ther 2002;7:89–94.

49. Lee DH, Claussen GC, Oh S. Clinical nerve conduction and needle electromyography studies. J Am Acad Orthop Surg 2004;12: 276–87.

50. Atroshi I, Gummesson C, Johnsson R, et al. Prevalence of carpal tunnel syndrome in a general population. JAMA 1999;282: 153–8.

51. Gorsche RG, Wiley JP, Renger RF, et al. Prevalence and incidence of carpal tunnel syndrome in a meat packing plant. Occup Environ Med 1999;56:417–22.

52. Descatha A, Leclerc A, Chastang JF, et al. Incidence of ulnar nerve entrapment at the elbow in repetitive work. Scand J Work Environ Health 2004;30:234–40.

53. Elvey RL. Treatment of arm pain associated with abnormal brachial plexus tension. Aust J Physiother 1986;32:225–30.

54. Butler D. The sensitive nervous system. Adelaide City West, South Australia: The NOI Group; 2000.

55. Coppieters MW, Stappaerts KH, Wouters LL, et al. The immediate effects of a cervical lateral glide treatment technique in patients with neurogenic cervicobrachial pain. J Orthop Sports Phys Ther 2003;33:369–78.

56. Nee RJ, Vicenzino B, Jull GA, et al. Neural tissue management provides immediate clinically relevant benefits without harmful effects for patients with nerve-related neck and arm pain: a randomised trial. J Physiother 2012;58:23–31.

57. Basson A, Olivier B, Ellis R, et al. The effectiveness of neural mobilization for neuro-musculoskeletal conditions: a systematic review and meta-Analysis. J Orthop Sports Phys Ther 2017; 1–76.

58. Fritz JM, Thackeray A, Brennan GP, et al. Exercise only, exercise with mechanical traction, or exercise with over-door traction for patients with cervical radiculopathy, with or without consideration of status on a previously described subgrouping rule: a randomized clinical trial. J Orthop Sports Phys Ther 2014;44: 45–57.

59. Borman P, Keskin D, Ekici B, et al. The efficacy of intermittent cervical traction in patients with chronic neck pain. Clin Rheumatol 2008;27:1249–53.

60. Chiu TT, Ng JK, Walther-Zhang B, et al. A randomized controlled trial on the efficacy of intermittent cervical traction for patients with chronic neck pain. Clin Rehabil 2011;25: 814–22.

61. Thoomes EJ, Scholten-Peeters W, Koes B, et al. The effectiveness of conservative treatment for patients with cervical radiculopathy: a systematic review. Clin J Pain 2013;29:1073–86.

62. Klaber Moffett JA, Hughes GI, Griffiths P. An investigation of the effects of cervical traction part 1: clinical effectiveness. Clin Rehabil 1990;4:205–11.

63. Jellad A, Ben Salah Z, Boudokhane S, et al. The value of intermittent cervical traction in recent cervical radiculopathy. Ann Phys Rehabil Med 2009;52:638–52.

64. Young IA, Michener LA, Cleland JA, et al. Manual therapy, exercise, and traction for patients with cervical radiculopathy: a randomized clinical trial. Phys Ther 2009;89:632–42.

65. Coppieters MW, Bartholomeeusen KE, Stappaerts KH. Incorporating nerve-gliding techniques in the conservative treatment of cubital tunnel syndrome. J Manipulative Physiol Ther 2004;27:560–8.

66. Shacklock MO. Clinical neurodynamics: a new system of musculoskeletal treatment. Edinburgh: Elsevier Health Sciences; 2005.

67. Coppieters MW, Hough AD, Dilley A. Different nerve-gliding exercises induce different magnitudes of median nerve longitudinal excursion: an in vivo study using dynamic ultrasound imaging. J Orthop Sports Phys Ther 2009;39:164–71.

68. Coppieters MW, Alshami AM. Longitudinal excursion and strain in the median nerve during novel nerve gliding exercises for carpal tunnel syndrome. J Orthop Res 2007;25:972–80.

69. Nee RJ, Butler D. Management of peripheral neuropathic pain: integrating neurobiology, neurodynamics, and clinical evidence. Phys Ther Sport 2006;7:36–49.

70. Finnerup NB, Attal N, Haroutounian S, et al. Pharmacotherapy for neuropathic pain in adults: a systematic review and meta-analysis. Lancet Neurol 2015;14:162–73.

18

CASE PRESENTATIONS
Clinical Reasoning and Clinical Decision Making

■ ■ ■ ■ ■ ■ ■ ■ ■ ■ ■ ■ ■ ■ ■ ■ ■ ■ ■ ■

Conservative physical therapies are the primary interventions for the management of neck pain disorders. However, neck pain presentations vary between patients as does the clinical reasoning processes underpinning management decisions. The text to this point has discussed clinical reasoning and considered the use of several interventions in relative isolation. In this chapter, we present patient cases to practically demonstrate the clinical reasoning processes underlying differential diagnosis and/or selection of integrated management approaches. Cases are used to illustrate how various therapies may be selected and integrated, based on the outcomes of clinical reasoning of findings of the patient interview, the physical examination and progressive assessments. The cases have different emphases to illustrate different components of examination and management and associated reasoning. The reader is referred to relevant chapters to refresh details of particular treatment techniques/regimes.

CASE 1: DIRECTIONALLY BIASED PERSISTENT NECK PAIN (FIG. 18.1)

For many patients, an informative relationship can be established between their movement behaviours and symptoms. The following case is a prime example of this relationship. The case highlights the need for a thorough patient interview, particularly with regard to the behaviour of symptoms and identification of aggravating factors to neck pain that share a common provocative movement component. This case also highlights the powerful impact that patient education, advice and compliance has on recovery.

Patient presentation and key examination findings

PS, a 28-year-old primary school teacher, presents with a 5-year history of daily left-sided neck and upper thorax pain that occasionally spreads into the left upper arm. This condition started when she returned to university to commence studies in education in her mid-twenties. PS reported that in the initial 2 to 3 years, her condition was episodic and seemingly related only to her study. However, symptoms persisted and progressively worsened well beyond the completion of her degree. They were now affecting multiple aspects of her life. Over the past 3 years she had sought treatment for her neck condition from many health professionals. Management strategies included manual therapy, exercise (predominantly stretches), acupuncture and dry needling, chronic pain education and pain management. To date, none of these interventions had been effective for any length of time, with no sustainable positive change in symptoms over time.

Reported aggravating factors and functional examination

The salient factor in this case was that PS reported key aggravating factors that had a common mechanical element relevant to her persisting symptoms, i.e., flexion of the lower cervical spine. These specific activities were computer work on a laptop, working with young children

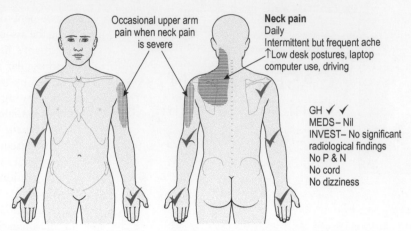

Fig. 18.1 ■ Case 1: Body chart. GH general health; MEDS medications, INVEST investigations, P & N pins and needles.

at schools on low desks, and driving her car with the head rest pushing her head forward. When asked to replicate these activities in the clinic as best as possible, it was evident that all activities positioned her in mid-range to end-range lower cervical flexion, a position that PS was required to function in for a large proportion of her days. Replication of these activities in the clinic resulted in a familiar feeling of strain to her neck that resolved when the neck was returned to a more neutral position.

Other examination findings

Examination of active movements revealed that, although mildly uncomfortable, there were no limitations to PS's cervical flexion range of motion, or any other motion direction. Manual segmental examination revealed marked pain provocation on palpation of the (L) C5–6 motion segment in the absence of any apparent intersegmental mobility loss. The most notable finding during formal examination of the cervical motor system was a marked reduction in cervical extensor muscle endurance, with self-reported fatigue after less than five repetitions of lower cervical extension. There were no apparent impairments in thoracic mobility or the neural system (nerve conduction or neurodynamics). Although the patient expressed frustration with the persistence of her disorder and the lack of improvement with previous treatment, these emotional responses were understandable based on the longevity of the condition and were not considered as potential barriers to recovery. Furthermore, the patient appeared very positive about

recovery once the link between her aggravating activities, physical findings and persistence of pain was established, providing her a sense of empowerment.

Diagnosis and clinical reasoning

The diagnosis considered the condition from both a movement-related and structure-related perspective. A diagnosis was made of a chronic flexion related C5–6 motion segment strain. The movement disorder aspect of the condition was driven by identifying the common element to all reported aggravating activities. Specific and comprehensive questioning that transferred to activity replication during the physical examination demonstrated that a flexed position of the lower region of the neck was related to the provocation of symptoms. Although it was uncertain as to what specific structure of the lower neck region was responsible for the persistence of symptoms, findings from the manual examination suggested the C5–6 segment may be implicated. Importantly, the examination findings indicated that this lower-neck condition was of a postural overuse strain nature, perpetuated by habitual loading to the neck *in* flexion and a deconditioned muscular system. The success of management would therefore require PS's full participation to change the habitual loading pattern and condition the muscular system.

Management approach

Advice and education

A key aspect of management was to adequately inform PS that her neck condition was not caused by a lack of neck flexibility, but rather habitual patterns of movement and muscle deconditioning. This was important because she had been told in the past that stretches would help her neck condition, which they did not. Instead it was reinforced that resolving the habitual movement pattern of her neck was the most relevant factor that would be complimented by conditioning exercises of her neck muscles. This included strategies to reduce the time and excursion of cervical flexion in which PS functioned by changing the work environment when able, as well as her work practices and behaviours. Strategies included use of a laptop holder and external keyboard, and an inclined reading board, to remove the need for excessive cervical flexion when working on the laptop computer, or reading documents, respectively. Although PS could not avoid sitting at lower desks while supervising school students, the need for more regular breaks during this work with children was emphasized and undertaken. PS also modified her car seat position so that her head felt comfortable and not in a flexed position.

Exercise therapy

Exercise included both postural correction training as well as specific conditioning of the cervical muscles. Postural correction training incorporated the practice and familiarity of attaining a neutral upright posture. PS incorporated this into work postures with use of memory joggers. A neutral posture was also facilitated with the use of the laptop holder and inclined reading board. Training also included progressive lower cervical extensor training. Training initially incorporated through-range coordination and low-load endurance training in the prone on elbows position. The exercise was subsequently progressed to resistance exercise directed towards higher load and sustained contractions to attain gains in muscular strength and endurance. Although PS was only seen over a 6-week period as her symptoms had markedly improved, she was encouraged to continue progression of her exercises for several months. This was justified to her based on the longevity of her condition and the expected time frame required to achieve sustainable changes in muscle conditioning, as well as the prevention of recurrence.

Reflection and clinical message

PS responded well to this intervention with substantial alleviation of pain and increased comfort during the relevant activities. The key element to the success of this intervention was identifying the association between the aggravating factors, the patient's habitual movement behaviour, and the neuromuscular impairments, that were collaboratively identified by the patient and the clinician. This was very motivating and empowering for PS because she could immediately implement the strategies (changes in movement behaviour, work practices and ergonomics, muscular training) that clearly complimented each other. It should be noted that such strong and consistent directionally based clinical presentations do not always exist. Many mechanical neck pain presentations are more clouded, with multiple aggravating directions of motion and more widespread motor impairments. However, even within these more clouded presentations there may be a certain pattern of movement disorder that is dominant and can be prioritized in management.

CASE 2: HEADACHE—DIFFERENTIATING THE ROLE OF THE NECK (FIG. 18.2)

Neck pain is a common feature of frequent intermittent headache types such as migraine, tension-type headache, cervicogenic headache, and headaches associated with craniomandibular dysfunction. The neck pain can arise from cervical musculoskeletal dysfunction or it may be part of the headache symptom complex. Thus cervical musculoskeletal dysfunction can be the primary cause of headache (cervicogenic headache), a contributor or comorbid feature of the headache symptomology, or have no role in the headache syndrome. The use of local treatments to the neck (e.g., manipulative therapy, therapeutic exercise) in headache management is relevant only when a link is established between the neck pain, relevant cervical musculoskeletal dysfunction and the headache.

This case presents a patient whose primary reason for seeking a physiotherapy consultation was to know if her headaches had a neck cause/component and, if so, what to do about it. The reasoning will be narrated through the examination to expose the clinician's thinking in determining the presence or not and possible role of cervical musculoskeletal dysfunction in this person's headache.

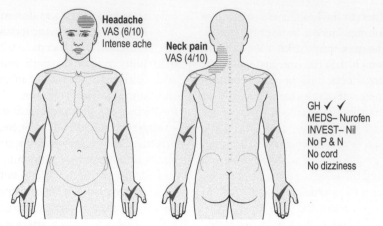

Fig. 18.2 ■ Case 2: Body chart. VAS visual analogue scale; GH general health; MEDS medications, INVEST investigations, P & N pins and needles.

Patient presentation

JD is a 62-year-old office manager. She reports a history of menstrual migraine since the age of 16 years. In the last 10 years or more, she reports feeling more neck pain with her headaches and is also getting headaches more frequently. They still feel like her usual migraines although the intensity has lessened, and she no longer experiences auras. JD has always found that if she pushes at the base of her skull, she can change the headache.

Reasoning. First thoughts are that JD has experienced an improvement in her menstrual migraines likely coinciding with the end of menopause and she may be describing a transition to either a frequent common migraine, tension-type or cervicogenic headache or is developing a mixed headache. Changing the headache by pushing on the base of the skull is not helpful in differential diagnosis. It is a non-specific sign because it is possible to do this with migraine, tension-type or cervicogenic headache.

JD reports a headache frequency of at least two headache days per week, their intensity at worst is a 6/10, and duration is several hours. She now takes Nurofen (an over the counter nonsteroidal antiinflammatory drug) to control the headache (up to 6 per day on headache days). The time of onset of headache is variable and does not appear to be related to any particular activity or posture. She can wake with a headache, or the headache comes on in the afternoon, either at work or at home, often on a Saturday.

Reasoning. Waking with a headache could be as a result of sleeping position of the neck, but it is also a common feature of migraine. Headaches on a Saturday could be suggestive of a stress-release migraine or tension-type headache. JD is not relating headache onset to any particular neck-related activity at this time, which is lessening thoughts about cervicogenic headache. She is managing headaches with Nurofen, which can assist some persons with any of migraine, tension-type or cervicogenic headache types.

JD describes her headaches as an intense ache, felt in the frontal region. They are usually worse on the left side but can involve the whole head and neck. Headaches usually start in her forehead and JD reports that the top part of her neck begins to ache when she has a headache. She really thinks that her neck is triggering her headaches. Her neck is usually more bothersome when she has the headache than when she is headache free. When she has a headache, JD reports she is sensitive to light and computer work can be aggravating.

Reasoning. Headaches are unilateral and seem to be relatively side consistent, which is consistent with cervicogenic headache but does not dismiss migraine. Cervicogenic headaches usually start in the neck and then spread to the head, but JD reports a pain onset in the head, which is more commonly a characteristic of migraine. Sensitivity to light and computer work while a headache is present are often generic complaints of headache sufferers. Of interest, JD's neck pain seems to be very closely related to the headache (i.e., it is not so bothersome on non-headache days), yet her view is that it appears that the neck is triggering the migraine. Although it is important to acknowledge her beliefs, the inconsistent presence of neck pain in the absence of headache further lessens thoughts about cervicogenic headache.

JD has a family history of migraine (mother). Apart from the headaches, JD reports no other health issues, has had no surgeries and takes no medication (with the exception of Nurofen). She is working full time, and manages on headache days with Nurofen, but would prefer not to rely on medication. Outside work, she is involved in several community organizations, and is rather busy. All children have left home, and she and her husband enjoy four grandchildren.

Hypotheses from the patient interview

There is well recognized symptomatic overlap between headache types and, as often occurs, JD is not presenting with classical features of one headache type. Based on information from the patient interview, it is reasoned that JD's headache is, in descending order of possibility, chronic migraine (the neck pain is part of the pain of migraine), a mixed headache or a cervicogenic headache. Tension-type headache was ruled out at this stage for lack of defining characteristics. This rather mixed symptomatic picture realizes the importance of the physical examination to determine whether or not the neck pain is associated with a pattern of musculoskeletal dysfunction to confirm or rule out a cervical cause or contributor to JD's headaches.

Physical examination: key findings

- Posture: JD demonstrated a generally mildly flexed spinal posture, with flexion of the cervicothoracic region and an associated slight forward head posture. Her scapulae were slightly downwardly rotated bilaterally. Correction of both spinal and scapular postures made no immediate difference to the test movement of (L) neck rotation (range or perceived stiffness).
- Articular system: Examination of cervical mobility revealed that cervical rotation was symmetrically restricted bilaterally (60 degrees) with no reproduction of symptoms. Cervical extension was limited to approximately 20 degrees but was also asymptomatic. The cervical flexion rotation test

(C1/2 rotation) was unremarkable. The cervicothoracic region was generally hypomobile. Manual examination revealed (L) C2/3 moderate hypomobility and slight pain provocation. There was general hypomobility in the lower cervical and upper thoracic regions.
- Neuromuscular system: Examination of the muscle system revealed that JD could achieve 24 mmHg in the craniocervical flexion test (CCFT) with good movement patterning and sustain a holding contraction at this level without difficulty. There was premature fatigue (5 repetitions) in the scapular holding test and no immediate change in palpation findings (reassess: passive accessory intervertebral movements (PAIVMs) C2–3—no major change) immediately afterwards. Testing of the cervical extensor muscles demonstrated a good pattern of motion in the craniocervical and cervical muscle tests but some premature fatigue in performing 10 repetitions of cervical extension.
- Examination of sensorimotor function and the neural system were unremarkable.

Clinical reasoning and reflections

The physical examination did reveal a pattern of musculoskeletal dysfunction consistent with a neck pain disorder. The examination revealed a slightly reduced (for age) range of active cervical movements, there were joint signs of moderate hypomobility but little pain at the (L) C2–3, and muscle function (e.g., CCFT achieved the 24 mmHg stage) was fair but not optimal. Given the frequency and severity of JD's headache, it was reasoned that the cervical musculoskeletal dysfunction was not comparable in severity to the headache complaint. This, in conjunction with the information from the patient's history, led to the conclusion that JD did not have a cervicogenic headache. Rather it was hypothesized that she continued to suffer from chronic migraines and as well, had a mild comorbid neck disorder. However, it was possible that the cervical musculoskeletal dysfunction was a contributor or augmenting the migraine. A trial of treatment might confirm or refute this hypothesis.

The findings and the reasoning behind the diagnosis and neck pain hypothesis was discussed with JD as was the various relationships between headaches and neck pain. She was keen to try a trial of treatment and to learn appropriate exercises for her neck. She attended for treatment on four occasions over a 4-week period. Management included manual therapy for the hypomobile C2–3 segment and cervicothoracic region and a comprehensive self-management program of neuromuscular training and mobility exercises was developed. Further discussions took place about different headache types and the role of the neck as JD was interested to know more. JD was followed-up by telephone 1 month after discharge, at which time she reported that the exercises had definitely helped her neck and it felt a lot freer. Headaches were at best, possibly a little less severe, but there had been no substantive change in their pattern.

The definite change in neck symptoms together with the lack of change in the headache pattern, confirmed retrospectively, the hypothesized diagnosis of chronic migraines and a comorbid mild neck disorder.

CASE 3: (1) LEARNING FROM PAST TREATMENT RESPONSE; (2) IMPORTANCE OF DIFFERENTIAL DIAGNOSIS TO GUIDE MANAGEMENT OF COMPLEX PATIENTS AFTER A WHIPLASH INJURY (FIG. 18.3)

Patient presentation and key examination findings

JR is a 35-year-old female who was involved in a motor vehicle crash on her way to work 4 months ago. She briefly lost consciousness and has little memory of the crash. Head and neck scans revealed no significant findings. All symptoms were severe in the first few weeks after the accident. They gradually improved, but in the last month, there had been no change. JR had 6 weeks off work and then commenced a graduated return to work. JR is a medical registrar at a large city hospital and she currently works 30 hours per week. She manages work by changing positions regularly but is now not doing any physical or specific exercise because she has found that this exacerbates her symptoms. She has no history of neck pain or trauma, has a history of intermittent mild migraine (2 per year) and her general health is good. Before the crash, JR worked full time and enjoyed regular ballet and jogging for fitness.

JR presented with bilateral neck and thoracic pain, daily moderate left occipital headache, once monthly left orbital migraines, regular sleep disturbance, intermittent unsteadiness, visual disturbances and general fatigue. Her neck, thoracic and headache symptoms were exacerbated by driving, sustained sitting, computer work, lifting and carrying and physical activity. Unsteadiness and visual disturbances were exacerbated when neck pain and headache increase. Symptoms eased temporarily when exacerbating activities were avoided and with heat, simple analgesics and rest. JR is anxious while driving and avoids driving if possible. She works on bi-monthly rotations in wards throughout the hospital and her work environment and tasks can differ between rotations.

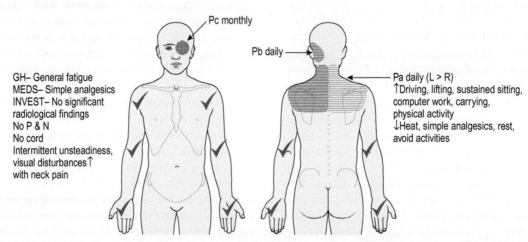

Pc monthly

Pb daily

Pa daily (L > R)
↑Driving, lifting, sustained sitting, computer work, carrying, physical activity
↓Heat, simple analgesics, rest, avoid activities

GH– General fatigue
MEDS– Simple analgesics
INVEST– No significant radiological findings
No P & N
No cord
Intermittent unsteadiness, visual disturbances↑ with neck pain

Fig. 18.3 ▪ Case 3: Body Chart. P pain; GH general health; MEDS medications, INVEST investigations, P & N pins and needles.

JR has attended physiotherapy. The focus was on strengthening and physical activity exercises which exacerbated symptoms. Subsequently, she stopped doing all types of exercise and is not sure of where to go from here. She consults her GP regularly and sees a psychologist to manage her posttraumatic stress symptoms. JR has also consulted a neurologist who prescribed medication for the migraines. JR takes simple analgesics and antiinflammatories as required.

Current levels of pain and disability were scored as followed:

Neck disability index (NDI): 30%
Pain visual analogue scale (VAS): 4/10
Patient specific functional scale (PSFS/10)
  Sleeping: 7
  Sustained sitting (40 minutes): 5
  Lifting/carrying: 7
Dizziness handicap inventory (DHIsf) score: 5/13.

Clinical reasoning

Important points to highlight in this case are that the previous treatment of strengthening and physical activity aggravated JR's symptoms, she is not getting better, and she has stopped doing any exercise at all as a result, which is a poor and undesirable outcome. It is important to determine the reasons for this outcome. JR's NDI and pain score (VAS) indicate moderate neck pain and disability. It is possible there is an element of sensory hypersensitivity that might explain this adverse reaction to strengthening exercises and it should be explored in the physical examination. JR has several symptoms other than pain, and a single focus modality, i.e., strengthening exercises, is unlikely to address all symptoms. The physical examination needs to include a full movement, neuromuscular and sensorimotor assessment, directed by her complaints to differentially diagnose symptoms particularly headache, dizziness and visual complaints, as a basis for developing a best practice management program.

Given JR's description of symptoms and relationship to activity, it could be hypothesized that her neck and thoracic pain and occipital headache arise from cervical musculoskeletal dysfunction. The trauma may have exacerbated JR's preexisting orbital migraine or now, may be an additional trigger. JR's description and behaviour of her unsteadiness, visual disturbances and

fatigue suggest they are related to cervical sensorimotor dysfunction. A vestibular pathology is unlikely, but the examination should screen for vestibular and oculomotor dysfunction, in light of the concussion that JR sustained at the time of the crash. JR has some symptoms of posttraumatic stress, which may impact on physical symptoms, but she is managing these with the help of a psychologist. The nature of JR's work and the potential long hours requires monitoring. Besides posttraumatic stress symptoms, JR has few yellow flag indicators and seems to have good self-efficacy and coping strategies.

Key physical examination findings

- Sensory testing: Tests of pressure pain thresholds revealed widespread mechanical hyperalgesia. There was no evidence of thermal hyperalgesia.
- Neural examination: Neurodynamic testing of the upper limbs (median biased) revealed marked bilateral elbow extension and pain provocation (unfamiliar arm pain) with no relevant symptom modification with the addition of sensitizing manoeuvres.
- Movement examination: There was a slight restriction overall in cervical range of motion and a positive (L) C1–2 flexion rotation test. The manual segmental examination determined joint dysfunction (palpable muscle spasm and pain provocation) in the (L) C0–1, C1–2 and (R) C5–6 segments, as well as general thoracic hypomobility.
- Neuromuscular examination: JR performed poorly in the CCFT as well as in the tests for the craniocervical and cervical extensors and right middle and lower trapezius. JR demonstrated poor movement patterns altered muscle activation and premature fatigue.
- Sensorimotor examination: Impaired performance was evident in tests of joint position sense, trunk-head and eye-head coordination, balance, and gaze stability. The visual oculomotor screen identified an abnormal near point of convergence (NPC) distance.

Diagnosis and clinical reasoning

JR's responses to sensory and neurodynamic testing suggested the presence of sensory hypersensitivity, which may be why previous high-load and general exercise approaches exacerbated her symptoms and were counter-productive. This highlights the importance of considering the potential for pain provocation when implementing and progressing exercise programs and implementing a program of graduated return to physical activity and work.

Differential tests supported the hypothesis of a cervicogenic basis of the daily headache dizziness, and visual symptoms. The diagnosis of cervicogenic headache is supported by the presence of a pattern of painful cervical (and thoracic) segmental joint dysfunction (C1–2), decreased range of cervical motion and altered neuromuscular function. Poor neuromuscular function appears to be relevant to the persistence of the disorder and requires management. JR's migraine exacerbation may have been triggered by the neck injury; its response to management strategies for the neck will need to be monitored. A neck trigger would be confirmed if migraines decrease as neck pain and dysfunction improve.

Signs of altered cervical sensorimotor control were consistent with symptoms of dizziness and visual disturbances. Treating sensorimotor deficits including NPC should address any central vestibular oculomotor contributions to symptoms as management methods for peripheral and central disturbances overlap. Prior treatment did not address these specific sensorimotor impairments, which might contribute to her lack of recovery.

Overall management approach

JR required multimodal management as directed by the impairments found in the physical examination in the articular, neuromuscular and sensorimotor systems. Advice and education for graduated return to physical activity and full-time work were important components of management. In addition, the psychologist's contribution to JR's stress management and modulation was a vital part of management.

Specific physiotherapy management included manual therapy (without pain provocation) to address pain and improve segmental motion. This was complimented with active segmental exercises for C1/2 and the cervicothoracic region to capitalize on the effect of manual therapy. These exercises were also included as part of the home program.

Extensive rehabilitation was undertaken to train neuromuscular control because the physical examination revealed impaired function of flexors, extensors and right axioscapular muscles. A comprehensive progressive training regime was undertaken (refer to Chapter 15), which progressed from training appropriate patterns of muscle use to challenging the muscle system with load. Training was undertaken over several weeks and was monitored carefully to avoid pain exacerbation. It was altered at times to cope with occasional relapses.

The impaired sensorimotor control found in the physical examination was addressed with exercises to challenge (L) eye-head coordination and gaze stability, trunk head coordination and tandem stance with eyes closed. As JR coped with these exercises, Joint position error (JPE) training in (L) rotation, walking with head rotations and flexion/extension as well as near-point convergence practice were added to the program and progressed accordingly (refer to Chapter 16).

Graded physical activity was commenced early in the program with specific instructions for the amount of activity. Over a 6-month period, JR progressed from walking, to water running, to walk/run progressing to running and eventually returned to ballet. As JR's work requirements changed when she went to a new hospital ward, attention was given to recognizing any foreseeable problems. Collaborating with JR on how to solve any issues was important. Advice and education regarding stress management and mindfulness were also provided as well as strategies for rescue management if pain exacerbation occurred.

Reflection and clinical message

The management of whiplash-associated disorders can be challenging with some patients not recovering well. JR did achieve a good outcome when initially she was on a projection for a poor outcome. The modification to exercise load, the addition of specific interventions to address sensorimotor impairments, and a sensible graduated approach to work and physical activity, were key aspects of the change in her path of recovery. Following a 6-month period of management (10 treatment sessions), JR had returned to full-time work with minimal neck pain and no headaches (NDI 10%). She self-manages her neck pain and continues regular maintenance exercise.

JR's presentation demonstrates the importance of avoiding pain exacerbation in the presence of sensory hypersensitivity. This applies to all aspects of management, but in JR's case this particularly pertained to high-load exercises and general physical activity that exacerbated her symptoms. Exercises for training cervical neuromuscular and sensorimotor control were vital in JR's case. They were directly relevant to her symptoms and reduced capacity for physical function. A particular advantage of these programs is that training commences with low-load exercises. All exercises were tailored and progressed within JR's capabilities and symptom tolerance. Nevertheless, graded physical activity was included as early as possible. It was vital that a specific collaborative plan was established with JR to progress a return to exercise and physical activity. Several months of an appropriately paced program was required, which is not unlike a time-frame for rehabilitation following for example, a major knee injury.

Different patients respond differently to physical rehabilitation. JR's response to the initial treatment (i.e., pain exacerbation) suggested that any further exercise and the return to physical activity had be progressed and planned carefully. In addition, JR needed to be equipped with the awareness, knowledge and strategies, to pre-empt and effectively self-manage any potential relapses. This case is a prime example that warns against assuming that a patient presenting with sensory hypersensitivity will not have a favourable outcome. Rather an unfavourable response may be a reflection of a misdirected management approach for that individual.

CASE 4: CLINICAL REASONING IN THE PHYSICAL EXAMINATION GUIDES TREATMENT DECISIONS (FIG. 18.4)

This case presents a patient with neck pain and headache related to office work to illustrate the importance of clinical reasoning in the physical examination to guide optimal treatment, rather than delivering a standard protocol of care. Even though patients may have a similar history and symptoms, slight variations in the findings of the physical examination can significantly modify the treatment approach as will be illustrated in this case presentation.

Patient presentation

SJ is aged 22 years, and he presented with a 3-month history of insidious onset neck pain. Occipital headaches began 1 month ago. He started work as a programmer 6 months ago after finishing his degree in information technology. He likes his job and is working within a good team to develop innovative applications. SJ has neck pain most days and it usually comes on around midday. The neck pain increases in the afternoon and on days when it gets quite bad, a headache develops on the same side. Recently, neck pain is coming on earlier in the day.

SJ sits at work, uses a three-screen set-up and mainly works on the screen directly in front. He admits that he tends to slump in his chair and usually has coffee breaks at his desk. Turning his head hurts his neck

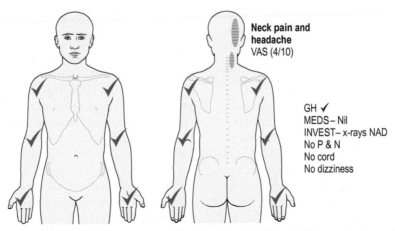

Neck pain and headache
VAS (4/10)

GH ✓
MEDS– Nil
INVEST– x-rays NAD
No P & N
No cord
No dizziness

Fig. 18.4 ■ Case 4: Body chart. VAS visual analogue scale; GH general health; MEDS medications, INVEST investigations, P & N pins and needles.

especially when he uses the right screen for a prolonged period. Neck pain generally eases with activity, although SJ admits he often uses electronic devices in the evenings as well. He used to get an odd ache in the neck when he was at university, but this is the first time his neck pain has really bothered him consistently. He is otherwise in good health.

Clinical reasoning from the patient interview

SJ's clinical presentation is consistent with a diagnosis of neck pain and cervicogenic headache. The headache fulfils the main criteria for cervicogenic headache, it is unilateral, without side shift, associated with ipsilateral neck pain, pain begins in the neck and headache is aggravated by neck movement or neck postures.

Work postures and work habits are likely contributors to his condition. For all case scenarios, education and training in better work postures and practices is an essential part of management as is a discussion on his use of electronic devices in the evenings.

Scenario 1

Physical examination—key findings

- Postural assessment: When replicating his working sitting posture, SJ slump sits in lumbopelvic flexion. His (R) scapula is downwardly rotated and anteriorly tilted. Movement to test for the effect of posture correction: (R) rotation, restricted to 50 degrees with neck pain (3/10).

Facilitation of a corrected spinal posture increased (R) rotation to 75 degrees with a concurrent reduction in neck pain (1/10). The addition of scapular posture correction resulted in no further changes in range of motion (i.e., remains 75 degrees) but it completely eliminated the pain (0/10).

- Articular system: Active cervical movements are painful and limited; extension 20 degrees; (R) lateral flexion (little head tilt) 30 degrees; and (R) rotation 50 degrees resulting in neck pain of 3/10. Upper cervical flexion and extension are unremarkable. The flexion-rotation test revealed normal mobility of (L) C1–2 rotation with (R) C1–2 rotation limited to 35 degrees (slightly hypomobile).

Manual examination added further confirmation, Passive accessory intervertebral movements (PPIVMs), C1–2, moderately hypomobile and PAIVMs, C1/2 moderately hypomobile with pain provocation (6/10). Tests of adjacent joints/regions (temporomandibular joint (TMJ); shoulder) were unremarkable.

- Neural system: No abnormality detected.
- Tests of muscle function: A poor retraction pattern of motion was noted during the CCFT. SJ could not extend beyond neutral during the cervical extension test and fatigued within 5 repetitions. Craniocervical extension and rotation muscle tests were unremarkable. Scapular holding tests revealed marked endurance deficits of the trapezius muscles with notable incapacity to sustain the test position for greater than 3 repetitions of 5 second holds. Reassessment of C1–2 PAIVMs (slight hypomobility, pain 1/10) immediately following the test revealed a notable improvement, despite a poor test performance.
- Sensorimotor function: No abnormality detected.

Clinical reasoning for diagnosis

The physical examination confirmed the pattern for cervicogenic headache (reduced motion, upper cervical joint signs, reduced cervical muscle function) and substantiates the diagnosis of cervicogenic headache.

Clinical reasoning for the initial treatment approach

The physical examination suggests that adverse strains from posture and attendant muscle loading are major provocative factors of the neck pain because correction of spinal and scapular posture significantly reduced neck pain and improved range of movement. In addition, reassessment of C1–2 PAIVMs following the scapular holding test significantly changed (but did not eliminate) joint signs and pain. The test targeting lower trapezius encourages reciprocal relaxation of the scapular elevators, suggesting that adverse muscle forces have a major role in aggravating the joint. Muscle tests indicated very poor neuromuscular control.

Based on these findings, it was hypothesized that poor posture and muscle function were the primary drivers of the condition. Thus management will have a strong focus on facilitating and reeducating correct sitting and working postures and neuromuscular training (cervical flexors [pattern initially], extensors and axioscapular muscles) to both help alleviate this episode of neck pain as well as prevent it reoccurring. It could be reasoned that the painful C1–2 joint dysfunction is a secondary consequence. Although manipulative therapy may have a role to address any residual joint dysfunction (depending on subsequent reassessment findings), its role is lesser than that of reeducating sitting, working postures and neuromuscular training.

Scenario 2

Physical examination

The patient has similar findings in the physical examination but there are some key differences from Scenario 1. The same findings are presented, and differences are **highlighted** and inform a different management focus for this patient.

Physical examination

- Postural assessment: When replicating his working sitting posture, SJ slump sits in lumbopelvic flexion. His (R) scapula is downwardly rotated and anteriorly tilted. Movement to test for the effect of posture correction: (R) rotation, restricted to 50 degrees with neck pain (3/10). *Neither correction of spinal posture or scapular posture resulted in changes in (R) rotation range or pain response*
- Articular system: Active cervical movements are painful and limited; extension 20 degrees; (R) lateral flexion (little head tilt) 30 degrees; and (R) rotation 50 degrees resulting in neck pain of 3/10. Upper cervical flexion and extension are unremarkable. The flexion-rotation test revealed normal mobility of (L) C1–2 rotation *with (R) C1–2 rotation limited to 25 degrees (moderately hypomobile).*
  Manual examination added further confirmation, PPIVMs, C1–2, moderately hypomobile and PAIVMs, C1/2 moderately hypomobile with pain provocation (6/10). Tests of adjacent joints/regions (TMJ; shoulder) were unremarkable.
- Neural system: No abnormality detected.
- Tests of muscle function: A poor retraction pattern of motion was noted during the CCFT. SJ could not extend beyond neutral during the cervical extension test and fatigued within 5 repetitions. Craniocervical extension was unremarkable.

Rotation muscle tests revealed a poor ability to perform C1–2 rotation, which improved with facilitation. Scapular holding tests revealed marked endurance deficits of the trapezius muscles with notable incapacity to sustain the test position for greater than 3 repetitions of 5 second holds. *Reassessment of C1–2 PAIVMs following the scapula hold test revealed little change (moderate hypomobility, pain (5/10).*
- Sensorimotor function: No abnormality detected.

Clinical reasoning for the initial treatment approach

Although the basic findings of the examination are similar in this scenario, an important difference was that strategies that may relieve joint and muscle loading (facilitating the neutral posture, placing the scapula in a neutral position and the effects of the scapular muscle test on manual examination of C1–2) had little effect on neck movement and pain. It could therefore be reasoned that C1–2 joint dysfunction is the primary problem. The poor ability to rotate in the craniocervical rotation test, and the improvement with facilitation suggests an element of poor joint proprioception at the C1–2 joint which supports the hypothesis of articular dysfunction.

Based on these findings, it was hypothesized that articular dysfunction at C1–2 was a stronger feature than in scenario 1, and more emphasis on manipulative therapy was needed to address this joint dysfunction. Active segmental exercises and exercises to improve C1–2 movement sense were included to augment the effects of manipulative therapy. The neuromuscular findings were still very relevant, but attention to them alone may not result in as rapid recovery if not undertaken in conjunction with techniques to address the C1–2 joint dysfunction.

Scenario 3

Physical examination

Again, the patient has similar findings in the physical examination but there are some key differences from Scenario 2. They are **highlighted** and inform yet another different management focus for this patient.

- Postural assessment: When replicating his working sitting posture, SJ slump sits in lumbopelvic flexion. His (R) scapula is downwardly rotated and anteriorly tilted. Movement to test for the effect of posture correction: (R) rotation, restricted to 50 degrees with neck pain (3/10).

Neither correction of spinal posture or scapular posture resulted in changes in (R) rotation range or pain response

■ Articular system: Active cervical movements are painful and limited; extension 20 degrees; (R) lateral flexion (little head tilt) 30 degrees; and (R) rotation 50 degrees resulting in neck pain of 3/10. *Upper cervical flexion reproduces a pulling feeling in the neck.* Upper cervical extension is unremarkable. The flexion-rotation test revealed normal mobility of (L) C1–2 rotation with (R) C1–2 rotation limited to 25 degrees (moderately hypomobile).

Manual examination added further confirmation, PPIVMs, C1–2, moderately hypomobile and PAIVMs, C1/2 moderately hypomobile with pain provocation (6/10). Tests of adjacent joints/regions (TMJ; shoulder) were unremarkable.

■ Neural system: *Upper cervical flexion with the addition of a straight leg raise reproduced neck pain and headache.*

■ Tests of muscle function: *The CCFT was not performed because of these positive signs of neural mechanosensitivity specific to upper cervical flexion.* SJ could not extend beyond neutral during the cervical extension test and fatigued within 5 repetitions. Craniocervical extension was unremarkable. Rotation muscle tests revealed a poor ability to perform C1–2 rotation, which improved with facilitation. Scapular holding tests revealed marked endurance deficits of the trapezius muscles with notable incapacity to sustain the test position for greater than 3 repetitions of 5 second holds. Reassessment of C1–2 PAIVMs following the scapula hold test revealed little change (moderate hypomobility, pain (5/10).

■ Sensorimotor function: No abnormality detected.

Clinical reasoning for the initial treatment approach

Despite similar basic findings of the examination in this scenario compared with scenario 2, the important variable is the positive response to the test of neural mechanosensitivity. Attention to neural tissue mechanosensitivity takes priority. Despite the importance of

rehabilitating neuromuscular control, exercises for the craniocervical flexors at least must be delayed or modified as the training movement stands to provoke the mechanosensitivity. Thus based on the examination findings, treatment in this case will be directed initially to resolve the neural mechanosensitivity. This may be achieved with a combination of manual therapy to address an interface possibly contributing to the sensitivity (i.e., the C1–2 joint arthropathy) and gentle active mobilizing exercise for the neural structures (sliding exercises).

CASE 5: NECK PAIN ASSOCIATED WITH NEUROPATHY (FIG. 18.5)

Identifying the presence and nature of neuropathy in neck pain disorders relies on a comprehensive structural differential examination that will subsequently guide management approaches. The most appropriate and safe course of conservative care depends on determining the relative presence of signs of nerve conduction and nerve mechanosensitivity. The following case describes a patient with cervical radiculopathy with dominant features of neural mechanosensitivity that directly guided a successful management approach.

Patient presentation and key examination findings

JL, a 46-year-old male, presented with discomfort on the right side of the neck and shoulder girdle accompanied by pain and paraesthesia in the right arm extending down to the lateral forearm and hand, particularly his fingers and thumb. These symptoms had been present for 3 weeks. Although no single event or incident could be recalled, JL suspected he had strained his neck while lifting heavy customer travel bags off the conveyer belt during his work as an international airline customer service officer. He reported that more recently, he would spend up to 5-hour shifts checking in bags, 4 to 5 days a week. JL reported that lifting heavy bags (with a tendency to use his dominant right arm) off the conveyer belt would often result in neck tightness. However, over the past 3 weeks, this had progressed to a discomfort in his neck and progressive symptoms into the right upper limb. His general medical practitioner had arranged a magnetic resonance imaging that revealed moderate levels of degenerative

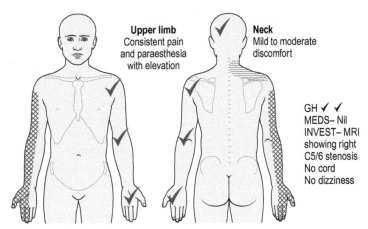

Upper limb
Consistent pain
and paraesthesia
with elevation

Neck
Mild to moderate
discomfort

GH ✓ ✓
MEDS– Nil
INVEST– MRI
showing right
C5/6 stenosis
No cord
No dizziness

Fig. 18.5 ■ Case 5: Body chart. GH general health; MEDS medications, INVEST investigations, MRI magnetic resonance imaging.

change including lateral stenosis at the C5–6 level on the right.

Examination findings strongly indicating neural mechanosensitivity

JL's main aggravating activity was elevation of the right upper limb. When replicated in the clinic, this reproduced the upper limb symptoms and feelings of strain to the neck. These symptoms were magnified if arm elevation was performed with the wrist and hand in extension suggesting neural mechanosensitivity. Structural differentiation during neurodynamic tests further implicated neural tissue mechanosensitivity. Familiar symptoms were reproduced during the median nerve biased neurodynamic test in a combined position of right shoulder abduction/external rotation/80-degree elbow flexion, with symptoms able to be altered (increased/reduced) with either the addition of sensitizing movements of the wrist (wrist extension/flexion) or cervical spine (lateral flexion left/right), respectively. The clinical neurological examination (for nerve conduction) revealed normal muscle strength and reflexes, and mild reduction in sensation to light touch (7/10) in the right C6 dermatome.

The patient had also reported some discomfort with right cervical rotation. When examined, this movement reproduced familiar discomfort locally at the neck only. Cervical extension was also mildly restricted and when combined with right lateral flexion reproduced neck pain and very mild arm symptoms. Manual examination revealed the presence of protective muscle spasm and mild segmental reduction in mobility evident on examination of (R) lateral flexion of C5–6. Cervical lateral glides directed at C5–6 were markedly restricted to the left (protective muscle spasm) when the (R) upper limb was prepositioned in the neural provoking position (shoulder abduction and external rotation), compared with when lateral glides were applied to the right with the left arm in the same posture.

Other relevant examination findings

In relaxed standing, the patient demonstrated downwardly rotated and protracted shoulder blades bilaterally, especially on the right side. This scapular posture on the right was magnified when arm elevation was lightly resisted. Examination of the craniocervical flexors (CCFT 26 mmHg) revealed a fair to good performance in the test whereas the cervical flexors and extensors revealed premature fatigue during the head lift test and cervical extensor test, respectively. Poor patterns of movement were observed after 3 to 4 repetitions of the tests, which worsened with further repetitions. These scapular and cervical muscle test findings were considered relevant to the pathomechanics of the disorder, potentially indicating suboptimal physical support to the cervical spine and brachial plexus structures at the neck when lifting. This thought process was further supported when manual elevation of the shoulder girdle to a more neutral posture relieved feelings of tension at the neck. A general lack of thoracic spine extension and rotation was noted which was of potential relevance to both scapular function and mobility demands at the lower neck. There were no apparent impairments of the glenohumeral joint or rotator cuff muscles.

Diagnosis and clinical reasoning

A diagnosis was made of a C6 radiculopathy associated with a strain of the right C5–6 motion segment. Examination findings suggested a predominant pattern of neural mechanosensitivity to motion (very positive neurodynamic tests including structural differentiation). Although there was some evidence of nerve conduction deficits (sensory changes) these were mild. The observed radiologic stenosis was probably present and asymptomatic before the injury, therefore it was considered a relevant finding. In particular, the presence of a degenerative stenosis may have increased the risk of developing a neuropathy when combined with the injury induced perineural inflammation.

Management approach

Advice and education

The patient had initially expressed concern regarding his "pinched nerve". Time was devoted initially to reassure JL that this was a completely reversible condition that would cease once the inflammation had resolved and pain-free motion restored. An emphasis was therefore placed on modifying any factors that were aggravating to the condition. In particular, this included the organization of suitable duties for a period in his workplace that did not involve lifting heavy bags.

Although the resolution of neural inflammation was the short-term goal of management, the patient was also advised that the long-term management would incorporate specific training of neuromuscular function of his shoulder girdle, neck and thorax to optimize the physical support of the neck and brachial plexus to prevent recurrence.

Manipulative therapy

Manual therapy targeted the restoration of a pain-free cervical lateral glide in progressive pre-set positions of the neurodynamic test position. This was targeted because it was the most substantial and relevant finding during the physical examination. Treatment was enhanced by the performance of daily neural sliding exercises. Diligent reassessment showed this approach to have positive effects on both the neural mechanosensitivity and cervical movement signs.

Exercise therapy

Exercise initially focused on the correction of habitual scapular posture (corrected towards upward rotation and retraction) incorporating the use of memory joggers and strapping tape. To train the capacity to lift baggage at work with minimal strain to the neck, specific daily strengthening of his scapular upward rotators using progressive resisted shrugging exercises were also commenced immediately. In subsequent sessions, this was combined with lifting practice specific to JL's work duties (i.e., removing baggage from the conveyer belt—arm in low-elevation position and controlling shoulder girdle and neck orientation under load) with progressive increase in load as able. Progressive resistance exercises with an emphasis on movement control for the cervical flexors and extensors were incorporated to foster optimal physical support of his neck particularly in light of the physical demands of his work. At discharge, the patient was encouraged to continue shoulder girdle and neck strengthening exercises 3 times a week as a maintenance program.

Initially, the exercise program also included thoracic mobility exercises (thoracic rotation and extension) and neural mobilization exercises (neural sliding—elbow flexion/extension in wrist extension in progressive shoulder elevation) 3 times daily. As no residual signs of neural mechanosensitivity were evident at discharge, neural mobilizing exercises were ceased and JL was encouraged to continue the thoracic mobility exercises as a work break for maintenance purposes.

Reflection and clinical message

Not all cervical pain disorders associated with neuropathy are the same and this case featured predominant signs of nerve mechanosensitivity that guided the management approach. If the presentation had implicated nerve conduction deficits, the management approach would have differed. In this case, the single mild sign of nerve conduction deficit (reduced sensation) resolved quickly with intervention. Neural mechanosensitivity progressively resolved over an 8-week period (mostly in the first 3–4 weeks) with milder fluctuating residual symptoms experienced over the last 4 weeks associated with the progressive return to normal work duties including lifting bags. Collaborative reasoning with the patient concerning the fluctuations in recovery associated with his progressive return to lifting over this final 4 weeks was paramount. This was particularly so because it reinforced to him the importance of the work-specific neuromuscular conditioning element of the management approach, which permitted his return to normal work duties while maintaining a healthy neck-nerve status.

CONCLUSION

Clinical practice is not an exact science and at present, research evidence although very informative, can only guide management approaches. As such best practice relies on a collaborative effort incorporating the perspectives of the patient, the clinical expertise of the therapist and the scientific evidence. With conservative care, the majority of patients with neck pain will gain some to complete relief of symptoms, gain improved function and acquire knowledge and strategies to self-manage their necks. Such patients have been presented in this chapter. Nevertheless, there are limitations to the benefits that conservative therapies can achieve, particularly for those patients who have very high pain states, severe or advanced pathology or neuropathic pain states. In these cases, multiprofessional management is required which includes adequate pharmacotherapeutics for pain relief, which might help facilitate rehabilitation. In some cases, interventional management may prove to be a suitable option. However, conservative management is the first treatment of choice.

19

CONCLUDING REMARKS
Focusing on Prevention

There would be little argument against a claim that knowledge has increased substantially over the last decade in the basic and clinical sciences pertinent to neck pain disorders. Yet during this same time, the burden of neck pain has increased worldwide.[1] Systematic reviews report that effect sizes of benefits for various interventions in the management of neck pain remain relatively small whether interventions are medical, educational, physical or psychological. The contrast between increasing knowledge yet increasing burden and lack of major change in treatment outcomes encourages thought about directions for future research (and its design) and health care practice.

The rate of increase in the burden of neck pain has been quite rapid. Its incidence globally, rose by 21% between 2005 and 2015, and in terms of the metric of years lived with a disability, neck pain ranked 4th of 301 chronic conditions in 2013, but rose to 1st of 310 chronic conditions by 2015, together with low-back pain.[1,2] Several factors undoubtedly contribute to this escalating problem. The ageing population is one factor. Even though ageing may not cause osteoarthritis, the frequency of osteoarthritis increases with age. The incidence of osteoarthritis increased by 33% in the last 10 years, which might, in part, account for the increase in neck pain.[1] Another factor impacting negatively on the neck is the technology revolution, which is transforming both the world of work and lifestyle. Workplaces have become more computerized and more sedentary across a spectrum of occupations. Computer work has been linked with the development of neck pain.[3–6]

Lifestyles are incorporating increasing use of various electronic devices and applications for communication, education and entertainment with the net result of more sedentary lifestyles outside work. Of most concern, is that this change in lifestyle is beginning in early childhood. This was well illustrated by Howie et al.[7] who measured the body movements of children from 3 to 5 years of age while they played games on tablet computers, watched television or played with toys. Compared with the other two conditions, playing with the tablet computer was linked with more neck and thoracic flexion, lesser postural variation, more time sitting and less physical activity—a potential recipe for the development of neck pain and other health concerns. A focus on prevention at primary, secondary and tertiary level is crucial.

PREVENTION

The adage that prevention is better than cure is certainly an aim to strive for, even though it may be idealistic. Neck pain is unlikely to ever be eliminated as, in the first instance, age is a non-modifiable factor and it would impossible to eliminate all trauma. Nevertheless, many adverse lifestyle, personal and work-related behaviours that may underlie neck pain are modifiable. The concept of prevention is not new, but systematic reviews suggest current workplace prevention and intervention programs are not providing the answers.[8] Further creative work in primary, secondary and tertiary prevention are key and critical to reduce the burden of neck pain.

Primary prevention

Primary prevention is an urgent area of need. New and inventive approaches are required to influence all people across their lifespan. At the current time, there is no effective, evidence-base primary public health prevention program for neck pain, despite the internet being full of advice from diverse perspectives. The desired endpoint is evidence-based primary prevention programs, but in the first instance research informed programs must be created, developed and tested. The development of a fresh and forward-thinking primary prevention strategy could be an initiative of a collaboration between international leaders in neck pain representing all relevant parties from the health sector and community. Such a strategy might consist of concerted, multiple and coordinated levels of educational and effective practical interventions. The world's connectivity via the internet could support a major international public health campaign, with targeted information on healthy work and lifestyle habits and a few simple, yet effective preventative active strategies for posture, muscles and movement that could easily be incorporated into the daily routines of all age groups, from children and their parents through to the aged. Any such internet campaign would need to be supplemented with work on the ground at all levels—in schools, in training colleges and universities[9] (where students need to learn not only about the nature of their chosen work but how to perform it safely from the perspective of their own neck/musculoskeletal health), in workplaces, as well as applications relevant to everyday life activities for all ages. Consistent education locally reinforces the global public health program and caters to local cultural, personal,[10] work and activity variables.

Secondary prevention

Recent decades have witnessed a focus on patient-centred care that is fully supported. This focus is evident in randomized controlled trials (RCT) and systematic reviews where the primary outcome is usually a patient self-rated, numerical measure of neck pain or a rating on a questionnaire of neck pain and disability. This focus on pain seems to have lessened the emphasis on rehabilitation to restore normal neuromuscular and sensorimotor function to reestablish safe function after an episode of neck pain. Exercise programs are frequently

trialled in the management of neck pain, but the primary outcome of interest is pain relief, not measures of the exercise effects on muscle or other physical functions.

Patients desire pain relief; it is frequently their primary goal. Neck pain is a recurrent disorder. It could be argued that an equally vital patient-centred outcome is to prevent recurrent episodes of pain. Yet the current model of care is principally concerned with relieving the presenting episode of neck pain, not on physical and functional rehabilitation towards lessening recurrence rates. Many personal and environmental factors are likely to contribute to neck pain recurrence. It would be naïve to suggest that rehabilitation of good posture, movement and neuro-muscular and sensorimotor control will provide the complete answer for prevention of recurrence. Likewise, it is naïve to continue a very narrow focus on management of current pain only and to pay no attention to whether physical function has been restored towards addressing the real burden, which is the recurrent episodes of pain.

There is always pressure to contain and even lessen costs of care and provide minimal intervention. Controlling costs is understandable—but is this false economy? The costs are not in a single episode of neck pain, they are in the costs of repeated episodes of neck pain, the costs of repeated demands on health care, the costs on productivity of absenteeism and presenteeism, the costs of harm (e.g., opioid addiction, side effects of non-steroidal antiinflammatory drugs), as well as the personal costs in quality of life. Reflection and reappraisal on several fronts is necessary towards providing appropriate treatment and secondary prevention for a presenting episode of neck pain. Three points are presented for thought and discussion.

Defining the desired outcomes of exercise prescription. Exercise has many different modes, physiological responses and benefits. It is important to clearly define what outcomes are being sought from the exercise intervention to direct both clinical practice and research. Take the example of two RCTs both of which are testing the intervention of a resistance training program. RCT 1 has the primary outcome of decreasing neck pain whereas the primary outcome of RCT 2 is to increase muscle strength to meet a patient's functional demand. The outcomes in these trials are underpinned by different neuroscience and physiological rationales and mechanisms of effect. It could be expected that the nature and dosage of a resistance training program for achieving a hypoalgesic effect without concern for changes in motor output would be quite different to a program for increasing cervical muscle strength. This example casts doubt on the wisdom of prescription of exercise without careful consideration of the desired outcome. Furthermore, several studies have already shown that quite specific modes of exercise are required to improve different cervical muscle behaviours and motor outputs and address sensorimotor deficits in patients with neck pain disorders.[11–15] More work regarding the physiological effects of various exercise modes and matching exercise with specific outcomes of interest is required to ensure we develop optimal exercise protocols for secondary prevention programs.

Prescribing appropriate exercise dosage. Dosages to achieve the desired outcomes of an exercise intervention have not been researched to any great extent in relation to neck pain disorders. It could be expected that different exercise applications and dosage would be required if the primary outcome is to modulate pain, versus it being to reach a certain level of muscle function. Unlike rehabilitation protocols for many extremity disorders, there is little information on dosage requirements to successfully address altered motor and sensorimotor behaviours in neck pain conditions. The diverse times used in RCTs to test various interventions suggest that dosage prescription in many cases is not scientifically based but rather is an arbitrary choice. Dosages of exercise to achieve an effect will vary between individuals but urgent areas of research are to determine if (1) all neuromuscular and sensorimotor impairments can be restored to a "normative" status and (2) the average exercise dosage (e.g., frequency, intensity, duration) to achieve a normative or satisfactory status. Once guidelines for dosage are established, RCTs can be conducted to determine the impact of a full rehabilitation program on recurrence rates. The evidence suggests that a progressive multimodal exercise program is required that is tailored to the individual patient (see Chapters 15 and 16).

Adequate treatment of the presenting episode of neck pain. Time to manage and settle the neck pain and to fully rehabilitate an individual who has suffered an episode of neck pain will vary greatly between different persons and different neck pain disorders. Judging by the time allowed

for rehabilitation protocols for disorders of the extremities, rehabilitation programs may range from a few weeks to 3 or even 6 months for some individuals. Pain will usually settle well within that time. Facilitating understanding that pain relief alone may be an inadequate outcome in the context of prevention of recurrence will require a change in mind set of health care providers, patients and funding bodies alike. Treatment may be over a prolonged period, but much will be within the context of self-management. Thus the number of occasions of care and costs of management of the episode of neck pain do not have to increase greatly. However, essential to success is consistent interest in and support of the patient, monitoring of adherence, evaluation of performance and progression of the program (see Chapters 15 and 16).

Tertiary prevention

A percentage of patients have persistent neck pain as a result of trauma, degenerative conditions or of undetermined aetiology. Tertiary prevention aims to assist the person manage the impact of their ongoing neck pain in order to maintain their function and quality of life. Tertiary prevention is topical with the ageing population and the increase in incidence of osteoarthritis and requires particular attention in practice and research. Tertiary prevention will include major components of self-management. Nevertheless, self-management does not mean "no" management from a health care provider. Provision of personnel resources or a clinical review intermittently can have positive benefits. The effects of booster sessions or occasional provision of treatment needs further investigation. Because a person is older and has persistent pain does not negate good outcomes from conservative management as was illustrated in a recent RCT evaluating the effectiveness of manual therapy and specific exercises for seniors with chronic neck pain and headaches.[16]

Tertiary management for some patients with persistent neck pain can be challenging to all health professionals. These include the relatively small cohort of patients who have a poor recovery following a whiplash injury (10%–15% of those seeking care).[17,18] Effective secondary and tertiary management of this group remains rather illusive. Likewise, patients who develop neuralgias in association with spondylitic changes remain a challenge. Patients in these categories sometimes require interventional management such as radiofrequency neurotomies albeit pain relief when attained is usually temporary.

CONCLUSION

Prevention at all levels is an important aim of practice. Outcomes at all levels of prevention have to be enhanced if the burden of neck pain is to be lessened. The effectiveness (effect sizes) of various interventions have to be improved. This is challenging because even though RCTs remain the gold standard, they have limitations for translation to clinical practice. Population mean outcomes of RCTs do not reflect an individual patient's needs and responses. Effect sizes reflect the average response to an intervention, and often suffer a wash out effect. Participants who actually benefit from the intervention trialled in the RCT are usually not identified. From another perspective, many RCTs test the effect of a single modality. This does not reflect real life practice where multimodal management is provided on an individual basis. Thus RCTs miss the cumulative and potentially interacting effects of a treatment program. All fault does not lie in the RCT design. Further research is needed to improve diagnostics and interventions.

Indications for certain management methods need to be clearly defined in future research and practice. For instance, despite the long history of use of manipulative therapy, there is a lack of international/interdisciplinary consensus on clear indications for its use.[19] It is possible that the common indications of impaired neck movement and associated symptomatic segmental joint dysfunction are appropriate. Clinicians may intuitively recognize associations between treatment and effects, but there needs to be an empirical demonstration that manipulative therapy does resolve symptomatic segmental joint dysfunction and restores impaired neck movement and that these changes are associated with relief of symptoms.[19] Clinical examination methods are the cornerstone to guide management of neck pain disorders. Clinical tests are proving to have diagnostic validity in identifying segmental sources of pain.[20,21] Further research into diagnostics is required in several areas. For instance, differential diagnosis of headache, visual disturbances, dizziness, light headedness and unsteadiness from the perspective of a cervical musculoskeletal cause or contributor is necessary to identify patients who will benefit from management of cervical spine

There is always room for improved application of current interventions whether in prescribing accurate dosages or improving ways to help clinicians develop high-level therapeutic skills to deliver the intervention. Research will lead to the development of new interventions and these may intervene at the periphery or directly on the central nervous system.[22] Neck pain will never be successfully managed by monotherapy. To further the understanding of mechanisms and capabilities of both current and new treatments, it is essential to assess their effect on outcomes representing relevant components within and across domains of the biopsychosocial model. This will improve knowledge about what an intervention can and cannot achieve, which will contribute to the development of best practice multimodal and multiprofessional programs.

Progressive experimentation both in the clinic as well as the laboratory will inform on best combinations of multimodal approaches towards optimal management of persons with neck pain disorders. There has been a rapid increase in knowledge in the last 2 decades in particular and with that foundation, the next decade promises more significant advances.

REFERENCES

1. GBD 2015 Disease and Injury Incidence and Prevalence Collaborators. Global, regional, and national incidence, prevalence, and years lived with disability for 310 diseases and injuries, 1990-2015: a systematic analysis for the Global Burden of Disease Study 2015. Lancet 2016;388:1545–602.
2. Global Burden of Disease 2013 Collaborators. Global, regional, and national incidence, prevalence, and years lived with disability for 301 acute and chronic diseases and injuries in 188 countries, 1990-2013: a systematic analysis for the Global Burden of Disease Study 2013. Lancet 2015;386:743–800.
3. Blatter B, Bongers P. Duration of computer use and mouse use in relation to musculoskeletal disorders of neck or upper limb. Int J Ind Ergon 2002;30:295–306.
4. Côté P, van der Velde G, Cassidy J, et al. The burden and determinants of neck pain in workers: results of the Bone and Joint Decade 2000-2010 Task Force on Neck Pain and Its Associated Disorders. Spine 2008;33(4 Suppl.):S60–74.
5. Shahidi B, Curran-Everett D, Maluf K. Psychosocial, physical, and neurophysiological risk factors for chronic neck pain: a prospective inception cohort study. J Pain 2015;16:1288–99.
6. Tornqvist E, Hagberg M, Hagman M, et al. The influence of working conditions and individual factors on the incidence of neck and upper limb symptoms among professional

computer users. Int Arch Occup Environ Health 2009;82: 689–702.

7. Howie E, Coenen P, Campbell A, et al. Head, trunk and arm posture amplitude and variation, muscle activity, sedentariness and physical activity of 3-to-5-year-old children during tablet computer use compared to television watching and toy play. Appl Ergon 2017;65:41–50.

8. Varatharajan S, Côté P, Shearer H, et al. Are work disability prevention interventions effective for the management of neck pain or upper extremity disorders? A systematic review by the Ontario Protocol for Traffic Injury Management (OPTIMa) collaboration. J Occup Rehabil 2014;24:692–708.

9. Hanvold T, Wærsted M, Mengshoel A, et al. A longitudinal study on risk factors for neck and shoulder pain among young adults in the transition from technical school to working life. Scand J Work Environ Health 2014;40:597–609.

10. Eijckelhof B, Huysmans M, Blatter B, et al. Office workers' computer use patterns are associated with workplace stressors. Appl Ergon 2014;45:1660–7.

11. Falla D, Jull G, Hodges P, et al. An endurance-strength training regime is effective in reducing myoelectric manifestations of cervical flexor muscle fatigue in females with chronic neck pain. Clin Neurophysiol 2006;117:828–37.

12. Falla D, Jull G, Russell T, et al. Effect of neck exercise on sitting posture in patients with chronic neck pain. Phys Ther 2007; 87:408–17.

13. Falla D, Lindstrøm R, Rechter L, et al. Effectiveness of an 8-week exercise programme on pain and specificity of neck muscle activity in patients with chronic neck pain: a randomized controlled study. Eur J Pain 2013;17:1517–28.

14. Jull G, Falla D, Vicenzino B, et al. The effect of therapeutic exercise on activation of the deep cervical flexor muscles in people with chronic neck pain. Man Ther 2009;14:696–701.

15. O'Leary S, Jull G, Kim M, et al. Training mode dependent changes in motor performance in neck pain. Arch Phys Med Rehabil 2012;93:1225–33.

16. Uthaikhup S, Assapun J, Watcharasaksilp K, et al. Effectiveness of physiotherapy for seniors with recurrent headaches associated with neck pain and dysfunction: a randomized controlled trial. Spine J 2017;17:46–55.

17. Elliott J, Walton D. How do we meet the challenge of whiplash? J Orthop Sports Phys Ther 2017;47:444–6.

18. Jull G. Whiplash continues its challenges. J Orthop Sports Phys Ther 2016;46:815–17.

19. Smith J, Bolton P. What are the clinical criteria justifying spinal manipulative therapy for neck pain? A systematic review of randomized controlled trials. Pain Med 2013;14:460–8.

20. Hall T, Briffa K, Hopper D, et al. Comparative analysis and diagnostic accuracy of the cervical flexion-rotation test. J Headache Pain 2010;11:391–7.

21. Schneider G, Jull G, Thomas K, et al. Derivation of a clinical decision guide in the diagnosis of cervical facet joint pain. Arch Phys Med Rehabil 2014;95:1695–701.

22. Harvie D, Smith R, Hunter E, et al. Using visuo-kinetic virtual reality to induce illusory spinal movement: the MoOVi Illusion. PeerJ 2017;5:e3023.

INDEX

Page numbers followed by "*f*" indicate figures, "*t*" indicate tables, and "*b*" indicate boxes.